Study and Review Guide to accompany

ANATOMY & PHYSIOLOGY

Fifth Edition

Gary A. Thibodeau
Kevin T. Patton

Written by: Linda Swisher, RN, EdD

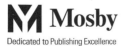 **Mosby**

Dedicated to Publishing Excellence

Mosby, Inc.
An Affiliate of Elsevier Science
St. Louis   London   Philadelphia   Sydney   Toronto

Mosby, Inc,
An Affiliate of Elsevier Science (USA)
11830 Westline Industrial Drive
St. Louis, Missouri 63146

ISBN 0-323-01668-5

Vice President, Publishing Director: Sally Schrefer
Senior Editor: Terri Wood
Associate Developmental Editor: Teena Ferroni
Developmental Editor: Catherine Ott
Project Manager: Gayle May
Illustrator: Barbara Cousins

Printed in the United States of America.

Last digit is the print number: 9 8 7 6 5 4 3 2 1

INTRODUCTION

This *Study and Review Guide to accompany Anatomy and Physiology,* fifth edition, is designed to help you be successful in learning anatomy and physiology. Before attempting to complete any chapter in the *Study and Review Guide,* thoroughly read the corresponding chapter in the textbook, learn the key terms listed at the beginning of each textbook chapter and study your lecture notes. You will then be prepared to complete the questions and exercises that are provided for each chapter.

Each chapter in the *Study and Review Guide* begins with a brief overview of the chapter concepts. A variety of questions is offered to help you cover the material effectively. These questions include multiple choice, true-false, matching, short answer, clinical challenges, labeling, and crossword puzzles.

Multiple Choice
For each multiple choice question, there is only one correct answer out of the choices given. Circle the correct choice.

True or False
Read each statement carefully and write *true* or *false* in the blank provided.

Matching
Match each numbered term or statement in the left-hand column with its corresponding lettered term or statement in the right-hand column. Write the correct letters in the blanks provided.

Fill in the Blanks
Fill-in-the-blank questions ask you to recall missing word(s) and insert it (them) into the answer blank(s) These questions may involve sentences or paragraphs.

Identify the Term that Does Not Belong
In questions that ask you to identify the incorrect term, three words are given that relate to each other in structure and function, and one more word is included that has no relationship to the other three terms. You are asked to circle the term that does not relate to the others. An example might be: iris, stapes, cornea, and retina. You would circle *stapes* because all other terms refer to the eye.

Application Questions
Application questions ask you to make a judgment based on the information in the chapter. These questions may ask you how you would respond to a situation or to suggest a possible diagnosis for a set of symptoms.

Labeling Exercises
Labeling exercises present diagrams with parts that are not identified. According to the directions given, fill in the appropriate labels on the numbered lines or match the numbers with the lettered list of terms provided.

Crossword Puzzles
Vocabulary words from the Key Terms section in each chapter of the text have been developed into crossword puzzles. This exercise encourages recall and proper spelling.

One Last Quick Check

This section selects questions from throughout the chapter to provide you with a final review of the chapter. This mini-test gives you an overview of your knowledge of the chapter after completing all of the other sections.

Finally, after completing the exercises in a chapter, check your answers. Answers can be found in the back of the book. Each answer is referenced to the appropriate text page. Additionally, questions are grouped into specific topics that correspond to the text. Each major topic of the *Study and Review Guide* provides references to specific areas of the text, so if you are having difficulty with a particular grouping of questions you have a specific reference area to assist you with remedial work. This allows you to identify your area of weakness accurately. Good luck!

FIGURE ACKNOWLEDGMENTS

Brundage, D.J.: *Renal disorders*, St. Louis, 1992, Mosby.
    Unn 28-1
    Unn 28-2

ACKNOWLEDGMENTS

I wish to express my appreciation to the staff at Elsevier, and especially to Terri Wood, Catherine Ott, and Teena Ferroni for their guidance and support. My continued admiration and thanks to Gary Thibodeau and Kevin Patton for another outstanding edition of their text. Your time and dedication to science education will, hopefully, create a better quality of health care for the future.

My thanks to Brian, whose encouragement kept me on task, whose discussions kept my creative juices flowing and whose love makes my life special.

My thanks, as well, to Bill Fortner who is always there whenever I need him.

To my mother, my daughter Amanda, and grandchildren Billy and Maddie this book is dedicated with gratitude and love. You are my roots and the fruit of my tree of life.

Linda Swisher, RN, EdD

CONTENTS

CHAPTER 1

ORGANIZATION OF THE BODY

The study of anatomy and physiology involves the structure and function of an organism and the relationship of its parts. It begins with a basic organization of the body into different structural levels. Beginning with the smallest level (the cell) and progressing to the largest, most complex level (the system), this chapter familiarizes you with the terminology and the levels of organization needed to facilitate the study of the body in parts or as a whole.

It is also important to be able to identify and describe specific body areas or regions as we progress in this field. The anatomical position is used as a reference when dissecting the body into planes, regions, or cavities. The terminology defined in this chapter allows you to describe the areas efficiently and accurately.

Finally, the process of homeostasis is reviewed. This state of relative constancy in the chemical composition of body fluids is necessary for good health. In fact, the very survival of the body depends on the successful maintenance of homeostasis.

I ANATOMY AND PHYSIOLOGY AND CHARACTERISTICS OF LIFE

Multiple Choice—select the best answer.

1. *Anatomy* refers to:
   a. using devices to investigate parameters such as heart rate and blood pressure.
   b. investigating human structure via dissection and other methods.
   c. studying the unusual manner in which an organism responds to painful stimuli.
   d. examining the chemistry of life.

2. *Systemic anatomy* refers to anatomical investigation:
   a. at a microscopic level.
   b. that begins in the head and neck and concludes at the feet.
   c. that approaches the study of the body by systems: groups of organs having a common function.
   d. at the cellular level.

3. *Physiology* refers to the:
   a. nature of human function.
   b. structure of the human form.
   c. evolution of human thought.
   d. accuracy of measuring the human physique.

4. The removal of waste products in the body is achieved by a process known as:
   a. secretion.   c. circulation.
   b. excretion.   d. conductivity.

5. *Metabolism* is the:
   a. exchange of gases in the blood.
   b. formation of new cells in the body to permit growth.
   c. sum total of all physical and chemical reactions occurring in the body.
   d. production and delivery of specialized substances for diverse body functions.

******If you had difficulty with this section, review pages **5-7**

1

II LEVELS OF ORGANIZATION

Multiple Choice—select the best answer.

6. Beginning with the smallest level, the levels of organization of the body are:
    a. cellular, chemical, tissue, organelle, organ, system, organism.
    b. cellular, chemical, organelle, organ, tissue, organism, system.
    c. chemical, cellular, organelle, organ, system, organism.
    d. chemical, organelle, cellular, tissue, organ, system, organism.

7. Molecules are:
    a. combinations of atoms forming larger chemical aggregates.
    b. electrons orbiting a nucleus.
    c. a complex of electrons arranged in orderly shells.
    d. composed of cellular organelles.

8. Mitochondria, Golgi apparatus, and endoplasmic reticulum are examples of:
    a. macromolecules.
    b. cytoplasm.
    c. organelles.
    d. nuclei.

9. Blood production is a function of which system?
    a. circulatory   c. skeletal
    b. respiratory   d. urinary

10. Support and movement are functions of which systems?
    a. respiratory, digestive, and urinary systems
    b. reproductive and urinary systems
    c. skeletal and muscular systems
    d. cardiovascular and lymphatic/immune systems

Matching—match the term on the left with the proper selection on the right.

11. _____ organelle

12. _____ cells

13. _____ tissue

14. _____ organ

15. _____ systems

a. many similar cells that act together to perform a common function
b. the most complex units that make up the body
c. a group of several different kinds of tissues arranged to perform a special function
d. collections of molecules to perform a function
e. the smallest "living" units of structure and function

Student Name_____

Matching—match each system with its corresponding functions.

16. _____ integumentary system
17. _____ skeletal system
18. _____ muscular system
19. _____ nervous system
20. _____ endocrine system
21. _____ digestive system
22. _____ respiratory system
23. _____ cardiovascular system
24. _____ lymphatic system
25. _____ urinary system
26. _____ reproductive system

a. support and movement
b. communication, control, and integration
c. outer protection
d. reproduction and development
e. transportation and defense
f. respiration, nutrition, and excretion

******If you had difficulty with this section, review pages **7-10**

III ANATOMICAL POSITION, BODY CAVITIES, BODY REGIONS, ANATOMICAL TERMS, AND BODY PLANES

Multiple Choice—select the best answer.

27. In the anatomical position the subject is:
    a. seated with the head facing forward.
    b. standing with the arms at the side and palms facing forward.
    c. seated with arms parallel to the ground.
    d. standing with the arms at the side and palms facing backward.

28. The dorsal body cavity contains the:
    a. brain and spinal cord.
    b. abdominal organs.
    c. pelvic organs.
    d. thoracic organs.

29. The ventral body cavity contains the:
    a. thoracic and abdominopelvic cavities.
    b. thoracic cavity only.
    c. abdominopelvic cavity only.
    d. brain and spinal cord.

30. The axial portion of the body consists of:
    a. arms, neck, and torso.
    b. neck, torso, and legs.
    c. torso, arms, and legs.
    d. head, neck, and torso.

31. The abdominopelvic cavity contains all of the following *EXCEPT* the:
    a. kidneys.   c. lungs.
    b. pancreas.   d. urinary bladder.

32. The mediastinum contains all of the following *EXCEPT* the:
    a. esophagus.   c. lungs.
    b. aorta.   d. trachea.

33. Visceral peritoneum would cover which of the following organs?
    a. heart.   c. lungs.
    b. liver.   d. brain.

34. A sagittal section would divide the body into:
    a. upper and lower parts.
    b. right and left sides.
    c. front and back portions.
    d. none of the above.

35. A coronal section would divide the body into:
    a. upper and lower parts.
    b. right and left sides.
    c. front and back portions.
    d. none of the above.

36. *Inguinal* is a term referring to which body
     region?
     a.   anterior portion of elbow
     b.   armpit
     c.   posterior knee
     d.   groin

Circle the correct answer.

37. The stomach is (superior or inferior) to the diaphragm.

38. The nose is located on the (anterior or posterior) surface of the body.

39. The lungs lie (medial or lateral) to the heart.

40. The elbow lies (proximal or distal) to the forearm.

41. The skin is (superficial or deep) to the muscles below it.

42. A midsagittal plane divides the body into (equal or unequal) parts.

43. A frontal plane divides the body into (anterior and posterior or superior and inferior) sections.

44. A transverse plane divides the body into (right and left or upper and lower) sections.

45. A coronal plane may also be referred to as a (sagittal or frontal) plane.

Select the correct term from the choices given and insert the letter in the answer blank.

46. _____ thoracic

47. _____ cranial

48. _____ abdominal

49. _____ pelvic

50. _____ mediastinum

51. _____ pleural

a.   ventral cavity
b.   dorsal cavity

Student Name_____

Labeling—using the terms provided, label the anatomical directions on the illustration below.

anterior	posterior	ventral	dorsal
distal	proximal	superior	inferior
lateral	medial	midline	sagittal plane
coronal plane	frontal plane	transverse plane	cross section

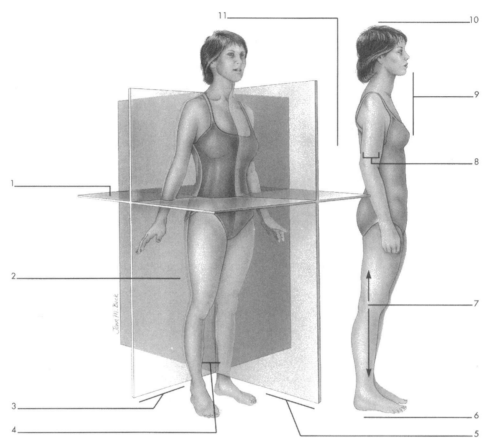

Labeling—label the various body cavities on the diagram below.

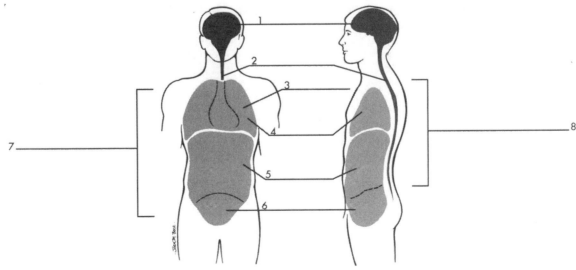

******If you had difficulty with this section, review pages **11-16**

IV   HOMEOSTASIS AND HOMEOSTATIC MECHANISMS OF CONTROL

Multiple Choice—select the best answer.

52. *Homeostasis* can be defined as the:
    a.   relatively constant state maintained by the body.
    b.   overall contribution of an organ system.
    c.   external stimuli that evoke a disruption to an organism.
    d.   lack of cytoplasm within a plasma membrane.

53. Which of the following is *NOT* a component of a feedback control loop?
    a.   sensory mechanism
    b.   integrating, or control center
    c.   effector mechanism
    d.   stressor stimulator

54. Negative feedback control systems:
    a.   oppose a change.
    b.   accelerate a change.
    c.   ignore a change.
    d.   none of the above

55. Positive feedback control systems:
    a.   oppose a change.
    b.   accelerate a change.
    c.   ignore a change.
    d.   none of the above.

True or false

56. _____   Any given physiological parameter will never deviate beyond the set point.

57. _____   In the thermostatically regulated furnace example of negative feedback, the furnace functions as the sensor.

58. _____   Negative feedback systems are inhibitory.

59. _____   The process of childbirth, in which the baby's head causes increased stretch of the reproductive tract, which in turn feeds back to the brain, thus triggering the release of oxytocin, is an example of positive feedback.

******If you had difficulty with this section, review pages **20-25**

V   HEALTH MATTERS

Matching—match the term on the left with the proper selection on the right.

60. _____   pathology
61. _____   signs
62. _____   symptoms
63. _____   etiology
64. _____   syndrome
65. _____   idiopathic
66. _____   acute
67. _____   pandemic
68. _____   endemic
69. _____   pathogenesis

a.   subjective abnormalities
b.   study of disease
c.   collection of different signs and symptoms that present a clear picture of a pathological condition
d.   study of factors involved in causing a disease
e.   objective abnormalities
f.   undetermined causes
g.   disease native to a local region
h.   symptoms appear suddenly and for a short period
i.   affects large geographic regions
j.   actual pattern of a disease's development

Student Name _____

Fill in the blanks.

70. _____ is the organized study of the underlying physiological processes associated

with disease.

71. Many diseases are best understood as disturbances of _____.

72. Altered or _____ genes can cause abnormal proteins to be made.

73. An organism that lives in or on another organism to obtain its nutrients is called a

_____.

74. Abnormal tissue growths may also be referred to as _____.

75. Autoimmunity literally means _____.

******If you had difficulty with this section, review pages **26-30**

Crossword Puzzle

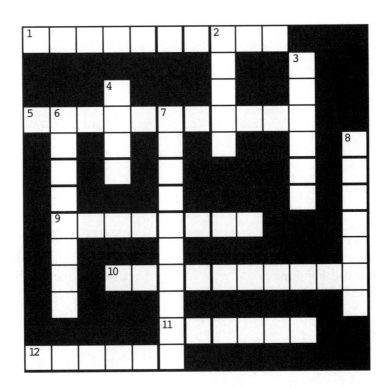

Across

1. Study of body function
5. "Staying the same"
9. _____ feedback is inhibitory
10. Total of chemical and physical reactions
11. Divides the body into sections
12. Group of similar cells

Down

2. Heart is an example
3. Organs arranged to perform a function
4. Basic unit of the body
6. Sum of its parts
7. Physique
8. Study of body systems

APPLYING WHAT YOU KNOW

76. Laurie has had an appendectomy. The nurse is preparing to change the dressing. She knows that the appendix is located in the right iliac inguinal region, the distal portion extending at an angle into the hypogastric region. Place an X on the diagram where the nurse will place the dressing.

77. Penny noticed a lump in her breast. Dr. Reeder noted on her chart that a small mass was located in the left breast medial to the nipple. Place an X where Penny's lump would be located.

78. Madison was injured in a bicycle accident. X-ray films revealed that she had a fracture of the right patella. A cast was applied beginning at the distal femoral region and extending to the pedal region. Place an X where Madison's cast begins and ends.

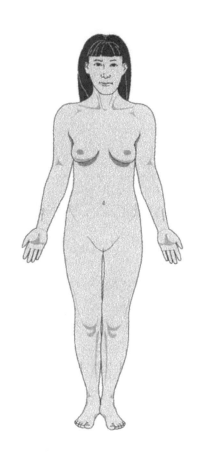

DID YOU KNOW?

- Many animals produce tears but only humans weep as a result of emotional stress.

ONE LAST QUICK CHECK ✔

Multiple Choice—select the best answer.

79. The body's ability to continuously respond to changes in the environment and maintain consistency in the internal environment is called:
    a. homeostasis.
    b. superficial.
    c. structural levels.
    d. none of the above.

80. The regions frequently used by health professionals to locate pain or tumors divides the abdomen into four basic areas called:
    a. planes.
    b. cavities.
    c. pleural.
    d. quadrants.

81. A lengthwise plane running from front to back that divides the body into right and left sides is called:
    a. transverse.
    b. coronal.
    c. frontal.
    d. sagittal.

82. A study of the functions of living organisms and their parts is called:
    a. physiology.
    b. chemistry.
    c. biology.
    d. none of the above.

83. Which of the following structures does *NOT* lie within the abdominopelvic cavity?
    a. right iliac region
    b. left antecubital region
    c. left lumbar region
    d. hypogastric region

84. The dorsal body cavity contains components of the:
    a. reproductive system.
    b. digestive system.
    c. respiratory system.
    d. nervous system.

85. If your reference point is "nearest the trunk of the body" vs. "farthest from the trunk of the body," where does the elbow lie in relation to the wrist?
    a. anterior
    c. distal
    b. posterior
    d. proximal

86. The buttocks are often used as injection sites. This region can also be called:
    a. sacral.
    c. cutaneous.
    b. buccal.
    d. gluteal.

87. Which of the following is *NOT* a component of the axial subdivision of the body?
    a. upper extremity
    b. neck
    c. trunk
    d. head

88. A synonym for medial is:
    a. toward the side.
    c. midline.
    b. in front of.
    d. anterior.

CHAPTER 2

CHEMICAL BASIS OF LIFE

Although anatomy can be studied without knowledge of chemistry, it is hard to imagine an understanding of physiology without a basic comprehension of chemical reactions in the body. Trillions of cells make up the various levels of organization in the body. Our health and survival depends upon the proper chemical maintenance in the cytoplasm of our cells.

Chemists use the terms *elements* or *compounds* to describe all of the substances (matter) in and around us. Distinguishing these two terms is the fact that an element cannot be broken down. A compound, on the other hand, is made up of two or more elements and has the ability to be broken down into the elements that form it.

Organic and inorganic compounds are equally important to us. Without organic compounds such as carbohydrates, proteins, and fats and inorganic compounds such as water, we could not sustain life.

Because we cannot see many of the chemical reactions that take place daily in our bodies, it is sometimes difficult to comprehend the principles involved in initiating them. Chemicals are responsible for directing virtually all of our bodily functions. It is therefore important to master the fundamental concepts of chemistry.

I BASIC CHEMISTRY

Multiple Choice—select the best answer.

1. Which of the following is *NOT* one of the major elements present in the human body?
   a. oxygen
   b. carbon
   c. iron
   d. potassium

2. Which of the following is *NOT* a subatomic particle?
   a. proton
   b. electron
   c. isotope
   d. neutron

3. The total number of electrons in an atom equals the number of:
   a. neutrons in its nucleus.
   b. electrons in its nucleus.
   c. protons in its nucleus.
   d. ions in its nucleus.

4. An atom can be described as chemically inert if its outermost electron shell contains:
   a. three electrons.
   b. five electrons.
   c. six electrons.
   d. eight electrons.

5. Isotopes are atoms of elements that differ in their number of:
   a. protons.
   b. electrons.
   c. neutrons.
   d. nuclei.

6. Ionic bonds are chemical bonds formed by the:
   a. sharing of electrons between atoms.
   b. donation of protons from one atom to another.
   c. transfer of electrons from one atom to another.
   d. acceptance of protons from one atom to another.

7. Chemical bonds formed by the sharing of electrons are called:
    a. ionic.
    b. covalent.
    c. hydrogen.
    d. electronic.

8. A chemical reaction in which substances combine to form more complex substances is called:
    a. synthesis.
    b. decomposition.
    c. exchange.
    d. reversible.

True or false

9. ___T___   *Matter* is a term used by chemists to describe all the materials or substances around us.

10. ___T___   *Atomic weight* refers to the number of protons plus the number of neutrons in an atom.

11. ___F___   Sodium chloride is an example of a covalent bond.

12. ___F___   Hydrogen bonds form from an equal charge distribution within a molecule.

13. ___T___   The digestion of food is an example of a decomposition reaction.

Identify the following elements:

14. ___Oxygen___   O

15. ___Calcium___   Ca

16. ___Potassium___   K

17. ___Sodium___   Na

18. ___Magnesium___   Mg

19. ___Iron___   Fe

20. ___Selenium___   Se

******If you had difficulty with this section, review pages **36-43**

II   INORGANIC MOLECULES

Multiple Choice—select the best answer.

21. Water comprises approximately what percentage of body weight?
     a. 50%
     b. 70%
     c. 80%
     d. 90%

22. Which of the following is *NOT* a property of water?
     a. strong polarity
     b. high specific heat
     c. high heat of vaporization
     d. strong acidity

23. Acids:
     a. are proton donors.
     b. dye litmus blue.
     c. release hydrogen ions when in an aqueous solution.
     d. accept electrons when in an aqueous solution.

24. Substances that accept hydrogen ions are referred to as:
     a. acids.
     b. bases.
     c. buffers.
     d. salts.

25. pH homeostatic mechanism is caused by the presence of substances called:
    a. salts.
    c. buffers.
    b. bases.
    d. acids.

True or false

26. ___T___ The pH scale indicates the degree of acidity or alkalinity of a solution.

27. ___F___ Milk is acid on the pH scale.

28. ___T___ Litmus will turn red in the presence of an acid.

29. ___T___ The basic substance of each cell is water.

30. ___F___ Oxygen and carbon dioxide are examples of organic compounds.

******If you had difficulty with this section, review pages **44-47**

III   ORGANIC MOLECULES

Multiple Choice—select the best answer.

31. Which of the following is *NOT* a type of carbohydrate?
    a. monosaccharides
    b. disaccharides
    c. megasaccharides
    d. polysaccharides

32. Which of the following is *INCORRECT* in reference to carbohydrates?
    a. They include substances referred to as *sugars.*
    b. They serve critical structural roles in RNA and DNA.
    c. They represent a primary source of chemical energy for body cells.
    d. They are replete with nitrogen atoms.

33. Proteins are composed of ____ commonly occurring amino acids.
    a. 8
    c. 20
    b. 12
    d. 24

34. Amino acids frequently become joined by:
    a. peptide bonds.
    b. phospholipid reactions.
    c. degradation synthesis.
    d. none of the above.

35. Which of the following is *NOT* an example of proteins?
    a. hormones
    c. urine
    b. antibodies
    d. enzymes

36. A structural lipid found in a cell membrane is:
    a. triglyceride.
    c. steroid.
    b. phospholipid.
    d. prostaglandin.

37. Which of the following is the correct example of DNA base pairing?
    a. adenine-cytosine
    b. guanine-adenine
    c. adenine-thymine
    d. guanine-thymine

38. A DNA molecule contains each of the following *EXCEPT:*
    a. sugar.
    b. nitrogenous base.
    c. phosphate.
    d. lipid.

39. DNA differs from RNA in that:
  a. RNA contains ribose instead of deoxyri-
       bose.
  b. RNA contains thymine instead of uracil.
  c. RNA contains a double polynucleotide
       strand.
  d. There is no structural difference between
       DNA and RNA.

True or false

40. ___F___   Steroids are poorly distributed throughout the body.

41. ___T___   High-density lipoprotein (HDL) is also called the "good" cholesterol.

42. ___F___   Protein compounds have no role in defending the body against harmful agents.

43. ___T___   The nonessential amino acids can be produced from the other amino acids or from
                simple organic molecules.

44. ___T___   Enzymes are proteins that function by the "lock and key" model.

******If you had difficulty with this section, review pages **48-59**

IV   METABOLISM

Multiple Choice—select the best answer.

45. Catabolism consists of chemical reactions
     that:
  a. break down compounds and release
       energy from them.
  b. participate in dehydration synthesis.
  c. unite smaller molecules into larger
       molecules.
  d. none of the above.

46. The bonds that exist between phosphate
     groups of the ATP molecules are:
  a. hydrogen bonds.
  b. high-energy bonds.
  c. electronic bonds.
  d. ionic bonds.

47. The energy of ATP is released by splitting it
     into:
  a. ATP and an inorganic phosphate.
  b. ADP and an organic phosphate.
  c. ADP and an inorganic phosphate.
  d. ATP and an organic phosphate.

Student Name _____

True or false

48. _____T_____ Anabolic reactions join monosaccharide units to form larger carbohydrates.

49. _____T_____ ATP is often referred to as the "energy currency of cells."

50. _____F_____ ATP is rarely consumed during exercise.

******If you had difficulty with this section, review pages **61-62**

Crossword Puzzle

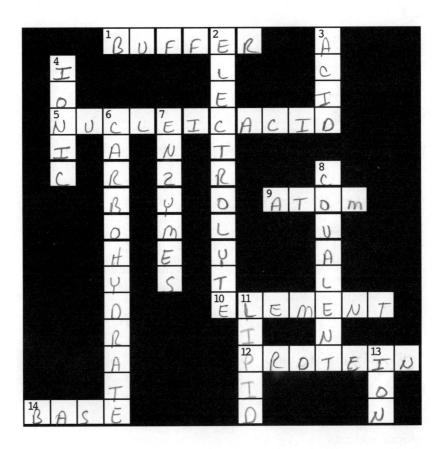

Across

1. Acts as a reservoir for H ions
5. DNA or RNA (two words)
9. Small particle of an element
10. Simple form of matter
12. Amino acid
14. Tastes bitter

Down

2. Dissociates in solution to form ions
3. Releases hydrogen when in solution
4. _____ bond/electrocovalent bond
6. Sugar or starch
7. Chemical catalysts
8. _____ bond/shares electron pairs between atoms
11. Fat
13. Electrically charged atom

APPLYING WHAT YOU KNOW

51. Amanda and Bill own a home that was recently discovered to contain very high levels of radon. Where in the house would these levels be greatest? What could be done to eliminate the radon? What is the family at greatest risk for?

52. Kim just finished preparing a meal of pan-fried hamburgers for her family. While the frying pan was still hot, she poured the liquid grease into a metal container to cool. Later she noticed that the liquid oil had solidified as it cooled. Explain the chemistry of why the now room-temperature fat was solid.

DID YOU KNOW?

- After a vigorous workout, your triglycerides fall 10 to 20% and your HDL increases by the same percentage for 2–3 hours.

ONE LAST QUICK CHECK ✓

Matching—identify each term with its corresponding description or definition.

53. ___e___ Atoms of the same element but with different atomic weights (because their nuclei contain different numbers of neutrons).

54. ___b___ Adenine-thymine and guanine-cytosine are examples of _____ present in DNA.

55. ___g___ Atoms with fewer than eight electrons in their valence shell will attempt to lose, gain, or share electrons with other atoms to achieve stability.

56. ___a___ The number of protons in an atom's nucleus.

57. ___i___ Any large molecule made up of many identical small molecules.

58. ___f___ Components of DNA and RNA that are composed of sugar, a nitrogenous base, and a phosphate group.

59. ___h___ Chemical property that allows water to act as an effective solvent.

60. ___c___ Large group of inorganic compounds including acids, bases, and salts.

a. atomic number
b. base pairs
c. electrolyte
d. high-energy bonds
e. isotopes
f. nucleotide
g. octet rule
h. polarity
i. polymers

Student Name _____

Matching—select the best answer.

61. ___b___ ribose

62. ___c___ steroids

63. ___a___ amino acid

64. ___c___ glycerol

65. ___b___ monosaccharides

66. ___c___ phospholipids

67. ___a___ enzymes

a. protein
b. carbohydrate
c. lipid

Matching—select the best answer.

68. ___b___ litmus turns blue

69. ___a___ "proton donor"

70. ___b___ bitter taste

71. ___b___ "proton acceptor"

72. ___a___ releases a hydrogen ion

a. acid
b. base

CHAPTER 3

ANATOMY OF CELLS

Cells are the smallest structural units of living things. Therefore, because we are living, we are made up of a mass of cells. Human cells, which vary in shape and size, can only be seen under a microscope. The three main parts of a cell are the cytoplasmic membrane, the cytoplasm, and the nucleus. As you review this chapter, you will be amazed at the resemblance of a cell to the body as a whole. You will identify a miniature circulatory system, reproductive system, digestive system, lymphatic system, skeletal system, and many other structures that will aid in your understanding of these and other body systems in future chapters.

I FUNCTIONAL ANATOMY OF CELLS

Multiple Choice—select the best answer.

1. Which of the following is *NOT* a main cellular structure?
    a. plasma membrane
    b. interstitial fluid
    c. cytoplasm (including organelles)
    d. nucleus

2. All of the following are examples of the plasma membrane function *EXCEPT*:
    a. boundary of cell
    b. self-identification
    c. receptor sites
    d. "power plants" of cell

3. Which of the following is a functional characteristic of ribosomes?
    a. provision of ATP
    b. protein synthesis
    c. DNA replication
    d. binding site for steroid hormones

4. Production of ATP occurs within which organelle?
    a. smooth endoplasmic reticulum
    b. Golgi apparatus
    c. lysosomes
    d. mitochondria

5. Preparation of protein molecules for cellular exportation is the function of which of the following organelles?
    a. Golgi apparatus   c.   peroxisomes
    b. microvilli   d.   mitochondria

6. In nondividing cells, DNA appears as threads that are referred to as:
    a. chromatin.
    b. nucleoplasm.
    c. nucleolus.
    d. none of the above.

7. The nucleolus is composed chiefly of:
    a. DNA.
    b. rRNA.
    c. tRNA.
    d. none of the above.

True or false

8. ___F___ The plasma membrane can be described as a triple layer of phospholipid molecules.

9. ___F___ Contrary to popular belief, the cytoskeleton really provides little supporting framework to the cell.

10. ___F___ Each and every cell always has one nucleus.

11. ___T___ Generally, the more active a cell is, the more mitochondria it will contain.

12. ___F___ Light microscopy is far superior to electron microscopy.

Matching—identify each cell structure with its corresponding function.

13. ___a___ forms ribosomes

14. ___d___ separates cell from environment

15. ___b___ acts as cell's "digestive system"

16. ___f___ acts as "protein factory"

17. ___c___ contains organelles

18. ___h___ contains DNA

19. ___g___ acts as "power plants" of the cell

20. ___e___ causes cellular locomotion

a. nucleoli
b. lysosome
c. cytoplasm
d. plasma membrane
e. flagella
f. ribosome
g. mitochondria
h. nucleus

Student Name _____

Labeling—label the following microscope diagram using the terms provided.

fine focus ~~~~   coarse focus   mechanical stage ~~~~
light source ~~~~   objective lens ~~~~   condensor lens ~~~~
specimen on slide ~~~~   ocular lens

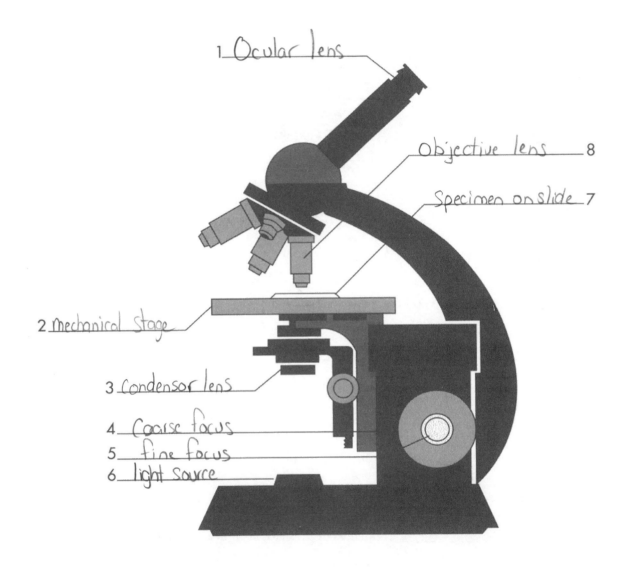

1 Ocular lens

Objective lens 8

Specimen on slide 7

2 Mechanical stage

3 Condensor lens

4 Coarse focus

5 fine focus

6 light source

Labeling—from memory, label the parts of the typical cell on the diagram below.

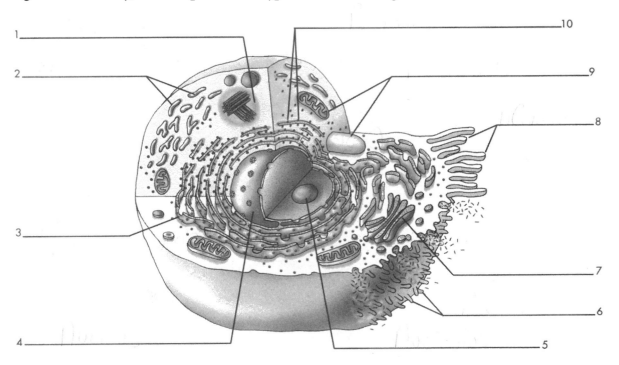

******If you had difficulty with this section, review pages **71-83**

II CYTOSKELETON

Fill in the blanks.

21. _Cytoskeleton_ is the cell's internal supporting framework.

22. _Microfilaments_ are the smallest cell fibers.

23. The thickest of the cell fibers are tiny, hollow tubes called _microtubules_.

24. The _Centrosome_ is an area of the cytoplasm near the nucleus that coordinates the building and breaking of microtubules in the cell.

25. _Microvilli_, _Cilia_, and _flagella_ are cell extensions that appear on certain types of cells.

26. When membrane channels of adjacent plasma membranes adhere to others, the formation is known as _gap_ _junctions_.

27. _Desmosomes_ hold skin together.

******If you had difficulty with this section, review pages **83-86**

Student Name_____

Crossword Puzzle

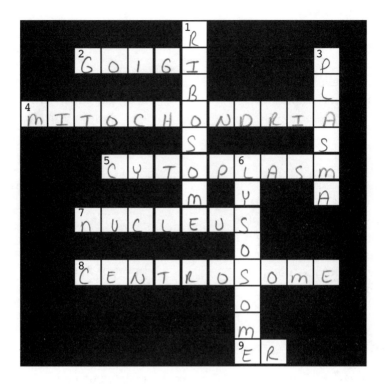

Across

2. _____ apparatus/synthesizes carbohydrates
4. Power plants
5. Gel-like substance within the cell
7. Contains DNA
8. Area of cytoplasm near the nucleus
9. Rough and smooth (abbrev.)

Down

1. Protein factory
3. _____ membrane/surrounds the cell
6. Cell's digestive system

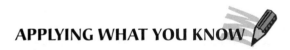

APPLYING WHAT YOU KNOW

28. Brian is a sedentary, overweight cigarette smoker who has chest pain whenever he exerts himself. Upon examination, his cardiologist determines that Brian is suffering from heart disease. Which receptors in the cells that line the blood vessels of his heart are responsible? What type of cholesterol is responsible? What other diseases may he be at risk for?

29. After several weeks of exercising in the weight room, Valerie notices that she has not only become stronger, but quite muscular as well. Which organelle has increased its density in the cytoplasm of her muscles in response to a greater demand for ATP production?

DID YOU KNOW?

• The largest single cell in the human body is the female sex cell, the ovum. The smallest single cell in the human body is the male sex cell, the sperm.

ONE LAST QUICK CHECK ✔

Multiple Choice—select the best answer.

30. Which of the following cellular extensions is required when absorption is important?
    a. cilia
    b. microvilli
    c. flagella
    d. none of the above

31. Movement of the ovum within the female reproductive tract is largely as a result of:
    a. the flagella extending from the ovum.
    b. the cilia extending from the ovum.
    c. the cilia lining the uterine tubes.
    d. none of the above.

32. Skin cells are held tightly together by:
    a. gap junctions.   c. tight junctions.
    b. desmosomes.   d. adhesions.

33. Ribosomes are attached to:
    a. lysosomes.
    b. rough endoplasmic reticulum.
    c. peroxisomes.
    d. cilia.

34. The phospholipid area of the plasma membrane of a cell is:
    a. single layered.   c. trilayered.
    b. bilayered.   d. multilayered.

Matching—identify each term with its corresponding definition.

35. __e__ nerve cells
36. __d__ muscle cells
37. __b__ red blood cells
38. __a__ gland cells
39. __c__ immune cells

a. release hormones
b. transport oxygen
c. destroy bacteria
d. contract for movement
e. detect changes in environment

Fill in the blanks.

40. A typical or ___Composite___ cell exhibits the most important characteristics of cell types.

41. ___Hydrophilic___ is the term used to describe "water loving."

42. ___Signal Transduction___ is the process that allows a message to be carried across a membrane.

43. ___Peroxisomes___ detoxify harmful substances that enter cells.

44. The ___Nucleus___ is one of the largest cell structures and occupies the central portion of the cell.

Student Name_____

CHAPTER 4

PHYSIOLOGY OF CELLS

Cells, just like humans, require water, food, gases, elimination of wastes, and numerous other substances and processes in order to survive. Cells must transport the substances within the cytoplasm and across cell membranes. The movement of these substances in and out of the cell is accomplished by two primary methods: passive transport and active transport. In passive transport, no cellular energy is required to effect movement through the cell membrane. However, in active transport, cellular energy is necessary to provide movement through the cell membrane.

Cell reproduction completes the study of cells. A basic explanation of DNA, the "hereditary molecule," gives us a proper respect for the capability of the cell to transmit physical and mental traits from generation to generation. Reproduction of the cell—mitosis—is a complex process requiring several stages. These stages are outlined and diagrammed in the text to facilitate learning. An understanding of cell physiology will assist you in your comprehension of the physiology of the body as a whole.

I MOVEMENT OF SUBSTANCES THROUGH CELL MEMBRANES

Multiple Choice—select the best answer.

1. Which of the following is *NOT* a passive transport process?
   a. dialysis
   c. filtration
   b. osmosis
   d. pinocytosis

2. Diffusion of water through a selectively permeable membrane in the presence of at least one impermeant solute is referred to as:
   a. diffusion.
   c. phagocytosis.
   b. osmosis.
   d. dialysis.

3. The trapping of bacteria by specialized white blood cells is an example of:
   a. pinocytosis.
   b. exocytosis.
   c. phagocytosis.
   d. none of the above.

4. A hypertonic solution is one that contains:
   a. a greater concentration of solute than the cell.
   b. the same concentration of solute as the cell.
   c. a lesser concentration of solute as the cell.
   d. none of the above.

5. The force of a fluid pushing against a surface could be described as:
   a. facilitated diffusion.
   b. hydrostatic pressure.
   c. hypostatic pressure.
   d. none of the above.

True or false

6. _____ Facilitated diffusion is a metabolically expensive process.

7. _____ The sodium-potassium pump is an example of an active transport process.

8. _____ Cellular secretion can be achieved by exocytosis.

9. _____ Solutes are particles dissolved in a solvent.

10. _____ Osmosis is a form of filtration that results in the separation of small and large solute particles.

Matching—identify each item with its corresponding description.

11. _____ solution that draws water from a cell

12. _____ solution with a net diffusion of zero

13. _____ solution that causes cells to swell

14. _____ passive transport

15. _____ active transport

a. isotonic solution
b. hypertonic solution
c. hypotonic solution
d. diffusion
e. endocytosis

Labeling—match each term with its corresponding number in the following diagram of cellular respiration.

_____ aerobic   _____ anaerobic   _____ lactic acid   _____ transition

_____ glucose   _____ pyruvic acid   _____ O_2 _____ H_2O

_____ mitochondrion   _____ citric acid cycle   _____ ATP   _____ acetyl CoA

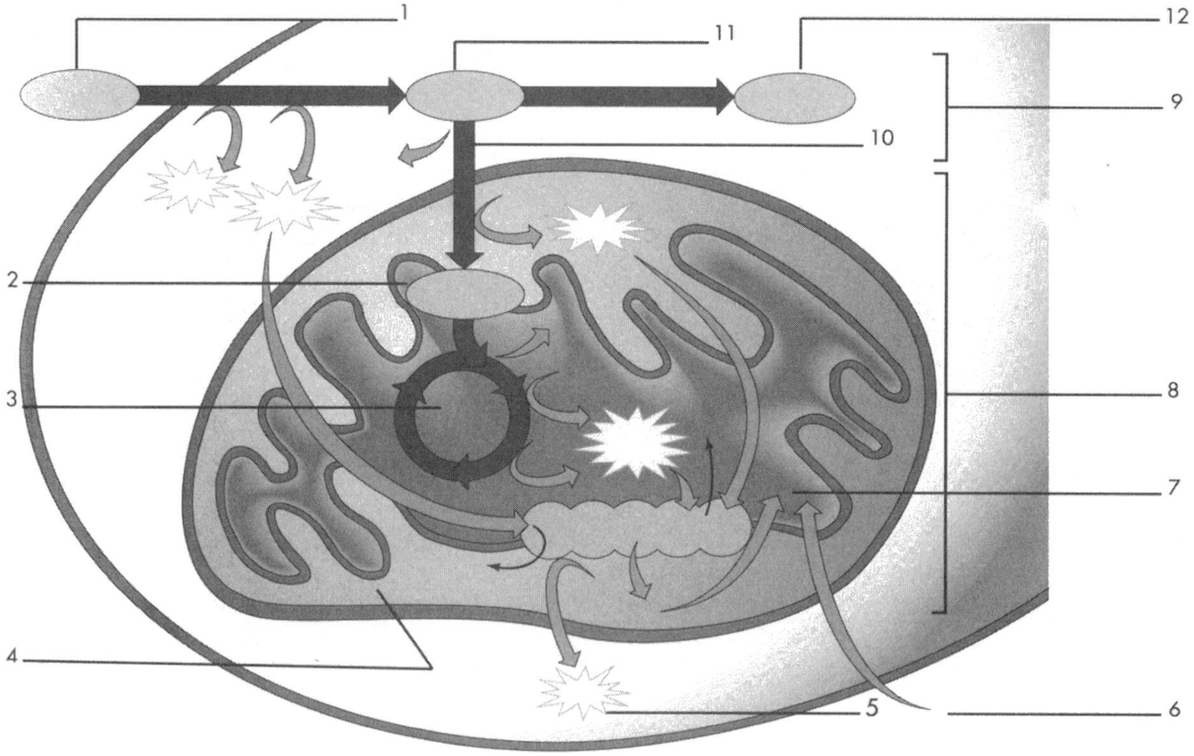

******If you had difficulty with this section, review pages **91-98** and page **103**

Student Name_____

II CELL METABOLISM

Multiple Choice—select the best answer.

16. Enzymes that cause essential chemical reactions to occur are called:
    a. metabolic agents.
    b. catalysts.
    c. substrates.
    d. initiators.

17. In the DNA molecule, a sequence of three base pairs forms a(n):
    a. codon.
    b. anticodon.
    c. polymerase.
    d. none of the above.

18. Transcription can best described as the:
    a. synthesis of tRNA.
    b. reading of mRNA codons by tRNA.
    c. synthesis of mRNA.
    d. synthesis of polypeptides at a ribosomal site.

19. Which of the following statements is true?
    a. Complex polypeptide chains form tRNA.
    b. The site of transcription is within the nucleus, whereas the site of translation is in the cytoplasm.
    c. Uracil is present in DNA in the place of thymine.
    d. None of the above is true.

20. A DNA molecule is characterized by all of the following *EXCEPT*:
    a. double-helix shape.
    b. obligatory base pairing.
    c. ribose sugar.
    d. phosphate groups.

21. Which of the following is *NOT* a characteristic of RNA?
    a. It is single-stranded.
    b. It contains uracil and not thymine.
    c. The obligatory base pairs are adenine-uracil and guanine-cytosine.
    d. Its molecules are larger than those of DNA.

True or false

22. _____ The three processes that comprise cellular respiration are glycolysis, the citric acid cycle, and the electron transport system.

23. _____ The portion of an enzyme molecule that chemically "fits" the substrate molecule(s) is referred to as the *active site*.

24. _____ One significant similarity between RNA and DNA is that they both are shaped as a double helix.

25. _____ The "lock and key" model is used to describe how DNA base pairs align.

26. _____ Protein anabolism is a major cellular activity.

27. _____ The citric acid cycle is also known as the *Krebs cycle*.

28. _____ Glycolysis is aerobic.

Labeling—label the following DNA molecule.

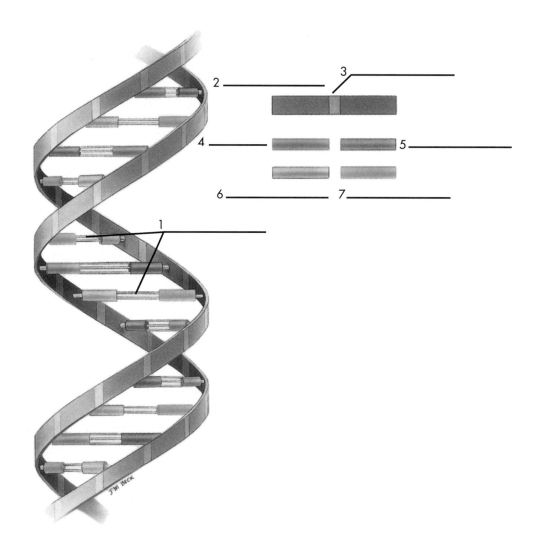

******If you had difficulty with this section, review pages **99-108**

III GROWTH AND REPRODUCTION OF CELLS

Multiple Choice—select the best answer.

29. An individual's entire set of DNA can be referred to as:
    a.   a genome.
    b.   a chromosome.
    c.   cytokinesis.
    d.   none of the above.

30. The correct order of mitosis is:
    a.   prophase, metaphase, anaphase, telophase.
    b.   anaphase, telophase, metaphase, prophase.
    c.   prophase, anaphase, metaphase, telophase.
    d.   none of the above.

31. The total of 46 chromosomes per cell is referred to as:
    a. haploid.
    b. diploid.
    c. myoid.
    d. none of the above.

32. Which of the following terms is synonymous with *tumor*?
    a. anaplasia   c. neoplasm
    b. hyperplasia   d. benign

True or false

33. _____ *Gamete* is a term referring to the point of attachment of newly replicated DNA molecules.

34. _____ Normal mitosis results in daughter cells that are genetically identical to the parent cell.

35. _____ It is during meiosis II that the number of chromosomes are halved.

36. _____ Telophase is the "completion phase" of mitosis.

37. _____ *Hyperplasia* refers to an increase in cell size, whereas *hypertrophy* refers to an increase in cell number.

Matching—identify the term related to protein synthesis with its corresponding definition.

38. _____ process that occurs when the double strands of a DNA segment separate and RNA nucleotides pair with the DNA nucleotides

a. mRNA
b. ribosome
c. tRNA
d. translation
e. transcription
f. complimentary base pair

39. _____ the type of RNA that carries information in groups of three nucleotides called codons, each of which codes for a specific amino acid

40. _____ the type of RNA that has an anticodon and binds to a base pair specific amino acid

41. _____ the process involving the movement of mRNA with respect to the ribosome

42. _____ uracil-adenine

43. _____ the site of translation

******If you had difficulty with this section, review pages **106-115**

IV   MECHANISMS OF DISEASE

True or false

44. _____   Diabetes mellitus is a disorder of cell membrane receptors.

45. _____   Genetic disorders are mutations in a cell's genetic code.

46. _____   Cystic fibrosis is a condition in which chloride ion pumps in the plasma membrane are missing.

47. _____   Viruses do not contain DNA or RNA.

48. _____   A blood disease caused by the production of abnormal hemoglobin is known as *sickle-cell anemia*.

Labeling—on the following diagram, label the phases of mitosis. Remember that interphase and DNA replication occur before mitosis begins!

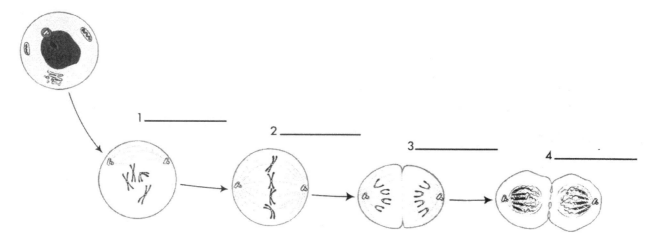

1 _____

2 _____

3 _____

4 _____

******If you had difficulty with this section, review pages **112-117**

Student Name _____

Crossword Puzzle

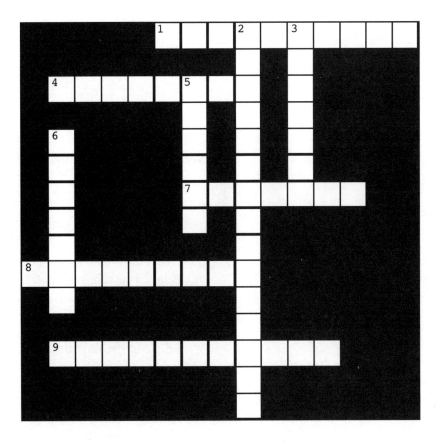

Across

1. Sum of chemical reactions in a cell
4. Concentration _____ measures difference from one area to another
7. Cell reproduction
8. Passive process
9. "Traps" extracellular material and brings it into cell

Down

2. Movement that requires cell energy (two words)
3. Diffusion of water
5. Chemical catalyst
6. Sex cell reproduction

APPLYING WHAT YOU KNOW

49. Nurse Bricker was instructed to dissolve a pill in a small amount of liquid medication. As she dropped the capsule into the liquid, she was interrupted by the telephone. On her return to the medication cart, she found the medication completely dissolved and apparently scattered evenly through out the liquid. This phenomenon did not surprise her since she was aware from her knowledge of cell transport that _____ had created this distribution.

50. Bobbi ran in the Boston marathon. During the race she lost a lot of fluids through perspiration and became dehydrated. Would you expect her cells to shrink, swell, or remain the same?

DID YOU KNOW?

- A human can detect one drop of perfume diffused throughout a three-room apartment.

ONE LAST QUICK CHECK ✔

Multiple Choice—select the best answer.

51. In which stage of mitosis do chromosomes move to opposite ends of the cells along the spindle fibers?
    a. anaphase
    c. prophase
    b. metaphase
    d. telophase

52. The synthesis of proteins by ribosomes using information coded in the mRNA molecule is called:
    a. translation.
    c. replication.
    b. transcription.
    d. crenation.

53. The energy required for active transport processes is obtained from:
    a. ATP.
    c. diffusion.
    b. DNA.
    d. osmosis.

54. Movement of substances from a region of high concentration to a region of low concentration is:
    a. active transport.
    b. passive transport.
    c. cellular energy.
    d. concentration gradient.

55. Osmosis is the _____ of water across a selectively permeable membrane.
    a. filtration
    c. active transport
    b. equilibrium
    d. diffusion

56. _____ involves the movement of solutes across a selectively permeable membraneby the process of diffusion.
    a. osmosis
    b. permease system
    c. filtration
    d. all of the above

57. A specialized example of diffusion is:
    a. osmosis.
    b. permease system.
    c. filtration.
    d. all of the above.

58. This movement always occurs down a hydrostatic pressure gradient.
    a. osmosis
    b. filtration
    c. dialysis
    d. facilitated diffusion

59. The uphill movement of a substance through a living cell membrane is:
    a. osmosis.
    c. active transport.
    b. diffusion.
    d. passive transport.

60. The ion pump is an example of this type of movement.
    a. gravity
    b. hydrostatic pressure
    c. active transport
    d. passive transport

61. An example of a cell that uses phagocytosis is the:
    a. white blood cell.
    c. muscle cell.
    b. red blood cell.
    d. bone cell.

62. A saline solution that contains a higher concentration of salt than living red blood cells would be:
    a. hypotonic.
    c. isotonic.
    b. hypertonic.
    d. homeostatic.

63. A red blood cell becomes engorged with water and will eventually lyse, releasing hemoglobin into the solution. This solution is _____ to the red blood cell.
    a. hypotonic
    c. isotonic
    b. hypertonic
    d. homeostatic

Student Name_____

Circle the word or phrase that does not belong.

64. DNA   adenine   uracil   thymine

65. RNA   ribose   thymine   uracil

66. translation   protein synthesis   mRNA   interphase

67. cleavage furrow   anaphase   prophase   2 daughter cells

68. metaphase   prophase   telophase   gene

CHAPTER 5

TISSUES

After successfully completing the study of the cell, you are ready to progress to the next level of anatomical structure: tissues. Four principal types of tissue—epithelial, connective, muscle, and nervous—perform multiple functions to assure that homeostasis is maintained. Among these functions are protection, absorption, excretion, support, insulation, conduction of impulses, movement of bones, and destruction of bacteria. This variety of functions gives us a real appreciation for the complexity of this level.

A macroscopic view confirms this statement as we marvel at the fact that soft, sticky, liquid blood and sturdy compact bone are both considered tissues. Our study continues with the discussion of body membranes and their function for the body. Membranes are thin layers of epithelial and/or connective tissue that cover and protect the body surfaces, line body cavities, and cover the internal surfaces of hollow organs. These major membranes—cutaneous, serous, mucous, and synovial—are also critical to homeostasis and body survival. An understanding of tissues and membranes is necessary to successfully bridge your knowledge between the cell and the study of body organs.

I   PRINCIPAL TYPES OF TISSUES

Multiple Choice—select the best answer.

1. A tissue is:
   a. a membrane that lines body cavities.
   b. a group of similar cells that perform a common function.
   c. a thin sheet of cells embedded in a matrix.
   d. the most complex organizational unit of the body.

2. The four principal types of tissues include all of the following *EXCEPT*:
   a. nervous.   c. cartilage.
   b. muscle.   d. connective.

3. The most complex tissue in the body is:
   a. muscle.   c. connective.
   b. blood.   d. nervous.

4. The nonliving intercellular material that surrounds tissues is called:
   a. intercellular material.
   b. matrix.
   c. lacunae.
   d. none of the above.

5. The hollow ball of cells that forms after fertilization is referred to as:
   a. primary germ layer.
   b. blastocyst.
   c. gastrulation.
   d. none of the above.

6. Which tissue lines body cavities and protects body surfaces?
   a. epithelial   c. muscular
   b. connective   d. nervous

True or false

7.   ___T___   The biology of tissues is referred to as *histology.*

8.   ___F___   The process of the primary germ layers of the embryo differentiating into specific tissues is called *gastrulation.*

9.   ___F___   Sweat and sebaceous glands are formed by connective tissue.

10.   ___T___   The three primary germ layers are endoderm, ectoderm, and mesoderm.

******If you had difficulty with this section, review pages **123-125**

II EPITHELIAL TISSUE

Multiple Choice—select the best answer.

11.   Which of the following is *NOT* a function of membranous epithelium?
    a.   secretion
    b.   protection
    c.   absorption
    d.   all are functions of the membranous epithelium

12.   Which of the following is *NOT* a structural example of epithelium?
    a.   stratified squamous
    b.   simple transitional
    c.   stratified columnar
    d.   pseudostratified columnar

13.   The simple columnar epithelium lining the intestines contains plasma membranes that extend into thousands of microscopic extensions called:
    a.   villi.   c.   cilia.
    b.   microvilli.   d.   flagella.

14.   Epithelial cells can be classified according to shape. Which of the following is *NOT* a characteristic shape of epithelium?
    a.   cuboidal   c.   squamous
    b.   rectangular   d.   columnar

15.   Keratinized stratified squamous epithelium is found in the:
    a.   mouth.   c.   epidermis.
    b.   vagina.   d.   all of the above.

16.   Endocrine glands discharge their products into:
    a.   body cavities.
    b.   blood.
    c.   organ surfaces.
    d.   none of the above.

17.   Which of the following is *NOT* a functional classification of exocrine glands?
    a.   alveolar   c.   holocrine
    b.   apocrine   d.   merocrine

18.   The functional classification of salivary glands is:
    a.   endocrine.   c.   holocrine.
    b.   apocrine.   d.   merocrine.

19.   This epithelial tissue readily allows diffusion, as in the linings of blood and lymphatic vessels.
    a.   simple squamous
    b.   stratified squamous
    c.   simple columnar
    d.   pseudostratified columnar

Student Name _____

True or false

20. ___T___ Epithelial tissue is attached to an underlying layer of connective tissue called the *basement membrane*.

21. ___F___ Epithelium is rich with blood supply.

22. ___F___ Exocrine glands discharge their products directly into the blood.

Matching—identify the arrangement of epithelial cells with its corresponding description.

23. ___b___ single layer of cube-shaped cells

24. ___e___ multiple layers of cells with flat cells at the outer surface

25. ___d___ single layer of cells in which some are tall and thin and able to reach the free surface and others are not

26. ___h___ layers of cells that appear cubelike when an organ is relaxed and flat or distended by fluid

27. ___a___ single layer of flat, scalelike cells

28. ___c___ single layer of tall, thin cells

    a. simple squamous
    b. simple cuboidal
    c. simple columnar
    d. pseudostratified columnar
    e. stratified squamous
    f. stratified cuboidal
    g. stratified columnar
    h. transitional

Labeling—label the following images and identify the principal tissue type of each. Be as specific as possible. Consult your textbook if you need assistance.

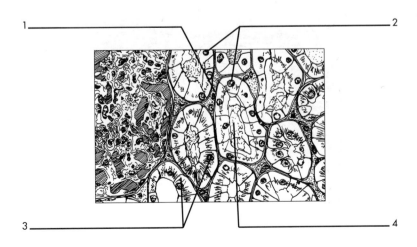

Tissue type: _____

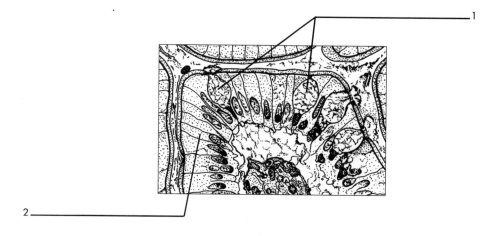

Tissue type: _____

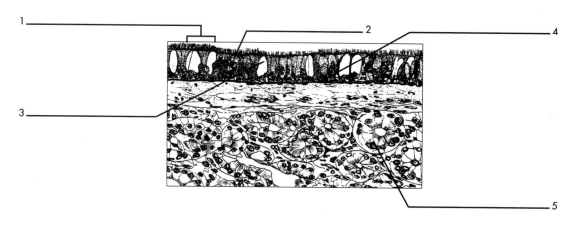

Tissue type: _____

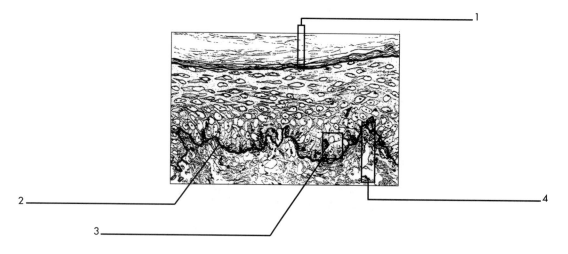

Tissue type: _____

******If you had difficulty with this section, review pages **124-131**

Student Name _____   _____

III CONNECTIVE TISSUE

Multiple Choice—select the best answer.

29. Which of the following is *NOT* an example of connective tissue?
    - a. transitional
    - b. reticular
    - c. blood
    - d. bone

30. Which of the following fibers is *NOT* found in connective tissue matrix?
    - a. collagenous
    - b. elastic
    - c. fibroblastic
    - d. reticular

31. Fibroblasts are usually present in the greatest numbers in:
    - a. adipose.
    - b. areolar.
    - c. reticular.
    - d. dense.

32. Adipose tissue performs each of the following functions *EXCEPT*:
    - a. insulation.
    - b. protection.
    - c. support.
    - d. immune protection

33. Which of the following connective tissue types forms the framework of the spleen, lymph nodes and bone marrow?
    - a. loose
    - b. adipose
    - c. reticular
    - d. areolar

34. The mature cells of bone are called:
    - a. fibroblasts.
    - b. osteoclasts.
    - c. osteoblasts.
    - d. osteocytes.

35. The basic structural unit of bone is the microscopic:
    - a. osteon.
    - b. lacunae.
    - c. lamellae.
    - d. canaliculi.

36. Mature bone grows and is reshaped by the simultaneous activity of which two cells?
    - a. osteoblasts and osteocytes
    - b. osteoblasts and osteoclasts
    - c. osteocytes and osteoclasts
    - d. none of the above

37. The most prevalent type of cartilage is:
    - a. hyaline cartilage.
    - b. fibrous cartilage.
    - c. elastic cartilage.
    - d. none of the above.

38. Which of the following is *NOT* released by injured tissues?
    - a. histamine
    - b. serotonin
    - c. kinins
    - d. all of the above are released

True or false

39. ___T___   The most prevalent types of cells in areolar connective tissue are fibroblasts and macrophages.

40. ___T___   The terms *osteon* and *haversian system* are synonymous.

41. ___F___   The long bones of the body are formed through the process of intramembranous ossification.

42. ___F___   Cartilage is perhaps the most vascular tissue in the human body.

43. ___T___   Many researchers believe that one of the most basic factors in the aging process is the change in the molecular structure of collagen.

44. ___F___   The greater a person's weight while immersed, the higher the body-fat percentage.

Labeling—label the following images and identify the principal tissue type of each. Be as specific as possible. Consult your textbook if you need assistance.

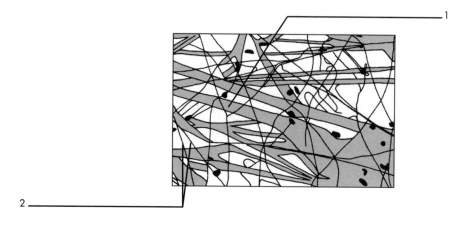

Tissue type: _____

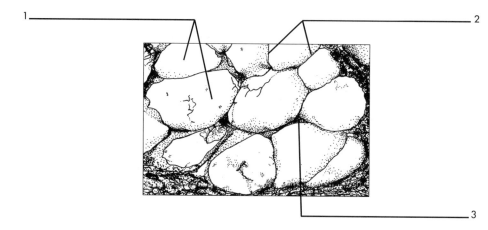

Tissue type: _____

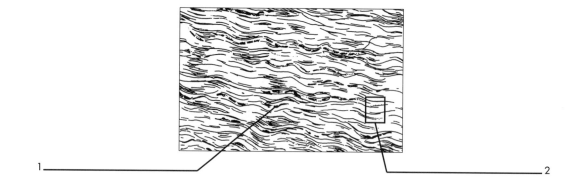

Tissue type: _____

Student Name_____

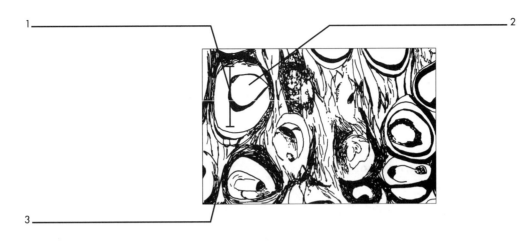

1 _____

2 _____

3 _____

Tissue type: _____

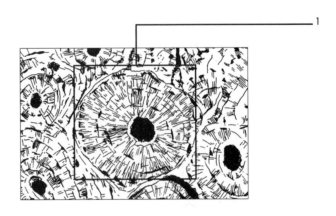

1 _____

Tissue type: _____

******If you had difficulty with this section, review pages **132-143**

IV   MUSCLE TISSUE

Matching—identify the type of muscle tissue with its corresponding definition.

45. ___b___   cylindrical, striated, voluntary cells

46. ___c___   nonstriated, involuntary, narrow fibers with only one nucleus per fiber

47. ___a___   striated, branching, involuntary cells with intercalated disks

48. ___b___   responsible for willed body movements

49. ___c___   also called *visceral muscle*

50. ___c___   found in the walls of hollow internal organs

a.   cardiac muscle
b.   skeletal muscle
c.   smooth muscle

Labeling—label the following images and identify the principal tissue type of each. Be as specific as possible. Consult your textbook if you need assistance.

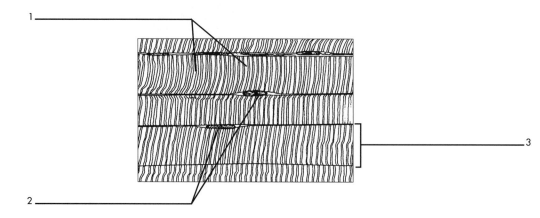

Tissue type: _____

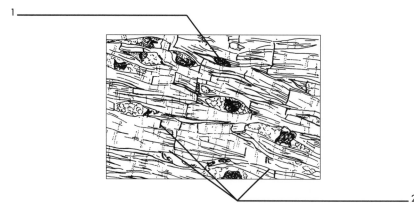

Tissue type: _____

******If you had difficulty with this section, review pages **143-145**

Student Name_____

V   NERVOUS TISSUE

Matching—identify each term with its corresponding description.

51. ___d___ the cell body of the neuron

52. ___b___ supportive cells

53. ___c___ cell process that transmits nerve impulses away from the cell body

54. ___a___ the conducting cells of the nervous system

55. ___e___ cell process that carries nerve impulses toward the cell body

A. neuron
B. neuroglia
C. axon
D. soma
E. dendrite

Labeling—label the following image and identify the principal tissue type. Be as specific as possible. Consult your textbook if you need assistance.

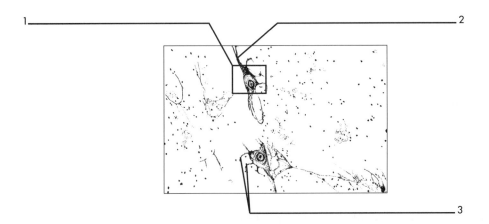

Tissue type: _____

******If you had difficulty with this section, review pages **145-146**

VI   TISSUE REPAIR

Matching—identify each term with its corresponding description.

56. ____/____   process by which white blood cells engulf and destroy bacteria

57. _____   redness indicating increased blood flow and pooling of blood following injury

58. _____   growth of new tissue (as opposed to scarring)

59. _____   heat resulting from the increased blood flow to the area of injury

60. _____   attraction of leukocytes

61. _____   pain

62. _____   chemical causing increased blood vessel permeability

63. _____   an unusually thick scar

64. _____   increased number of white blood cells

65. _____   the presence of abnormally large amounts of fluid in intercellular tissue spaces

a.   calor
b.   regeneration
c.   edema
d.   rubor
e.   histamine
f.   dolor
g.   keloid
h.   phagocytosis
i.   leukocytosis
j.   chemotaxis

******If you had difficulty with this section, review pages **142-147**

VII   BODY MEMBRANES

Multiple Choice—select the best answer.

66. Which of the following is *NOT* an example of epithelial membrane?
    a.   synovial membrane
    b.   cutaneous membrane
    c.   serous membrane
    d.   mucous membrane

67. Pleurisy is a condition that affects which membrane?
    a.   cutaneous membrane
    b.   serous membrane
    c.   mucous membrane
    d.   none of the above

Student Name_____

True or false

68. _____ Parietal membranes cover the surface of organs.

69. _____ Synovial membrane and bursae are examples of connective tissue membrane.

******If you had difficulty with this section, review pages **147-149**

VII   MECHANISMS OF DISEASE

Circle the correct answer.

70. Benign tumors usually grow (slowly or quickly).

71. Malignant tumors (are or are not) encapsulated.

72. An example of a benign tumor that arises from epithelial tissue is (papilloma or lipoma).

73. Malignant tumors that arise from connective tissues are generally called (melanoma or sarcoma).

74. A cancer specialist is an (osteologist or oncologist).

75. Chemotherapy uses (cytotoxic or cachexic) compounds to destroy malignant cells.

******If you had difficulty with this section, review pages **149-151**

Crossword Puzzle

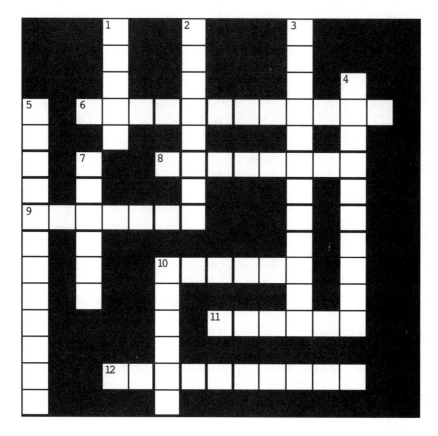

Across

6. Response to a tissue irritant
8. Provides strength for connective tissue
9. Tissue that contains neurons and neuroglia
10. Membrane that lines surfaces that lead to the exterior
11. Cells that perform a common function
12. Tissue that includes glandular

Down

1. Exocrine
2. "Scaly"
3. Process of primary germ layer's tissue development
4. Tissue that includes adipose
5. Growth of new tissue
7. Membrane that lines body cavities
10. Nonliving intercellular material

APPLYING WHAT YOU KNOW

76. Holly is a body builder who is obsessed with her physique. She exercises daily and eats a very low-fat diet. A personal fitness trainer has assessed her body fat at 12%. Determine whether she is too lean or too fat. Explain the relationship between her body-fat percentage and lifestyle.

77. Bruce is a sedentary, cigarette smoking, middle-aged man who is complaining of chest pain. Ultimately, he is diagnosed with lung cancer. What tests may have been utilized to determine his diagnosis? Which type of tissues would be involved?

Student Name _____

DID YOU KNOW?

- As many as 500,000 Americans die from cancer each year making it the second leading cause of death in the United States after cardiovascular disease. Half of all cancers are diagnosed in people under the age of 67.

ONE LAST QUICK CHECK ✔

Labeling—label the following images and identify the principal tissue type of each. Be as specific as possible. Consult your textbook if you need assistance.

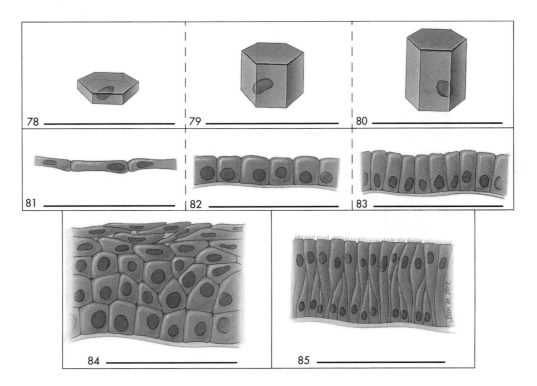

78 _____ 79 _____ 80 _____

81 _____ 82 _____ 83 _____

84 _____ 85 _____

Multiple Choice—select the best answer.

86. Which of the following is *NOT* an example of connective tissue?
    a. glands   c. fat
    b. blood   d. bone

87. Stratified squamous (nonkeratized) epithelium can be found in all of the following *EXCEPT*:
    a. vagina.   c. esophagus.
    b. mouth.   d. skin.

88. The most abundant and widespread tissue is:
    a. epithelial.   c. muscle.
    b. connective.   d. nervous.

89. Loose connective tissue is also known as:
    a. voluntary.   c. areolar.
    b. hyaline.   d. visceral.

90. Tissue that insulates to conserve body is:
    a. reticular.   c. adipose.
    b. fibrous.   d. osseous.

91. What statement regarding blood is true?
    a. Erythrocytes are white blood cells.
    b. Thrombocytes are also known as *platelets*.
    c. Leukocytes are red blood cells.
    d. Formed elements are known as *plasma*.

92. Cutaneous membrane:
     a.   covers body surfaces that are exposed to
          the external environment.
     b.   lines cavities that lead to the outside.
     c.   lines closed body cavities.
     d.   none of the above.

93. An example of mucous membrane is:
     a.   synovial fluid.
     b.   bursae.
     c.   lining of the respiratory tract.
     d.   peritoneum.

CHAPTER 6

SKIN AND ITS APPENDAGES

More of our time, attention, and money are spent on this system than any other. Every time we look into a mirror we become aware of the integumentary system, as we observe our skin, hair, nails, and the appendages that give luster and comfort to this system. The discussion of the skin begins with the structure and function of the two primary layers called the *epidermis* and *dermis*. It continues with an examination of the appendages of the skin, which include the hair, receptors, nails, sebaceous glands, and sudoriferous glands.

Your study of skin concludes with a review of one of the most serious and frequent threats to the skin—burns. An understanding of the integumentary system provides you with an appreciation of the danger that severe burns or trauma can pose to this system.

I SKIN FUNCTION AND STRUCTURE

Multiple Choice—select the best answer.

1. Beneath the dermis lies a loose layer of skin rich in fat and areolar tissue called the:
   a. dermal-epidermal junction.
   b. subcutaneous layer.
   c. hypodermis.
   d. none of the above.

2. The hypodermis:
   a. connects the dermis to underlying tissue.
   b. is the layer of skin where hair is produced.
   c. connects the dermis and the epidermis.
   d. is the skin layer where nails are produced.

3. The order of the cells of the epidermis, from superficial to deep, are:
   a. stratum corneum, stratum lucidum, stratum spinosum, stratum granulosum, stratum basale.
   b. stratum corneum, stratum spinosum, stratum lucidum, stratum granulosum, stratum basale.
   c. stratum basale, stratum corneum, stratum lucidum, stratum spinosum, stratum granulosum.
   d. stratum corneum, stratum lucidum, stratum granulosum, stratum spinosum, stratum basale.

4. In which area of the body would you expect to find an especially thick stratum?
   a. back of the hand
   b. thigh
   c. abdomen
   d. sole of the foot

5. In which layer of the skin do cells divide by mitosis to replace cells lost from the outermost surface of the body?
   a. stratum basale
   b. stratum corneum
   c. stratum lucidum
   d. stratum spinosum

6. Smooth muscles that produce "goose pimples" when they contract are:
   a. papillary muscles.
   b. hair muscles.
   c. follicular muscles.
   d. arrector pili muscles.

7. The most common type of skin cancer is:
   a. malignant melanoma.
   b. squamous cell carcinoma.
   c. basal cell carcinoma.
   d. Kaposi's sarcoma.

8. Meissner corpuscles are specialized nerve endings that make it possible for skin to detect:
    a. heat.
    b. cold.
    c. light touch.
    d. deep pressure.

9. The basic determinant of skin color is the quantity of:
    a. keratin.
    b. melanin.
    c. albinin.
    d. none of the above.

10. Which of the following is *NOT* a contributing factor to skin color?
    a. exposure to sunlight
    b. genetics
    c. place of birth
    d. volume of blood in skin capillaries

True or false

11. __F__   Most of the body is covered by thick skin.

12. __T__   A surgeon would most likely prefer to make an incision parallel to Langer cleavage lines.

13. __T__   If the enzyme tyrosinase is absent from birth because of a congenital defect, a condition called *albinism* results.

14. __F__   Both benign moles and malignant melanomas are outlined by a distinct border.

15. __T__   *Subcutaneous layer* and *hypodermis* are synonymous terms.

Labeling—match each term with its corresponding label on the following diagram of a cross section of skin.

_____ Meissner corpuscle

_____ stratum granulosum

_____ epidermis

_____ hair shaft

_____ sebaceous (oil) gland

_____ stratum basale

_____ hypodermis

_____ opening of sweat ducts

_____ dermal papilla

_____ stratum corneum

_____ dermis

_____ hair follicle

******If you had difficulty with this section, review pages **161-169**

Student Name_____

II   FUNCTIONS OF THE SKIN

Multiple Choice—select the best answer.

16. Which of the following is *NOT* a function of the skin?
    a.   sensation
    b.   excretion
    c.   immunity
    d.   all of the above are skin functions

17. Which of the following vitamins is synthesized by the skin?
    a.   vitamin A   c.   vitamin C
    b.   vitamin B   d.   vitamin D

18. Which of the following is *NOT* a mechanism of heat loss by the skin?
    a.   evaporation   c.   vasoconstriction
    b.   radiation   d.   convection

19. Langerhans cells are the mechanism of action of which function of skin?
    a.   immunity   c.   excretion
    b.   endocrine   d.   sensation

20. Which structure compares actual body temperature with set point temperature and then sends out appropriate correction signals to effectors?
    a.   pituitary
    b.   hypothalamus
    c.   thalamus
    d.   none of the above

True or false

21. ___F___   Skin is a minor factor in the body's thermoregulatory mechanism.

22. ___F___   Skin plays a major role in the overall excretion of body wastes.

23. ___T___   To help dissipate heat during exercise, sweat production can reach as much as 3 liters per hour.

******If you had difficulty with this section, review pages **170-173**

III   BURNS

Multiple Choice—select the best answer.

24. The "rule of palms" assumes that the palm size of a burn victim equals about _____ of total body surface area.
    a.   1%
    b.   2%
    c.   5%
    d.   none of the above

25. Blisters, severe pain, and generalized swelling are characteristic of which type of burn?
    a.   first-degree burns
    b.   second-degree burns
    c.   third-degree burns
    d.   none of the above

True or false

26. _____F_____ According to the "rule of nines," the body is divided into nine areas of 9%.

27. _____T_____ Immediately after injury, third-degree burns hurt less than second-degree burns.

Matching—identify each term with its corresponding description.

28. _____C_____ full-thickness burn

29. _____a_____ involves only the epidermis

30. _____d_____ another name for first- and second-degree burns

31. _____b_____ damage to epidermis and upper layers of dermis with blisters

32. _____e_____ destroys both epidermis and dermis and may involve underlying tissue; also called *third-degree burn*

a. first-degree burn
b. second-degree burn
c. third-degree burn
d. partial-thickness burn
e. full-thickness burn

Labeling—using the "rule of nines" method, label the following diagram to estimate the amount of skin surface for each area.

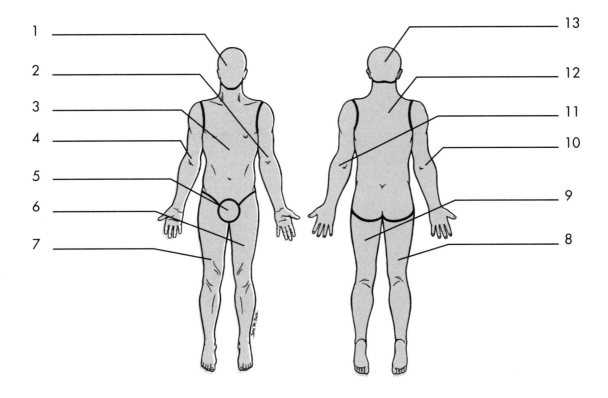

******If you had difficulty with this section, review pages **174-176**

Student Name_____

IV APPENDAGES OF THE SKIN

Multiple Choice—select the best answer.

33. The developing fetus is covered by an extremely fine, soft hair coat called:
    a. vellus.
    b. lanugo.
    c. fatalis follicle.
    d. none of the above.

34. Which of the following is associated with hair?
    a. sebaceous glands
    b. ceruminous glands
    c. eccrine glands
    d. none of the above

35. Ceruminous glands are found in:
    a. axilla.
    b. soles of feet.
    c. ear canal.
    d. none of the above.

36. The most numerous, important, and widespread sweat glands in the body are:
    a. apocrine.   c. ceruminous.
    b. eccrine.   d. sebaceous.

37. Hair growth is stimulated by:
    a. cutting it frequently.
    b. shaving.
    c. increasing melanin production.
    d. none of the above.

True or false

38. ___T___ The hair follicle is an extension of the epidermis into the dermis, forming a small tube.

39. ___F___ The inner core of the hair is called the *cortex*.

40. ___T___ Sweat or sudoriferous glands are the most numerous of the skin glands.

41. ___T___ One of the factors associated with male pattern baldness is testosterone.

42. ___T___ Growth of nails is due to mitosis in the stratum germinativum.

******If you had difficulty with this section, review pages **176-181**

IV MECHANISMS OF DISEASE

Matching—identify the term on the left with the corresponding description.

43. _____ impetigo

44. _____ tinea

45. _____ warts

46. _____ boils

47. _____ decubitus ulcers

48. _____ urticaria

49. _____ scleroderma

50. _____ eczema

a. papilloma
b. furuncle
c. ringworm
d. hard skin
e. symptom of underlying condition
f. staph or strep infection
g. bedsores
h. hives

Fill in the blanks.

51. _____ is the term associated with an unusually high body temperature.

52. _____ _____occurs when the body loses a large amount of fluid

    resulting from heat-loss mechanisms.

53. _____ _____ is also known as *sunstroke*.

54. Local damage caused by extremely low temperatures is referred to as _____.

******If you had difficulty with this section, review pages **181-184**

Crossword Puzzle

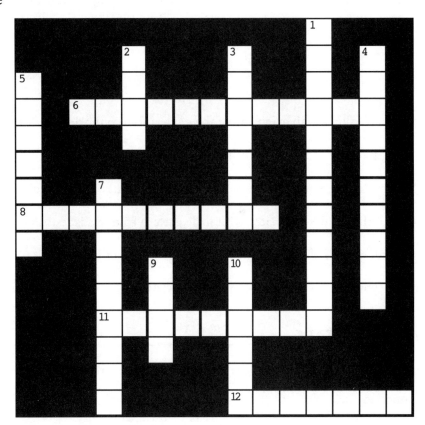

Across

6. Tube that contains the hair root (two words)
8. Skin
11. Outer layer of skin
12. "Layer"

Down

1. Layer beneath the dermis
2. Appendage of skin
3. Determines skin color
4. Sudoriferous gland (two words)
5. Water-repellent protein
7. Gland that secretes oil
9. Keratinized epithelial cells form this structure
10. Inner layer of skin

APPLYING WHAT YOU KNOW

55. Mr. Ziven was admitted to the hospital with second- and third-degree burns. Both arms, the anterior trunk, right anterior leg, and genital region were affected by the burns. The doctor quickly estimated that _____% of Mr. Ziven's body had been burned.

56. After investigating the scene of the crime, Officer Gorski announced that dermal papillae were found that would help solve the case. What did he mean?

57. Bernie is 65 and was recently diagnosed with melanoma. He finds this diagnosis difficult to believe because has lived in Alaska for the past 20 years and gets very little exposure to sun. Can you suggest a possible explanation for his diagnosis?

DID YOU KNOW?

- Because the dead cells of the epidermis are constantly being worn and washed away, we get a new outer skin layer every 27 days.
- The average person sheds 40 pounds of skin in a lifetime.

ONE LAST QUICK CHECK ✔

Multiple Choice—select the best answer.

58. Which of the following statements about hair follicles is true?
    a. Arrector pili muscles are associated with them.
    b. Sudoriferous glands empty into them.
    c. They arise directly from the epidermis layer of skin.
    d. All of the above.

59. Which of the following statements about apocrine glands is true?
    a. They can be classified as sudoriferous.
    b. They can be found primarily in armpit and genital regions.
    c. They secrete a thick substance that has a strong odor associated with it.
    d. All of the above.

60. Which of the following, if any, is *NOT* found in the dermis layer of the skin?
    a. nerves
    b. melanin
    c. blood vessels
    d. all of the above are found in the dermis

61. What characterizes second-degree burns?
    a. blisters   c. severe pain
    b. swelling   d. all of the above

62. Blackheads can result from the blockage of which of the following glands?
    a. lacrimal   c. ceruminous
    b. sebaceous   d. sudoriferous

63. Keratin is found in which layer of the skin?
    a. dermis   c. subcutaneous
    b. epidermis   d. serous

64. What is the fold of skin that hides the root of a nail called?
    a. lunula   c. cuticle
    b. body   d. papillae

65. Which of the following is *NOT* an important function of the skin?
    a. sense organ activity
    b. absorption
    c. protection
    d. temperature

66. Another name for the dermis is:
    a. corium.   c. subcutaneous.
    b. strata.   d. lunula.

67. The shedding of epithelial elements from the skin surface is called:
    a. desquamation.   c. cleavage lines.
    b. convection.   d. turnover.

Matching—identify the correct answer for each item on the left.

68. ___C___ melanin
69. ___b___ Pacinian corpuscle
70. ___e___ sebaceous
71. ___f___ hair
72. ___g___ lunula
73. ___a___ dermal papillae
74. ___d___ sudoriferous
75. ___h___ apocrine
76. ___i___ tinea
77. ___j___ psoriasis

a. fingerprint
b. pressure
c. brown pigment
d. perspiration
e. oil
f. follicle
g. little moon
h. axilla sweat glands
i. fungal infection
j. genetic inflammatory skin disorder

CHAPTER 7

SKELETAL TISSUES

How strange we would look without our skeleton! It is the skeleton that provides the rigid, supportive framework that gives shape to our bodies. But this is just the beginning, because the skeleton also protects the organs beneath it, maintains homeostasis of blood calcium, produces blood cells, and assists the muscular system in providing movement for us.

After reviewing the microscopic structure of bone and cartilage, you will understand how skeletal tissues are formed, their differences and their importance in the human body. Your micro-scopic investigation will make the study of this system easier as you logically progress from this view to macroscopic bone formation and growth and visualize the structure of long bones.

Bones are classified structurally by their shape: long bones, short bones, flat bones, and irregular bones. They are also classified by the types of cells that form the bone: compact bone and cancellous, or spongy, bone. Throughout life, bone formation (ossification) and bone destruction (resorption) occur concurrently to assure a firm and comfortable framework for our bodies.

I TYPES OF BONES

Matching—identify each structure with its corresponding description.

1. _____ the thin membrane that lines the medullary cavity
2. _____ an example of a flat bone
3. _____ the shaft of the long bone
4. _____ an example of a long bone
5. _____ the thin layer that cushions jolts and blows
6. _____ an example of a sesamoid bone
7. _____ an attachment for muscle fibers
8. _____ an example of a short bone
9. _____ the end of a long bone
10. _____ the tubelike, hollow space in the diaphysis of long bones
11. _____ an example of an irregular bone

a. epiphysis
b. medullary cavity
c. carpal
d. articular cartilage
e. femur
f. endosteum
g. vertebra
h. diaphysis
i. patella
j. periosteum
k. scapulae

******If you had difficulty with this section, review pages **189-190**

II BONE TISSUE STRUCTURE, FUNCTION, AND HOMEOSTASIS

Multiple Choice—select the best answer.

12. Which of the following is *NOT* a component of bone matrix?
    a. inorganic salts
    b. organic matrix
    c. collagenous fibers
    d. all of the above are components of bone matrix

13. Small spaces in which bone cells lie are called:
    a. lamellae.
    b. lacunae.
    c. canaliculi.
    d. interstitial lamellae.

14. The basic structural unit of compact bone is:
    a. trabeculae.
    b. cancellous bone.
    c. osteon.
    d. none of the above.

15. The cells that produce the organic matrix in bone are:
    a. chondrocytes.   c. osteocytes.
    b. osteoblasts.   d. osteoclasts.

16. The bones in an adult that include red marrow include all of the following *EXCEPT*:
    a. ribs.   c. pelvis.
    b. tarsals.   d. femur.

17. Low blood calcium evokes a response from:
    a. calcitonin.
    b. thyroid.
    c. parathyroid hormone.
    d. none of the above.

True or false

18. _____ Haversian canals run lengthwise, whereas Volkmann's canals run transverse to the bone.

19. _____ Giant, multinucleate cells that are responsible for bone resorption are called *osteocytes*.

20. _____ Bone marrow is found not only in the medullary cavities of certain long bones but also in the spaces of cancellous bone.

21. _____ Calcitonin functions to stimulate osteoblasts and inhibit osteoclasts.

22. _____ *Hematopoiesis* is a term referring to the formation of new haversian systems.

23. _____ Yellow marrow is found in almost all of the bones of an infant's body.

******If you had difficulty with this section, review pages **190-196**

III BONE DEVELOPMENT, GROWTH, RESORPTION, AND REPAIR

Multiple Choice—select the best answer.

24. The primary ossification center is located at the:
    a. epiphysis.
    b. diaphysis.
    c. articular cartilage.
    d. none of the above.

25. The primary purpose of the epiphyseal plate is:
    a. mending fractures.
    b. enlarging the epiphysis.
    c. providing bone strength.
    d. lengthening long bones.

Student Name _____

26. The epiphyseal plate is composed mostly of:
    a. chondrocytes.
    b. osteocytes.
    c. osteoclasts.
    d. none of the above.

27. Bone loss normally begins to exceed bone gain between the ages of:
    a. 30 and 35 years. c. 55 and 60 years.
    b. 35 and 40 years. d. 65 and 70 years.

28. The first step to healing a bone fracture is:
    a. callus formation.
    b. fracture hematoma formation.
    c. alignment of fracture.
    d. collar formation.

True or false

29. _____ The addition of bone to its outer surface resulting in growth in diameter is called *appositional growth.*

30. _____ Most bones of the body are formed by intramembranous ossification.

31. _____ Once an individual reaches skeletal maturity, the bones undergo years of metabolic rest.

32. _____ Lack of exercise tends to weaken bones through decreased collagen formation and excessive calcium withdrawal.

33. _____ When bones reach their full length, the epiphyseal plate disappears.

******If you had difficulty with this section, review pages **197-201**

IV CARTILAGE

Multiple Choice—select the best answer.

34. The fibrous covering of cartilage is:
    a. periosteum.
    b. perichondrium.
    c. chondroclast.
    d none of the above.

35. The external ear, epiglottis, and the auditory tube are composed of:
    a. hyaline cartilage.
    b. fibrocartilage.
    c. elastic cartilage.
    d. none of the above.

36. Vitamin D deficiency can result in:
    a. scurvy.
    b. rickets.
    c. osteochondroma.
    d. none of the above.

True or false

37. _____ Both bone and cartilage are well vascularized.

38. _____ The intervertebral discs are composed of fibrocartilage.

39. _____ The growth of cartilage occurs by both appositional and interstitial growth.

Labeling—label the following diagrams.

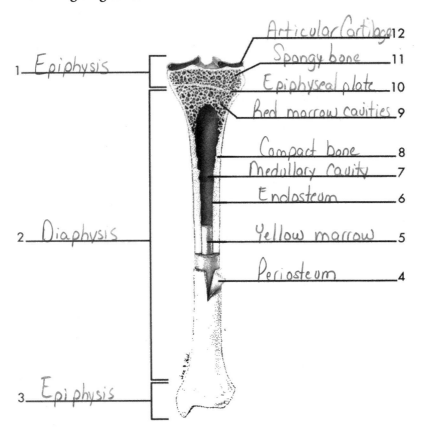

1 ___ Epiphysis

2 ___ Diaphysis

3 ___ Epiphysis

Articular Cartilage 12
Spongy bone 11
Epiphyseal plate 10
Red marrow cavities 9
Compact bone 8
Medullary Cavity 7
Endosteum 6
Yellow marrow 5
Periosteum 4

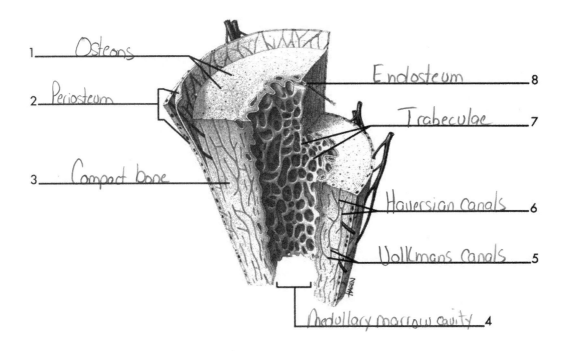

1 ___ Osteons

2 ___ Periosteum

3 ___ Compact bone

Endosteum 8
Trabeculae 7
Haversian Canals 6
Volkmans Canals 5
Medullary marrow cavity 4

******If you had difficulty with this section, review pages **191, 193, 202,** and **203**

Student Name_____

V   MECHANISMS OF DISEASE

Fill in the blanks.

40. _____ is the most common type of skeletal tissue tumor.

41. _____ is the most common primary malignant tumor of skeletal tissue.

42. _____ is a common bone disease often occurring in postmenopausal women and manifesting symptoms of porous, brittle, and fragile bones.

43. _____ _____ is also known as *osteitis deformans*.

44. _____ is a bacterial infection of the bone and marrow tissue.

******If you had difficulty with this section, review pages **204-206**

Crossword Puzzle

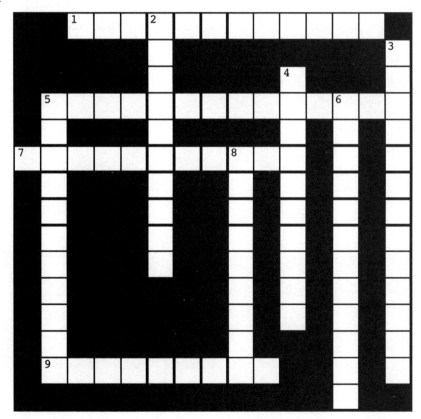

Across

1. Ossification that replaces cartilage with bone
5. Spongy bone (two words)
7. Contains osteons (two words)
9. Ends of long bone

Down

2. Bone-absorbing cell
3. Bone marrow (two words)
4. Bone-forming cell
5. Cartilage cell
6. Bone formation
8. Bone cell

APPLYING WHAT YOU KNOW

45. Mrs. Harris is a 60-year-old white woman. She has noticed in recent years that her height has slightly decreased. Recently, she fractured her wrist in a slight fall. Which skeletal system disorder might she be suffering from? What techniques could be used to diagnose her condition? What treatments are available?

46. Mrs. Perine had advanced cancer of the bone. As the disease progressed, Mrs. Perine required several blood transfusions throughout her therapy. She asked the doctor one day to explain the necessity for the transfusions. What explanation might the doctor give to Mrs. Perine?

47. Dr. Kennedy, an orthopedic surgeon, called the admissions office of the hospital and advised them that he would be admitting a patient in the next hour with an epiphyseal fracture. Without any other information, the patient is assigned to the pediatric ward. What prompted this assignment?

48. Ms. Strickland was in an auto accident. When the surgeon described the details of the surgery to her family, he stated that he was able to "patch" her fractures. Explain what he might have meant by "patching" the fractures.

DID YOU KNOW?

• Approximately 25 million Americans have osteoporosis. Four out of five are women.

ONE LAST QUICK CHECK ✔

Fill in the blanks.

49. There are _____ types of bones.

50. The _____ _____ is the hollow area inside the diaphysis of a bone.

51. A thin layer of cartilage covering each epiphysis is the _____ _____.

52. The _____ lines the medullary cavity of long bones.

53. _____ is used to describe the process of blood cell formation.

54. Blood cell formation is a vital process carried on in _____ _____

_____.

55. The _____ is a strong fibrous membrane that covers a long bone except at joint surfaces.

56. Bones may be classified by shape. Those shapes include _____, _____,

_____, and _____.

57. Bones serve as the major reservoir for _____, a vital substance required for normal

nerve and muscle function.

58. _____ is the most abundant type of cartilage.

Matching—identify the term on the left with the proper selection on the right.

59. _____ trabeculae

60. _____ compact

61. _____ spongy

62. _____ periosteum

63. _____ cartilage

64. _____ osteocytes

65. _____ canaliculi

66. _____ lamellae

67. _____ chondrocytes

68. _____ haversian system

a. outer covering of bone
b. dense bone tissue
c. fibers embedded in a firm gel
d. needlelike threads of spongy bone
e. ends of long bones
f. connect lacunae
g. cartilage cells
h. structural unit of compact bone
i. bone cells
j. ring of bone

CHAPTER 8

SKELETAL SYSTEM

The skeletal system may be compared to a large 206 piece puzzle. Each bone, as with each puzzle piece, is unique in size and shape. And again, just like with a puzzle, pieces or bones are not interchangeable. They have a lock-and-key concept that allows them to fit in only one area of the skeletal frame and perform functions necessary for that location.

The skeleton is divided into two main areas: the axial skeleton and the appendicular skeleton. All of the 206 bones of the human body may be classified into one of these two areas. And although we can divide them neatly by this system, there are subtle differences that exist between a man's and a woman's skeleton that provide us with insight to the functional differences between the sexes. An understanding of the skeletal system gives us an appreciation of the complex and interdependent functions that make this system essential for maintenance of homeostasis and sustaining life.

I   DIVISIONS OF THE SKELETON

Matching—identify each term with its associated division of the skeleton.

1. _____ coccyx
2. _____ 80 bones
3. _____ 126 bones
4. _____ vertebral column
5. _____ carpals
6. _____ scapulae
7. _____ auditory ossicles (ear bones)
8. _____ shoulder girdle
9. _____ skull
10. _____ clavicles

a.   axial skeleton
b.   appendicular skeleton

******If you had difficulty with this section, review pages **210-213**

II   THE SKULL

Multiple Choice—select the best answer.

11. The squamous suture connects which two bones?
    a.   frontal and parietal
    b.   parietal and temporal
    c.   temporal and sphenoid
    d.   sphenoid and frontal

12. The mastoid sinuses are found in which bone?
    a.   frontal   c.   parietal
    b.   sphenoid   d.   temporal

13. The skull bone that articulates with the first cervical vertebrae is the:
    a.   occipital.
    b.   sphenoid.
    c.   ethmoid.
    d.   none of the above.

14. A *meatus* can be described as:
    a.   a large bony prominence.
    b.   a shallow groove.
    c.   a tubelike opening or channel.
    d.   a raised, rough area.

15. Separation of the nasal and cranial cavities is achieved by the:
    a.   cribriform plate of the ethmoid bone.
    b.   sella turcica of the sphenoid bone.
    c.   foramen magnum of the occipital bone.
    d.   palatine process of the maxilla.

16. Which of the following is *NOT* a bone of the orbit?
    a.   ethmoid.   c.   lacrimal.
    b.   nasal.   d.   frontal.

True or false

17. _____   The sphenoid is a bone of the face.

18. _____   An immovable joint of the skull is called a *fontanel*.

19. _____   The largest paranasal sinus is the maxillary sinus.

20. _____   The hyoid is one of several bones that do not articulate with any other bones.

21. _____   The external auditory meatus is located within the temporal bone.

Student Name_____

Labeling—label the following diagrams.

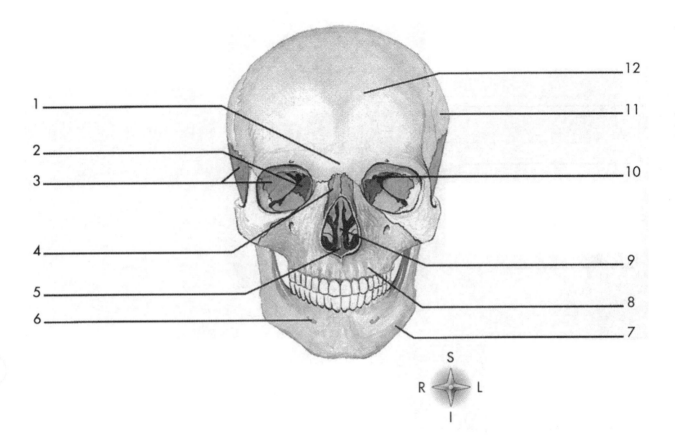

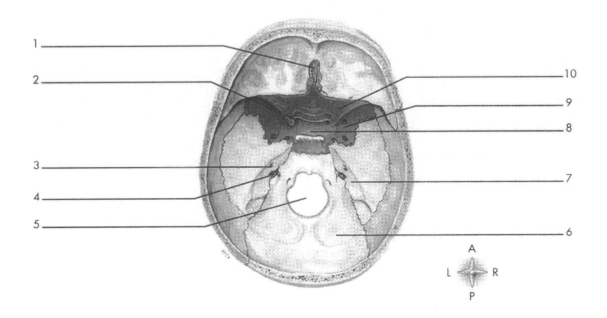

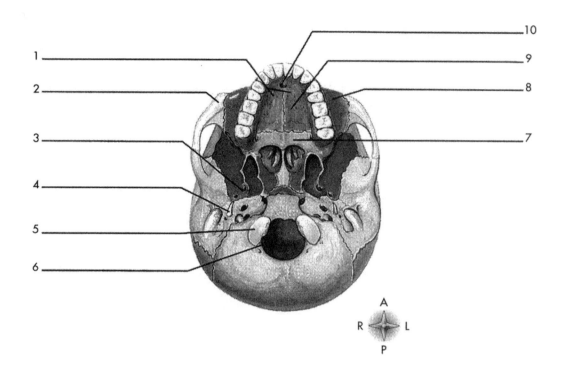

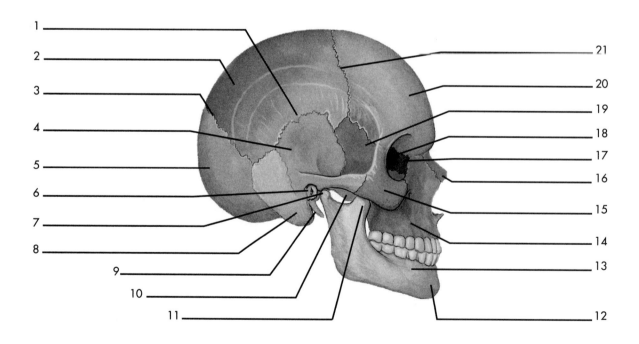

Student Name_____

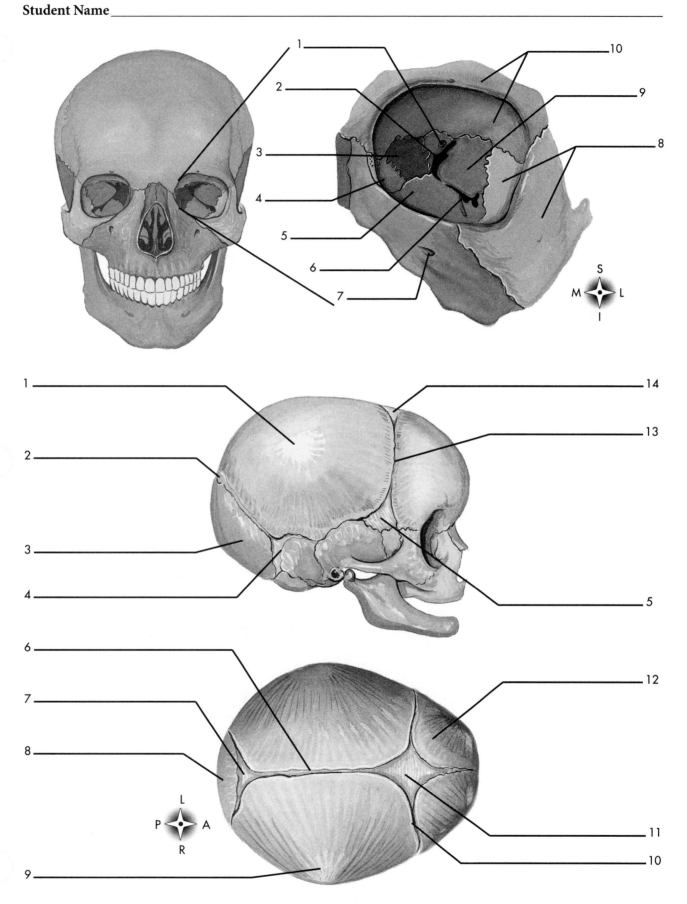

******If you had difficulty with this section, review pages **213-230**

III   VERTEBRAL COLUMN

Labeling—label the following diagrams of the vertebral column. Be sure to identify the spinal regions, spinal curves, and quantity of vertebrae for each region.

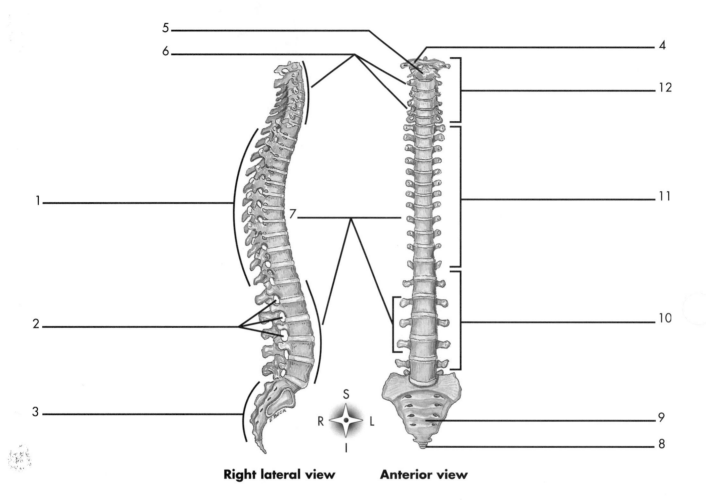

Right lateral view   **Anterior view**

Student Name_____

Labeling—label the following images of vertebrae.

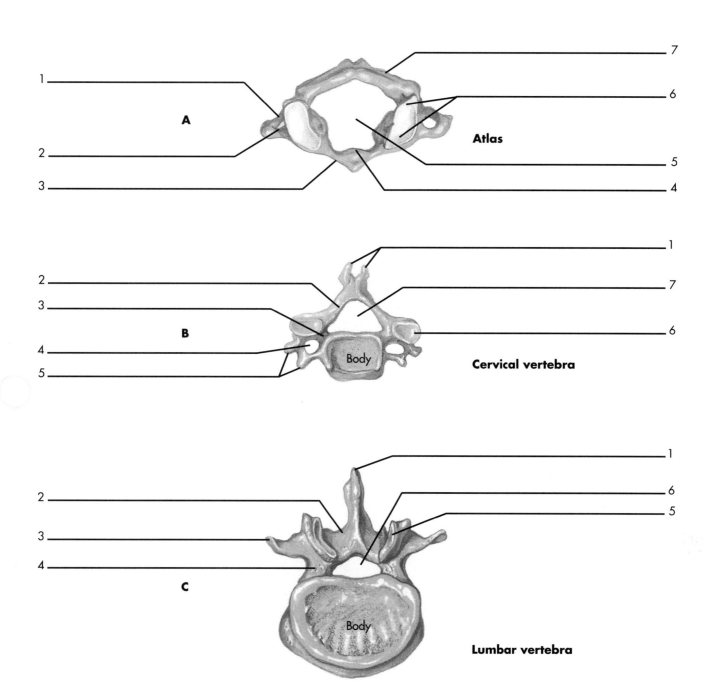

A

1

2

3

7

6

Atlas

5

4

B

2

3

4

5

Body

1

7

6

Cervical vertebra

C

2

3

4

Body

1

6

5

Lumbar vertebra

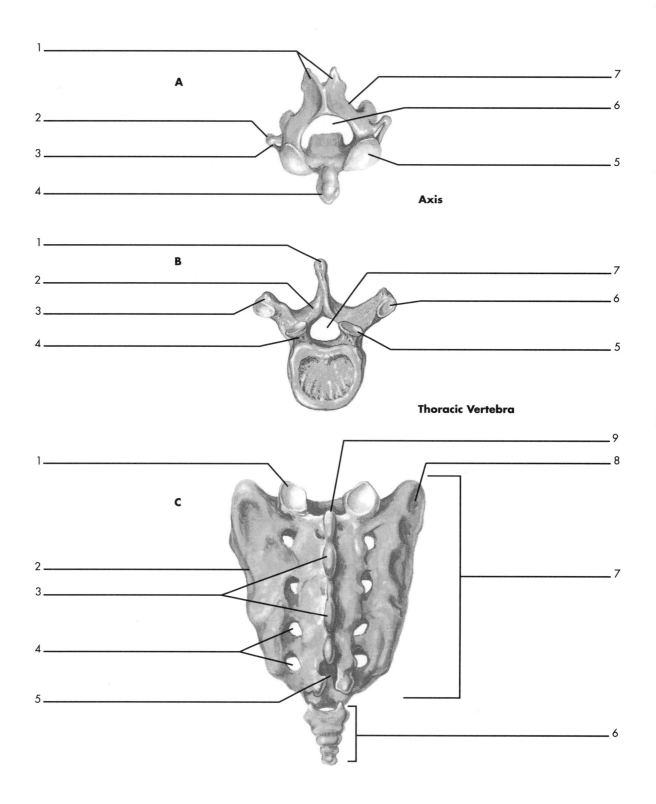

A

1
2
3
4

7
6
5

Axis

B

1
2
3
4

7
6
5

Thoracic Vertebra

C

1
2
3
4
5

9
8
7

6

******If you had difficulty with this section, review pages **231-234**

Student Name _____

IV   STERNUM AND RIBS

Matching—identify each term with its corresponding description.

22. _____ first seven pairs of ribs that attach directly to the sternum

23. _____ eleventh and twelfth ribs, which have no attachment to the sternum

24. _____ middle part of the sternum

25. _____ most superior part of the sternum

26. _____ the blunt, cartilaginous, lower tip of the sternum

27. _____ the five pairs of ribs that do not attach directly to the sternum

28. _____ tissue that attaches ribs directly or indirectly to the sternum

a.   body
b.   false ribs
c.   floating ribs
d.   manubrium
e.   true ribs
f.   xiphoid process
g.   costal cartilage

Labeling—label the following diagrams.

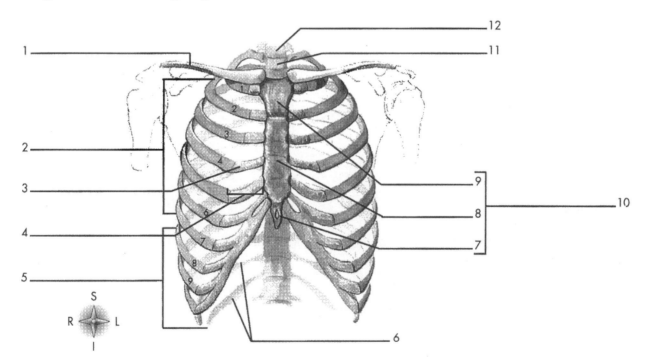

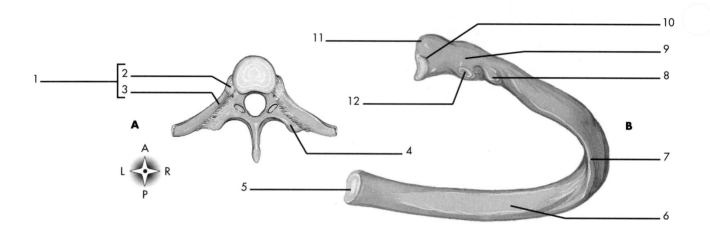

******If you had difficulty with this section, review pages **235-236**

V   THE APPENDICULAR SKELETON/UPPER EXTREMITY

Multiple Choice—select the best answer.

29. Which of the following is *NOT* part of the shoulder girdle?
     a.   clavicle
     b.   sternum
     c.   scapula
     d.   none of the above

30. The coronoid fossa is a:
     a.   depression on the thumb.
     b.   projection of the ulna.
     c.   region on the spine.
     d.   depression on the humerus.

31. The arm socket is the:
     a.   coronoid fossa.   c.   coracoid process.
     b.   olecranon fossa.   d.   glenoid cavity.

True or false

32. _____   The two bones that form the framework of the forearm are the radius and ulna.

33. _____   The wrist is composed of small bones called *metacarpals.*

34. _____   The medial forearm bone in the anatomical position is the ulna.

35. _____   The most evident carpal bone is the triquetrum.

Labeling—label the following diagrams.

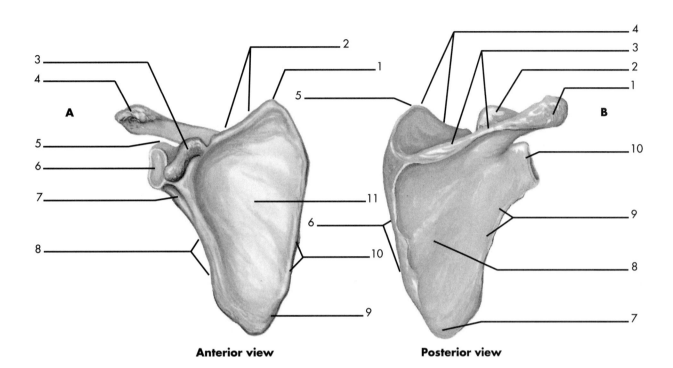

Anterior view

Posterior view

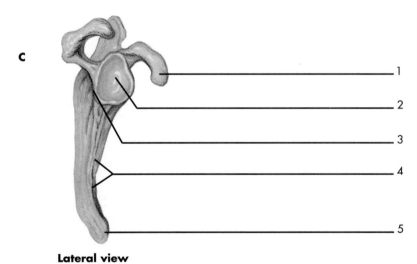

Lateral view

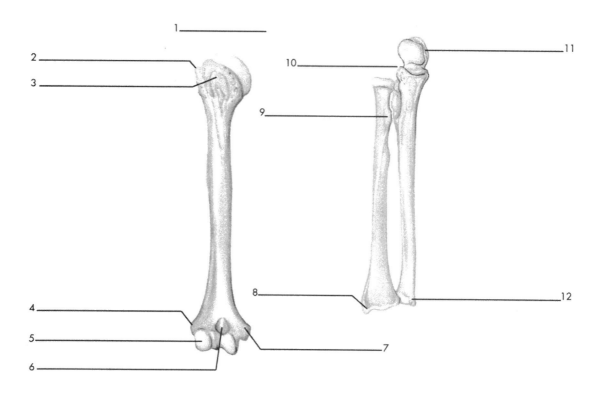

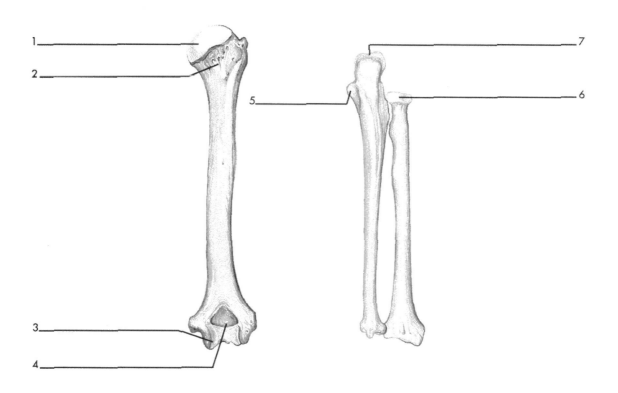

Student Name _____

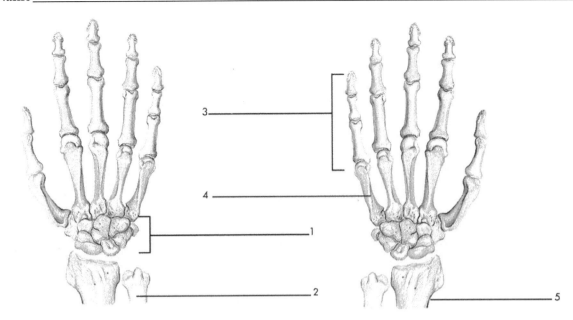

******If you had difficulty with this section, review pages **236-240**

VI   THE APPENDICULAR SKELETON/LOWER EXTREMITY

Multiple Choice—select the best answer.

36. Which of the following is *NOT* one of the bones of the pelvic girdle?
    a.   ilium   c.   ischium
    b.   acetabulum   d.   pubis

37. The greater trochanter is a bony landmark of the:
    a.   femur.   c.   pubis.
    b.   tibia.   d.   ramus.

38. During childbirth, the infant passes through an imaginary plane called the:
    a.   pelvic outlet.
    b.   symphysis pubis.
    c.   pelvic brim.
    d.   ilium.

39. Which of the following is *NOT* a tarsal bone?
    a.   talus   c.   scaphoid
    b.   cuneiform   d.   navicular

True or false

40. _____   The largest coxal bone is the ischium.

41. _____   The most distal portion of the fibula is composed of a bony landmark called the *medial malleolus.*

42. _____   The *longitudinal arch* refers to a structure within the pelvic inlet.

43. _____   Each toe contains three phalanges.

Labeling—label the following diagrams.

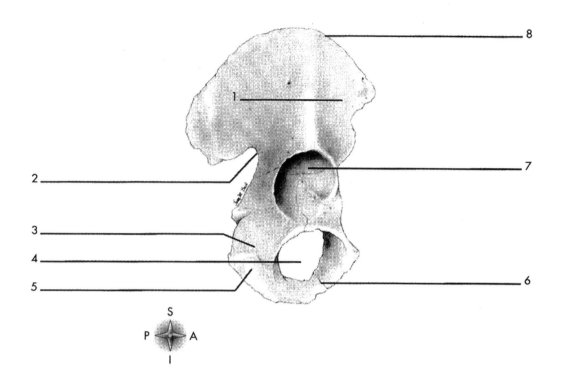

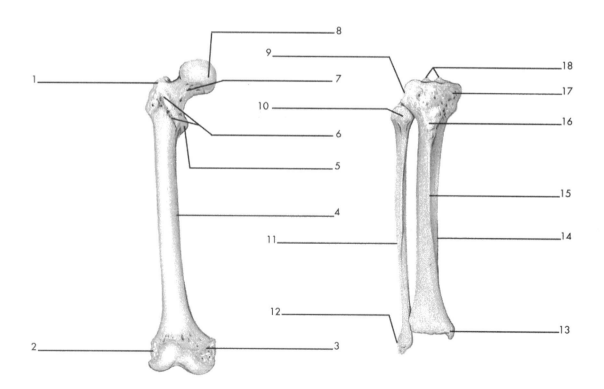

Student Name_____

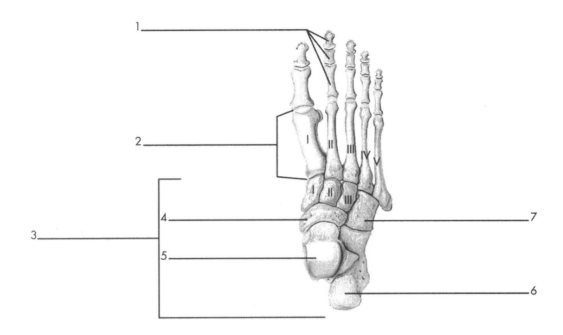

******If you had difficulty with this section, review pages **241-247**

VII   SKELETAL DIFFERENCES IN MEN AND WOMEN

Matching—identify the skeletal characteristics with the appropriate gender.

44. _____ elongated forehead

45. _____ small pelvic inlet

46. _____ subpubic angle less than 90 degrees

47. _____ wide sacrum

48. _____ more massive muscle attach-ment sites

49. _____ more movable coccyx

a.   male skeleton
b.   female skeleton

******If you had difficulty with this section, review pages **247-248**

VIII   CYCLE OF LIFE: MECHANISMS OF DISEASE

Multiple Choice—select the best answer.

50. All of the following are clinical signs and
     symptoms of a fracture *EXCEPT*:
     a.   soft tissue edema.
     b.   realignment of the bone.
     c.   loss of function.
     d.   pain.

51. An open fracture can be described as:
     a.   a complete separation of bones.
     b.   fractures in more than one area of a
          bone.
     c.   broken bone projecting through the
          skin.
     d.   none of the above.

True or false

52. _____   *Swayback* and *kyphosis* are synonymous terms.

53. _____   Normal curvature of the spine is convex posteriorly through the thoracic region and
                   concave posteriorly through the cervical and lumbar regions.

******If you had difficulty with this section, review pages **248-250**

Crossword Puzzle

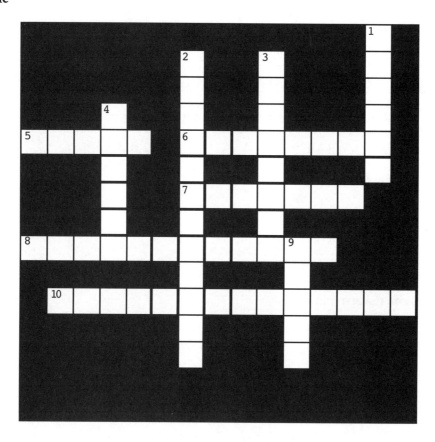

Across

5.   Cavity within a bone
6.   Bone that is part of the spinal column
7.   Encases the brain
8.   Section of skeleton that includes 126 bones
10. Clavicle and scapula (two words)

Down

1.   Bony cage
2.   Supports the trunk (two words)
3.   "Soft spot"
4.   Immovable joint in skull
9.   Section of skeleton that includes 80 bones

Student Name_____

APPLYING WHAT YOU KNOW

54. While playing football, Bill was involved in a tackle that caused a forced hyperextension of his elbow joint. Which skeletal structures could he have injured?

55. Amanda loves to wear extremely high-heeled shoes. How does this affect the weight distribution onto the bones of her feet? Which skeletal structures are at risk of being damaged?

DID YOU KNOW?

- The bones of the hands and feet make up more than half of the total 206 bones of the body.
- The bones of the middle ear are mature at birth.
- The skeleton of an average 160-pound body weighs about 29 pounds.

ONE LAST QUICK CHECK ✓

Circle the one that does NOT belong.

56. cervical	thoracic	coxal	coccyx
57. pelvic girdle	ankle	wrist	axial
58. frontal	occipital	maxilla	sphenoid
59. scapula	pectoral girdle	ribs	clavicle
60. malleus	vomer	incus	stapes
61. ulna	ilium	ischium	pubis
62. carpal	phalanges	metacarpal	ethmoid
63. ethmoid	parietal	occipital	nasal
64. anvil	atlas	axis	cervical

Matching—identify the bone with its marking. There may be more than one correct answer.

65. _____ occipital

66. _____ sternum

67. _____ coxal

68. _____ femur

69. _____ ulna

70. _____ temporal

71. _____ tarsals

72. _____ sphenoid

73. _____ ethmoid

74. _____ scapula

75. _____ tibia

76. _____ frontal

77. _____ mandible

a. mastoid
b. pterygoid process
c. foramen magnum
d. sella turcica
e. mental foramen
f. conchae
g. xiphoid process
h. glenoid cavity
i. olecranon process
j. ischium
k. acetabulum
l. symphysis pubis
m. ilium
n. greater trochanter
o. medial malleolus
p. calcaneus
q. acromion process
r. frontal sinuses
s. condyloid process
t. tibial tuberosity

CHAPTER 9

ARTICULATIONS

We conclude our study of bones with a chapter on joints, or articulations. A joint, or articulation, is a point of contact between bones. Sitting, walking, and running are just a few examples of movements that would not be possible without the successful functioning of articulations. Joints also permit us to lift heavy objects and perform fine motor skills such as needlepoint. The unusual and unique shape and size of articulations are responsible for the variety and degree of motion that we expect from our body.

Joints may be classified according to structure (fibrous and cartilaginous) or according to function (synarthrosis—immovable; amphiarthrosis—slightly movable; diarthrosis—freely movable). Proper functioning of articulations is necessary for us to adapt to our environment with controlled, smooth, and pain-free movements.

I CLASSIFICATION OF JOINTS

Multiple Choice—select the best answer.

1. The articulation between the root of a tooth and the alveolar process of the mandible or maxilla is called the:
   a. suture.
   b. gomphosis.
   c. synchondrosis.
   d. symphysis.

2. Immovable joints are called:
   a. synarthroses.
   b. amphiarthroses.
   c. diarthroses.
   d. none of the above.

3. The radioulnar articulation is classified as which type of articulation?
   a. syndesmosis
   b. synchondrosis
   c. symphysis
   d. diarthrosis

4. The most movable joints in the body are:
   a. symphyses.
   b. sutures.
   c. synovial joints.
   d. synchondroses.

5. An example of a symphysis is:
   a. the articulation between the pubic bones.
   b. the articulation between the bodies of adjacent vertebrae.
   c. both a and b.
   d. none of the above.

6. The inner surface of the joint capsule is lined with:
   a. bursae.
   b. a joint cavity.
   c. periosteum.
   d. synovial membrane.

7. The joint that allows for the widest range of movement is a _____ joint.
   a. gliding
   b. saddle
   c. ball and socket
   d. hinge

8. An example of a pivot joint is the:
   a. first metacarpal articulating with the trapezium.
   b. humerus articulating with the trapezium.
   c. interphalangeal joints.
   d. head of the radius articulating with the ulna.

True or false

9. _____   *Diarthrosis* and *synovial joint* refer to basically the same structure.

10. _____   The elbow joint is a ball and socket joint.

11. _____   The ability to oppose the fingers and thumb is achieved by a saddle joint.

12. _____   *Articulation* and *joint* are synonymous terms.

13. _____   Diarthrotic joints are the least common type of joint in the body.

14. _____   Articular cartilage is composed of fibrocartilage, providing ample cushioning inside a joint.

15. _____   Menisci are composed of hyaline cartilage.

16. _____   The shoulder joint is a ball and socket joint.

Matching—identify each joint or description with its corresponding classification.

17. _____   joint between bodies of vertebrae

18. _____   symphysis pubis

19. _____   hip joint

20. _____   fibrous joint

21. _____   immovable joint

22. _____   cartilaginous joint

23. _____   thumb

24. _____   joints between skull bones

25. _____   freely movable joint

26. _____   synovial joint

27. _____   slightly movable joint

28. _____   the most prevalent type of joint in the body

a.   amphiarthroses
b.   diarthroses
c.   synarthroses

Student Name_____

Matching—identify each joint with its corresponding functional classification.

29. _____ elbow

30. _____ joints between facets of
adjacent vertebrae

31. _____ ellipsoidal

32. _____ dens of axis/atlas joint

33. _____ knee joint

34. _____ atlantooccipital joint

35. _____ hip joint

36. _____ shoulder joint

37. _____ joint between first metacarpal
and trapezium

a. ball and socket
b. condyloid
c. gliding
d. hinge
e. pivot
f. saddle

Labeling—label the structures of the synovial joint on the following diagram.

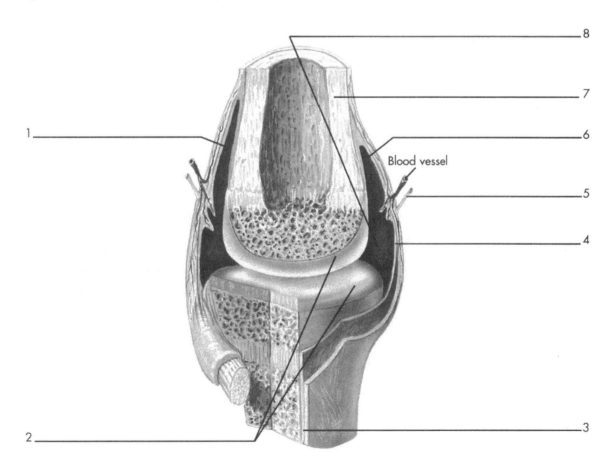

Blood vessel

******If you had difficulty with this section, review pages **255-267**

II   REPRESENTATIVE SYNOVIAL JOINTS

Multiple Choice—select the best answer.

38. The glenoid labrum is associated with which joint?
    a. hip   c. shoulder
    b. knee   d. vertebral

39. Perhaps the strongest ligament in the body is the:
    a. rotator cuff. c. pubofemoral.
    b. iliofemoral.   d. intertrochanteric.

40. The largest and most complex joint of the body is the:
    a. shoulder.   c. hip.
    b. knee.   d. ankle.

41. The anterior cruciate ligament of the knee connects the:
    a. anterior tibia with the posterior femur.
    b. posterior tibia with the anterior femur.
    c. anterior fibula with the posterior femur.
    d. anterior fibula with anterior femur.

42. Vertebral bodies are connected by:
    a. the anterior longitudinal ligament.
    b. the posterior longitudinal ligament.
    c. the ligamentum flavum.
    d. both a and b.

43. Protrusion of the nucleus pulposus through the annulus fibrosus results in:
    a. bursitis.
    b. housemaid's knee.
    c. herniated disk.
    d. none of the above.

44. The medial and lateral menisci are:
    a. ligaments.
    b. cartilage.
    c. bursae.
    d. none of the above.

45. "Joint mice" are structurally:
    a. impinged bursae.
    b. loose pieces of synovial membrane.
    c. loose pieces of articular cartilage.
    d. cracks in the articular cartilage.

Labeling—label the following diagrams of synovial joints.

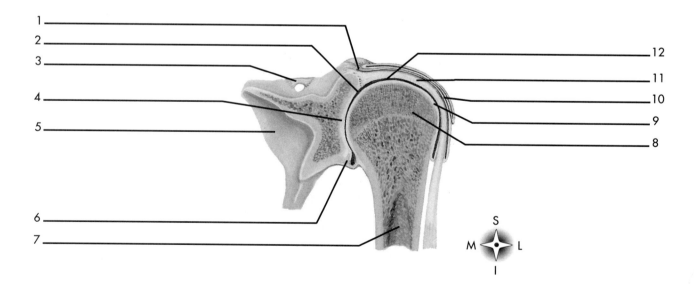

Shoulder joint.

Student Name_____

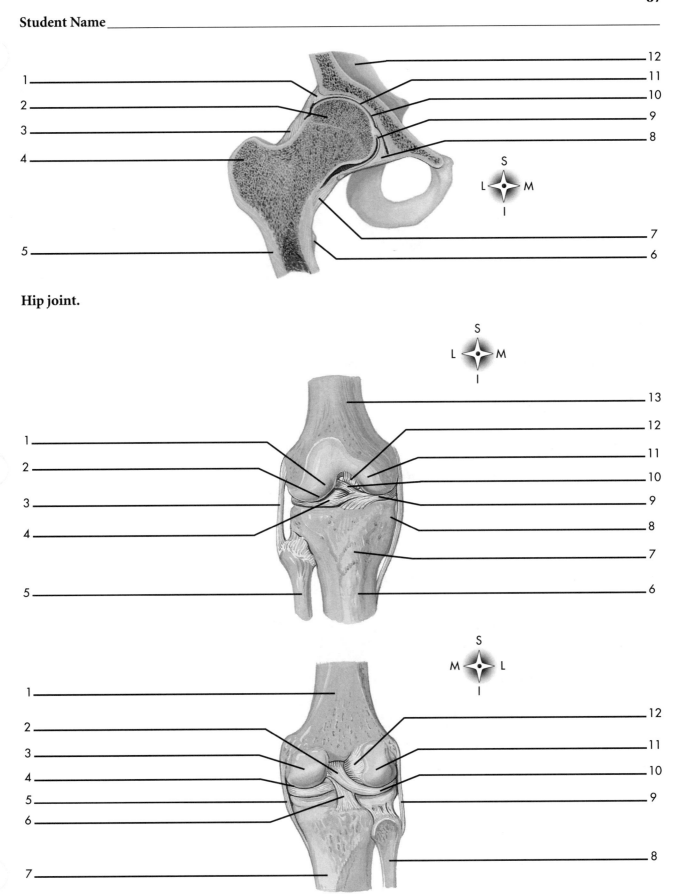

Hip joint.

1

2

3

4

5

12

11

10

9

8

7

6

S
L ✦ M
I

Knee joint. A, anterior view. **B,** posterior view.

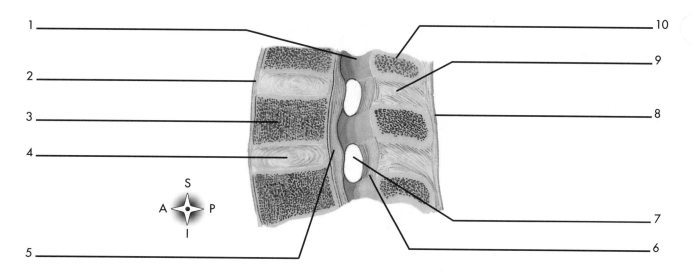

Vertebrae and their ligaments.

******If you had difficulty with this section, review pages **260-266**

III   TYPES AND RANGE OF MOVEMENT AT SYNOVIAL JOINTS

Matching—identify each term with its corresponding definition or description.

46. _____   instrument that measures ROM

47. _____   lifting the arms away from the midline

48. _____   turning the head as to say "no"

49. _____   elbow movement, as when lifting weights during a "bicep curl"

50. _____   increasing joint angle

51. _____   moving beyond extension

52. _____   causes extension of the leg as a whole

53. _____   turning sole of foot inward

54. _____   opening your mouth

55. _____   bringing fingers together

a.   plantar flexion
b.   extension
c.   abduction
d.   hyperextension
e.   goniometer
f.   rotation
g.   flexion
h.   inversion
i.   depression
j.   adduction

******If you had difficulty with this section, review pages **268-271**

Student Name _____

IV MECHANISMS OF DISEASE

Fill in the blanks.

56. _____ is an imaging technique that allows a physician to examine the internal

structure of a joint without the use of extensive surgery.

57. The most common noninflammatory joint disease is _____ or _____

_____ _____.

58. A general name for many different inflammatory joint diseases is _____.

59. A metabolic type of inflammatory arthritis is_____ _____

60. An acute musculoskeletal injury to the ligamentous structure surrounding a joint and disrupting the

continuity of the synovial membrane is a _____.

******If you had difficulty with this section, review pages **273-275**

Crossword Puzzle

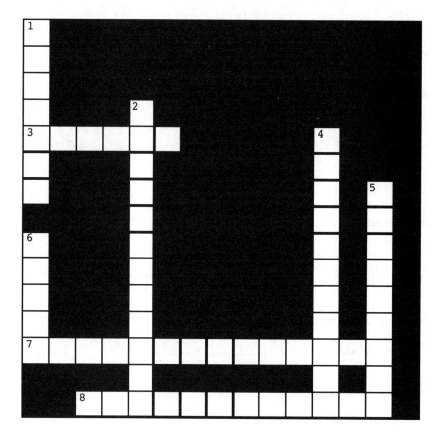

Across

3.   Immovable joint in skull
7.   Cartilaginous joint
8.   Fibrous joint

Down

1.   Articular disks
2.   Joint
4.   Synovial joint
5.   A joint where fibrocartilage connect two bones
6.   Pillowlike structure found between synovial joints

APPLYING WHAT YOU KNOW

61.   Mark is afflicted with severely inflamed joints—arthritis. If he is suffering from the chronic systemic version of this disease, what kind of symptoms would he be experiencing? Which joints are most likely involved and what is the most likely cause?

62.   Sam is suffering from a type of arthritis associated with excess blood levels of uric acid. What type of arthritis is this? What symptoms might he experience, which joints would be affected, and how is this form of arthritis treated?

DID YOU KNOW?

•   The average person uses their leg joints to walk an average of 115,000 miles during his or her lifetime.

Student Name_____

ONE LAST QUICK CHECK ✔

Circle the correct answer.

63. Freely movable joints are (amphiarthroses or diarthroses).

64. The sutures in the skull are (synarthrotic or amphiarthrotic).

65. All (diarthrotic or amphiarthrotic) joints have a joint capsule, a joint cavity, and a layer of cartilage over the ends of the two joining bones.

66. (Ligaments or tendons) grow out of periosteum and attach two bones together.

67. The (articular cartilage or epiphyseal cartilage) cushions surfaces of bones.

68. Gliding joints are the (least movable or most movable) of the diarthrotic joints.

69. The knee is the (largest or smallest) joint.

70. Hinge joints allow motion in (2 or 4) directions.

71. The saddle joint at the base of each of our thumbs allows for greater (strength or mobility).

72. When you rotate your head, you are using a (gliding or pivot) joint.

True or false

73. _____ A uniaxial joint is a synovial joint.

74. _____ Joints identified as synchondroses are synovial joints.

75. _____ Inflammation of the bursa is referred to as *pleurisy*.

76. _____ The main bursa of the shoulder joint is the subdeltoid bursa.

77. _____ Angular movements change the size of the angle between articulating bones.

78. _____ Pronation is a circular movement.

79. _____ Gliding movements are the most complex of movements.

80. _____ Protraction is an angular movement.

81. _____ Juvenile rheumatoid arthritis is more common in boys.

82. _____ The knee joint has a "baker's dozen" or 13 bursae which serve as protective pads around it.

Student Name_____

CHAPTER 10

ANATOMY OF THE MUSCULAR SYSTEM

The muscular system is often referred to as the "power system" and rightfully so, because it is this system that provides the force necessary to move the body and perform organic functions. Just as an automobile relies on the engine to provide motion, the body depends on the muscular system to perform both voluntary and involuntary types of movements. The power of this system is impressive indeed, for if we were able to direct all of our muscles in one direction, it is estimated that we would have the power to move 25 tons.

Over 600 skeletal muscles constitute 40 to 50% of our body weight. They are attached snugly over the skeletal frame to shape and mold the contours of our body. And while memorizing the names and locations of skeletal muscles appears to be an overwhelming task, it is comforting to learn that muscles are named and categorized quite simply. Classification and identification are focused upon location, function, shape, direction of fibers, number of heads or divisions, or points of attachment. This chapter assists you in understanding the structure of skeletal muscles and the logical approach to muscle recognition.

I SKELETAL MUSCLE STRUCTURE

Multiple Choice—select the best answer.

1. An entire skeletal muscle is covered by a coarse sheath called:
    a. endomysium.
    b. perimysium.
    c. epimysium.
    d. aponeurosis.

2. Muscles that are arranged like the feathers in a plume are described as:
    a. parallel.
    b. convergent.
    c. sphincter.
    d. pennate.

3. An aponeurosis is:
    a. broad and flat.
    b. tube-shaped.
    c. featherlike.
    d. none of the above.

4. Antagonists are muscles that:
    a. oppose prime movers.
    b. facilitate prime movers.
    c. stabilize muscles.
    d. directly perform movements.

5. A fixed point about which a rod moves is called a:
    a. lever.
    b. bone.
    c. belly.
    d. fulcrum.

6. In first-class levers the:
    a. fulcrum is between the load and force.
    b. load is between the fulcrum and force.
    c. force is between the fulcrum and load.
    d. load and force are equal.

True or false

7. ___F___   The origin of a muscle is the point of attachment that moves when the muscle contracts.

8. ___T___   Skeletal muscles usually act in groups rather than individually.

9. ___T___   *Prime mover* and *agonist* are synonymous.

10. ___F___   The optimum angle of pull of a muscle is generally parallel to the long axis of the bone.

11. ___T___   Tipping the head back, as in looking up at the sky, is an example of a first-class lever.

******If you had difficulty with this section, review pages **278-284**

II   HOW MUSCLES ARE NAMED

Matching—identify each muscle with the appropriate characteristic.

12. ___C___   deltoid
13. ___a___   brachialis
14. ___f___   sternocleidomastoid
15. ___e___   quadriceps
16. ___g___   gluteus maximus
17. ___b___   adductor
18. ___d___   rectus

a.   location
b.   function
c.   shape
d.   direction of fibers
e.   number of heads
f.   points of attachment
g.   size of muscle

******If you had difficulty with this section, review page **285**

III   IMPORTANT SKELETAL MUSCLES: MUSCLES OF THE FACE AND NECK

Matching—identify each muscle with its appropriate body movement.

19. ___b___   wrinkling the forehead verti- cally
20. ___e___   grating the teeth during mastication
21. ___a___   smiling
22. ___C___   raising the eyebrows
23. ___f___   flexing the head
24. ___d___   closing the eyes

a.   buccinator
b.   corrugator supercilii
c.   epicranius
d.   orbicularis oculi
e.   pterygoids
f.   sternocleidomastoid

Student Name_____

Labeling

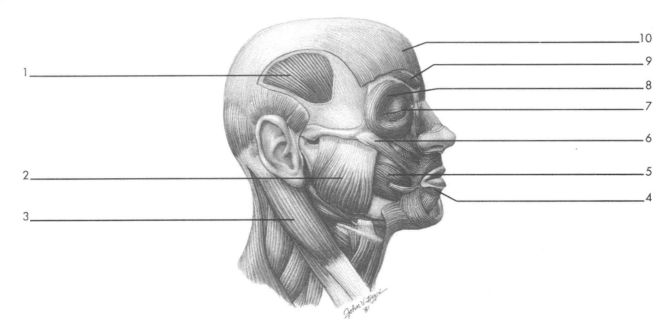

Facial muscles: (A) lateral view

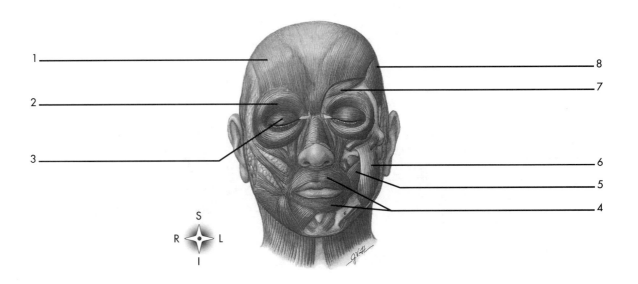

Facial muscles: (B) anterior view

******If you had difficulty with this section, review pages **286-288**

IV   IMPORTANT SKELETAL MUSCLES: TRUNK MUSCLES

True or false

25. _____   The external oblique compresses the abdomen.

26. _____   The rectus abdominis flexes the trunk.

27. _____   The levator ani closes the anal canal.

28. _____   The external intercostals function to elevate the ribs.

29. _____   The coccygeus muscles and levator ani form most of the pelvic floor.

Labeling

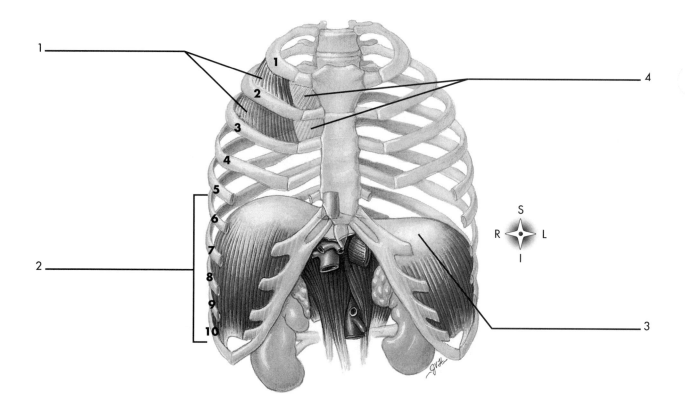

Muscles of the thorax.

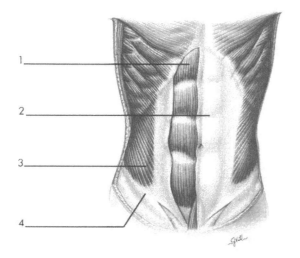 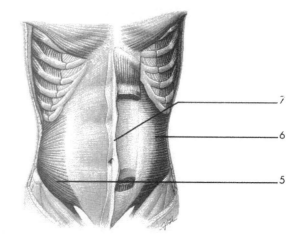

Muscles of the trunk and abdominal wall.

******If you had difficulty with this section, review pages **289-292**

V   IMPORTANT SKELETAL MUSCLES: UPPER LIMB MUSCLES

Multiple Choice—select the best answer.

30. All of the following are rotator cuff muscles *EXCEPT*:
    a. deltoid.   c. supraspinatus.
    b. infraspinatus.   d. teres minor.

31. The muscle that shrugs the shoulders is the:
    a. sternocleidomastoid.
    b. deltoid.
    c. trapezius.
    d. pectoralis minor.

32. The posterior arm muscle that extends the forearm is the:
    a. triceps brachii. c. brachialis.
    b. triceps surae.   d. biceps brachii.

33. The olecranon process of the ulna is a site of insertion for the:
    a. biceps brachii.   c. brachioradialis.
    b. brachialis.   d. triceps brachii.

True or false

34. _____ Intrinsic muscles of the hand originate on the forearm and insert on the metacarpals.

35. _____ Carpal tunnel syndrome affects the median nerve.

36. _____ The deltoid is a good example of a multifunction muscle.

37. _____ The pectoralis major flexes the upper arm.

38. _____ The biceps brachii is an extensor muscle

Labeling—using the terms provided, label the following illustrations.

levator scapulae	seventh cervical vertebra	trapezius
serratus anterior	teres major	pectoralis minor
rhomboideus major	latissimus dorsi	subscapularis
teres minor	rhomboideus minor	

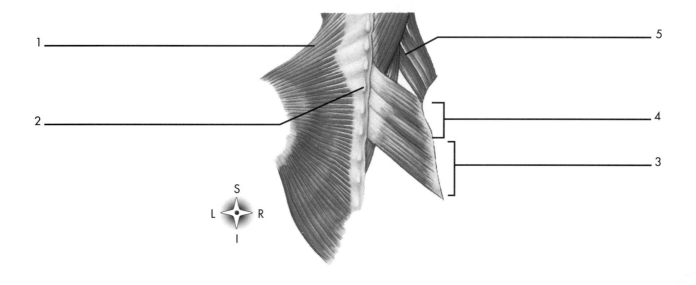

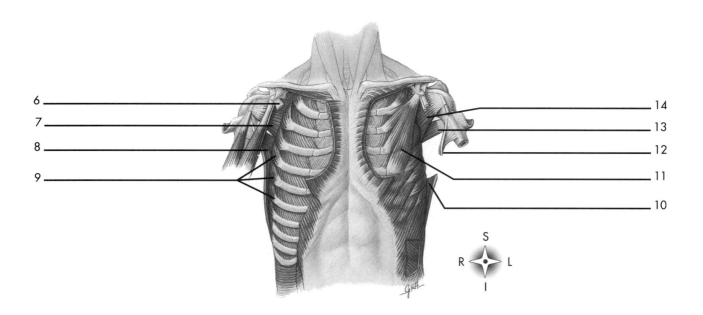

Muscles acting on the shoulder girdle.

Student Name_____

Labeling—using the terms provided, label the following illustration.

subscapularis   intertubercular (bicipital)   supraspinatus
acromion process   groove   lesser tubercle
coracoid process   teres minor   infraspinatus
greater tubercle   humerus   clavicle

Rotator cuff muscles.

Labeling—label the following illustrations

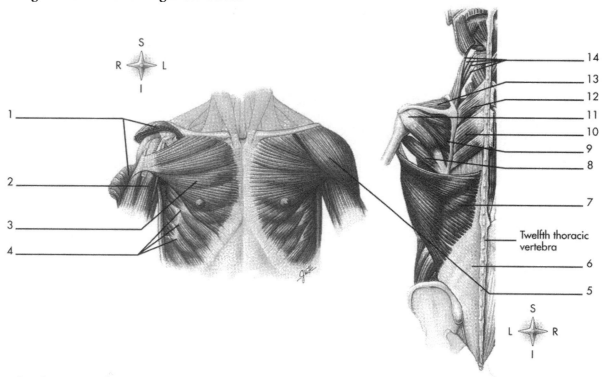

Muscles that move the upper arm.

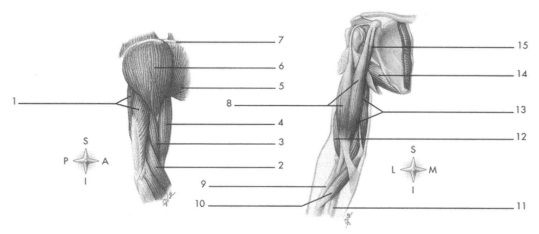

Muscles ot the upper arm.

Labeling—on the following illustrations, label the muscles that act on the forearm. Also label the origin and insertion point of each muscle.

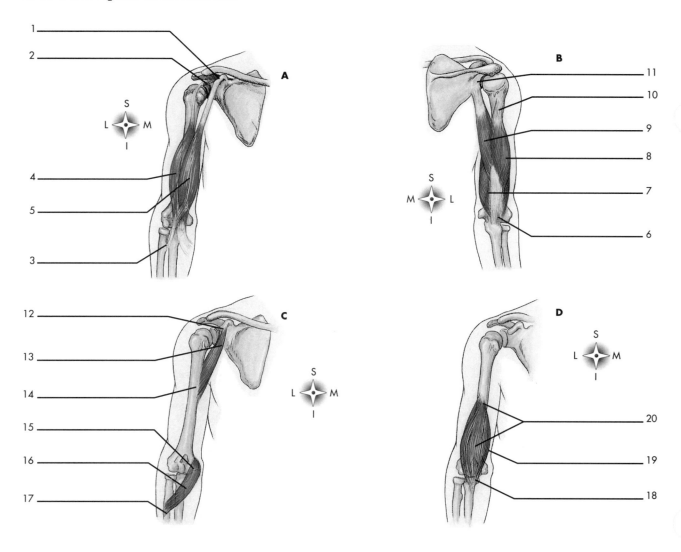

Muscles that act on the forearm.

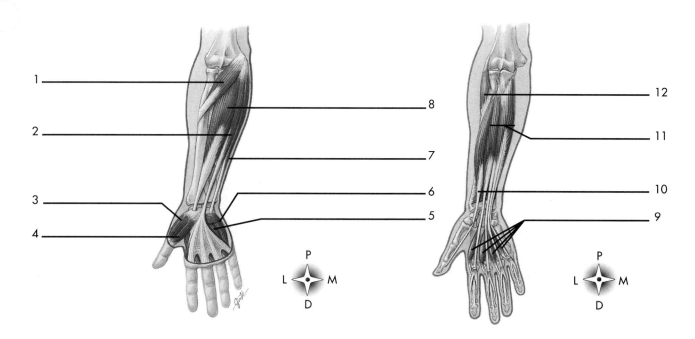

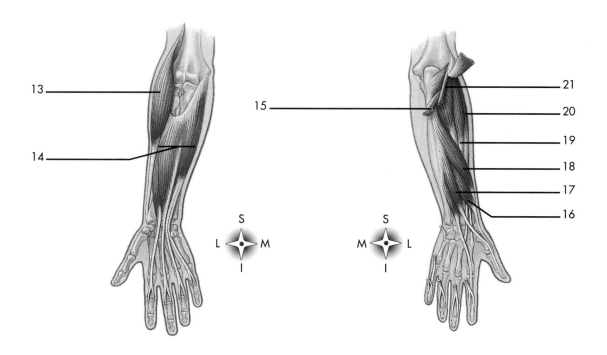

Muscles of the forearm.

******If you had difficulty with this section, review pages **293-300**

VI   IMPORTANT SKELETAL MUSCLES: LOWER LIMB MUSCLES

Multiple Choice—select the best answer.

39. The muscles of quadriceps femoris include all of the following *EXCEPT:*
    a.   vastus intermedius.
    b.   vastus medialis.
    c.   vastus lateralis.
    d.   vastus femoris.

40. The anterior superior iliac spine is the site of origin for the:
    a.   sartorius.   c.   gracilis.
    b.   rectus femoris.   d.   iliacus.

41. A common site for intramuscular injections is the:
    a.   gluteus maximus.
    b.   gluteus minimus.
    c.   gluteus medius.
    d.   tensor fasciae latae.

42. Plantar flexion of the foot is achieved by the:
    a.   tibialis anterior.
    b.   tibialis posterior.
    c.   peroneus brevis.
    d.   soleus.

43. The muscles of the hamstrings include all of the following *EXCEPT* the:
    a.   iliopsoas.
    b.   semitendinosus.
    c.   semimembranosus.
    d.   biceps femoris.

True or false

44. _____   The Achilles tendon is common to both the gastrocnemius and soleus.

45. _____   The iliopsoas is composed solely of the psoas major and the iliacus.

46. _____   The vastus intermedius originates on the posterior surface of the femur.

Student Name _____

Labeling

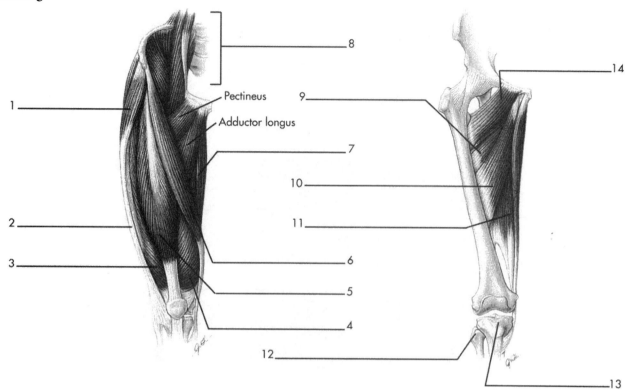

Muscles of the upper leg.

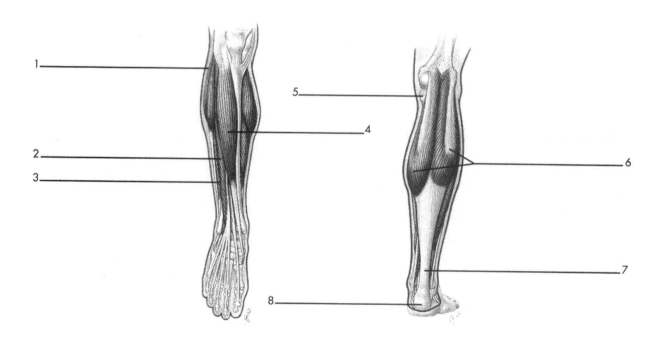

Muscles of the lower leg.

******If you had difficulty with this section, review pages **300-306**

Crossword Puzzle

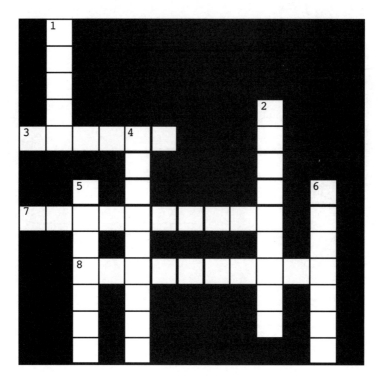

Across

3. Attachment that does not move
7. Agonist (two words)
8. Opposes prime mover

Down

1. Rigid bar free to turn about its fulcrum
2. Contracts at the same time as the prime mover
4. Attachment that moves
5. Joint stabilizer
6. Maintaining optimal body position

APPLYING WHAT YOU KNOW

47. Mr. Lynch spends hours typing on his computer. As of late, he is experiencing weakness, pain, and tingling in the palm and radial aspect of the hand. What condition may he be experiencing? Which anatomical structures are most likely involved? Which options for treatment are available?

48. The nurse was preparing an injection for Mrs. Tatakis. The amount to be given was 2 ml. What area of the body will the nurse most likely select for the injection?

49. Al is analyzing the musculature involved in the athletes he coaches. Today he is observing a basketball player executing a jump shot. Which muscles are involved at the hips, knees, and ankles as the athlete jumps? Which muscles are involved at the shoulders, elbows, and wrists as the athlete shoots the basketball?

Student Name_____

DID YOU KNOW?

- The muscles of the hand begin to grow rapidly between 6 and 7 years of age.
- A cat has 32 muscles in each ear.

ONE LAST QUICK CHECK ✔

Matching—choose the proper function(s) for the muscles listed. Muscles may have more than one answer.

50. _____	deltoid		a.	flexor
			b.	extensor
51. _____	tibialis anterior		c.	abductor
			d.	adductor
52. _____	gastrocnemius		e.	rotator
			f.	dorsiflexor or plantar flexor
53. _____	biceps brachii			

54. _____ gluteus medius

55. _____ soleus

56. _____ iliopsoas

57. _____ pectoralis major

58. _____ gluteus maximus

59. _____ triceps brachii

60. _____ sternocleidomastoid

61. _____ trapezius

62. _____ gracilis

Matching—identify the term on the left with the appropriate description.

63. __d__ origin		a.	contracts simultaneously with the prime mover
64. __b__ insertion		b.	attachment to the more movable bone
65. __a__ synergist		c.	functions as joint stabilizer
66. __e__ tendon		d.	attachment to more stationary bone
67. __c__ fixator		e.	anchors muscles to bones

CHAPTER 11

PHYSIOLOGY OF THE MUSCULAR SYSTEM

Although the muscular system has several functions, the primary purpose is to provide movement or power. Muscles produce power by contracting. The ability of a large muscle or muscle group to contract depends on the ability of microscopic muscle fibers to contract within the larger muscle. An understanding of these microscopic muscle fibers will assist you as you progress in your study to the larger muscles and muscle groups.

Three types of muscles provide us with a variety of motions. When skeletal or voluntary muscles contract, they provide movement of bones, heat production, and posture. Smooth muscles are found throughout the viscera of our body and assist with involuntary functions such as peristalsis. Cardiac muscle is the third and final type of muscle. It lines the wall of the heart and promotes the pumping action necessary for life. Our muscles must be used to keep the body healthy and in good condition. Scientific evidence keeps pointing to the fact that the proper use and exercise of muscles may prolong life. An understanding of the structure and function of the muscular system may, therefore, add quality and quantity to our lives.

I FUNCTION OF SKELETAL MUSCLE TISSUE

Multiple Choice—select the best answer.

1. Which of the following is *NOT* a general function of muscle tissue?
    a. movement
    c. heat production
    b. protection
    d. posture

2. The skeletal muscle fiber characteristic of excitability directly results in these cells being capable of:
    a. responding to nerve signals.
    b. shortening.
    c. returning to resting length after contracting.
    d. producing heat.

3. The correct order of arrangement of skeletal muscle cells, from largest to smallest, is:
    a. fiber, myofibril, myofilament.
    b. myofibril, myofilament, fiber.
    c. myofilament, myofibril, fiber.
    d. fiber, myofilament, myofibril.

4. Sarcoplasmic reticulum is:
    a. a system of transverse tubules that extend at a right angle to the long axis of the cell.
    b. a segment of the myofibril between two successive Z lines.
    c. a unique name for the plasma membrane of a muscle fiber.
    d. none of the above.

5. Which of the following are myofilament proteins?
    a. troponin
    b. tropomyosin
    c. a and b
    d. none of the above

6. The contractile unit of a myofibril is the:
    a. sarcomere.
    c. sarcolemma.
    b. triad.
    d. cross bridge.

107

7.   The chief function of the T tubule is to:
     a.   provide nutrients to the muscle fiber.
     b.   allow the fiber to contract.
     c.   allow the electrical signal to move deep into the cell.
     d.   allow the generation of new muscle fibers.

8.   Myosin heads are also called:
     a.   cross bridges.
     b.   motor endplates.
     c.   synapses.
     d.   motor neurons.

9.   During muscle contraction, Ca++ is released from:
     a.   synaptic cleft.
     b.   mitochondria.
     c.   sarcoplasmic reticulum.
     d.   sarcoplasm.

10. The region of a muscle fiber where a motor neuron connects to the muscle fiber is called the:
     a.   synaptic vesicle.
     b.   motor end-plate.
     c.   H band.
     d.   none of the above.

True or false

11.   _T_   The thick myofilament is myosin, whereas the actin is the thin myofilament.

12.   _F_   Skeletal muscle has a poor ability to stretch.

13.   _f_   A T tubule sandwiched between sacs of sarcoplasmic reticulum is called a *codon*.

14.   _T_   Actin, troponin, and tropomyosin are present on the thin myofilament.

15.   _T_   The I band resides within a single sarcomere.

16.   _T_   Rigor mortis is caused because of the lack of ATP to "turn off" muscle contraction.

17.   _F_   The cell membrane of a muscle fiber is called the *sarcoplasmic reticulum*.

18.   _F_   Anaerobic respiration is the first choice of the muscle cell for the production of ATP.

19.   _T_   Oxygen molecules in the sarcoplasm are bound to the myoglobin molecule.

20.   _T_   The all-or-none principle states that muscle fibers will contract with all possible force when stimulated to threshold, or they will not contract at all.

Student Name_____

Labeling—using the terms provided, label the structure of skeletal muscle on the following diagrams.

sarcomere
sarcoplasmic reticulum
myofibril
thin filament
bone
T tubule

Z line
fascicle
fascia
muscle fiber
perimysium
epimysium

Z disk
thick filament
tendon
endomysium
muscle

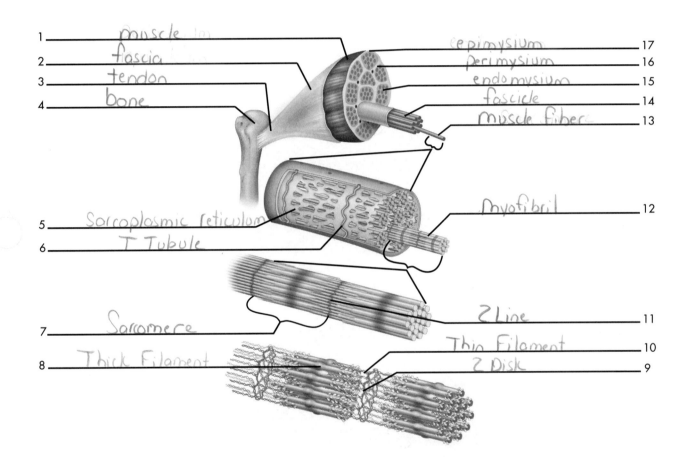

1. muscle
2. fascia
3. tendon
4. bone
5. Sarcoplasmic reticulum
6. T Tubule
7. Sarcomere
8. Thick Filament

17. epimysium
16. perimysium
15. endomysium
14. fascicle
13. muscle fiber
12. Myofibril
11. Z Line
10. Thin Filament
9. Z Disk

Labeling—using the terms provided, label the following diagrams.

sarcoplasm
synaptic vesicle
sarcoplasmic reticulum
motor neuron fiber
acetylcholine receptor sites

Schwann cell
motor endplate
sarcomere
sarcolemma
triad

myelin sheath
synaptic cleft
myofibril
mitochondria
T tubule

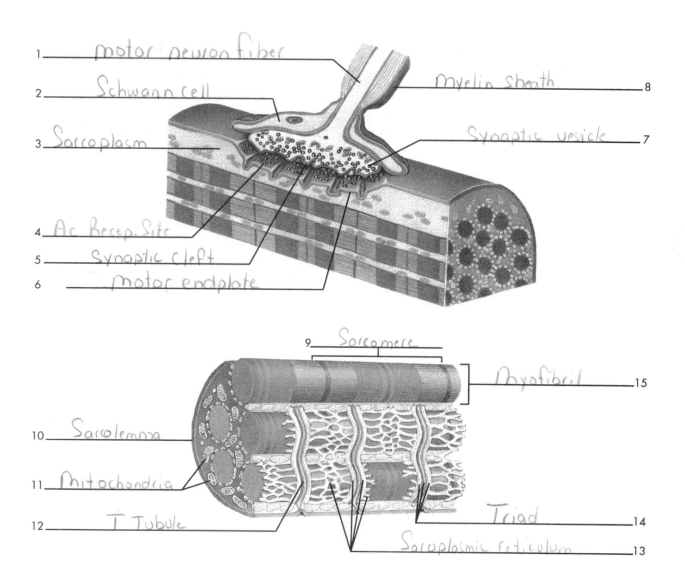

1. motor neuron fiber
2. Schwann cell
3. Sarcoplasm
4. Ac Recep. Site
5. Synaptic cleft
6. motor endplate
7. Synaptic vesicle
8. myelin sheath

9. Sarcomere
10. Sarcolemma
11. Mitochondria
12. T Tubule
13. Sarcoplasmic reticulum
14. Triad
15. Myofibril

******If you had difficulty with this section, review pages **312-322**

Student Name_____

II FUNCTION OF SKELETAL MUSCLE ORGANS

Multiple Choice—select the best answer.

21. The principal component(s) of a motor unit is/are:
    a. one somatic motor neuron.
    b. the muscle fibers supplied by a somatic motor neuron.
    c. none of the above.
    d. both a and b.

22. The staircase phenomenon is also known as:
    a. tetanus.
    b. electromyography.
    c. wave summation.
    d. treppe.

23. Skeletal muscles are innervated by:
    a. somatic motor neurons.
    b. autonomic motor neurons.
    c. both a and b.
    d. internal stimulation.

24. Which of the following statements concerning isometric contractions is true?
    a. The length of the muscle changes.
    b. Muscle tension decreases.
    c. Joint movements are swift.
    d. Muscle length remains constant.

25. Physiological muscle fatigue is caused by:
    a. relative lack of ATP.
    b. oxygen debt.
    c. lack of will.
    d. none of the above.

26. Increase in muscle size is called:
    a. hyperplasia.   c. hypertrophy.
    b. atrophy.   d. treppe.

27. Endurance training is also called:
    a. isometrics.
    b. hypertrophy.
    c. aerobic training.
    d. anaerobic training.

True or false

28. ___F___ A muscle contracts the instant it is stimulated.

29. ___T___ Isotonic contraction is a contraction in which the tone or tension within a muscle remains the same, but the length of the muscle changes.

30. ___T___ The longer a muscle is stretched prior to contraction, the more tension it will be able to generate.

31. ___F___ Muscles with more tone than normal are described as *flaccid*.

Labeling—using the terms provided, label the following illustration.

myofibrils   motor neuron   muscle fibers
neuromuscular junction   myelin sheath   Schwann cell
nucleus

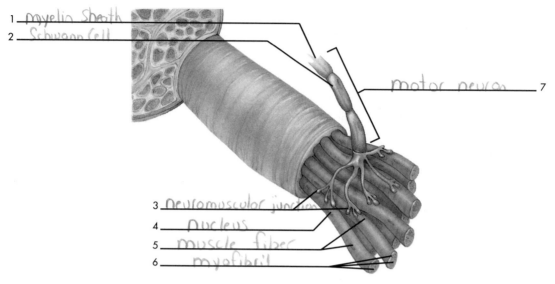

1. *myelin sheath*
2. *Schwann cell*
7. *motor neuron*
3. *neuromuscular junction*
4. *nucleus*
5. *muscle fiber*
6. *myofibril*

******If you had difficulty with this section, review pages **322-326**

III   FUNCTION OF CARDIAC AND SMOOTH MUSCLE TISSUE

Matching—identify each muscle tissue with its corresponding characteristics.

32. _____   located in the walls of the   a.   cardiac muscle tissue
                digestive tract   b.   skeletal muscle tissue
                                                        c.   smooth muscle tissue
33. _____   contains many nuclei near the
                sarcolemma

34. _____   voluntary

35. _____   not striated

36. _____   striated; contains a single
                nucleus

37. _____   a principal function: peristalsis

38. _____   has larger (in diameter) T
                tubules that form diads with
                sarcoplasmic reticulum

39. _____   principal functions: movement
                of bones, heat production, and
                posture

40. _____   contains intercalated disks

41. _____   has poorly developed sarco-
                plasmic reticulum

Student Name _____

Labeling—label the following diagram of a cardiac muscle fiber.

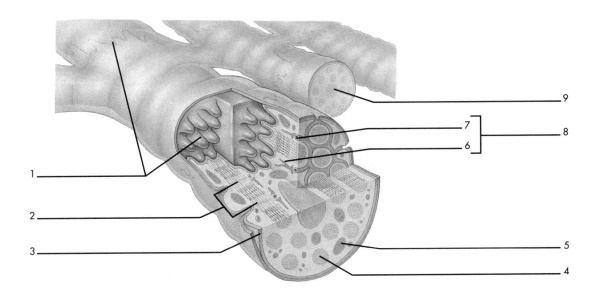

******If you had difficulty with this section, review pages **328-332**

IV MECHANISMS OF DISEASE

Circle the correct answer.

42. Muscle strains are characterized by (myalgia or fibromyositis).

43. Crush injuries can cause (hemoglobin or myoglobin) to accumulate in the blood and result in kidney failure.

44. A viral infection of the nerves that controls skeletal muscle movement is known as (poliomyelitis or muscular dystrophy).

45. (Muscular dystrophy or myasthenia gravis) is a group of genetic diseases characterized by atrophy of skeletal muscle tissues.

46. (Muscular dystrophy or myasthenia gravis) is an autoimmune disease in which the immune system attacks muscle cells at the neuromuscular junction.

******If you had difficulty with this section, review pages **332-334**

Crossword Puzzle

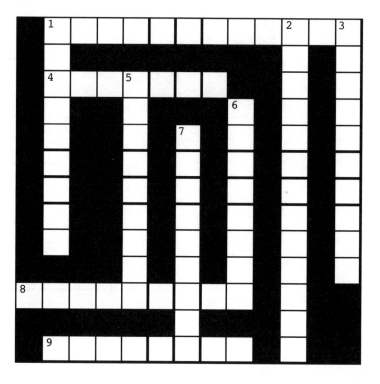

Across

1. Thick and thin
4. Smooth, sustained muscle contraction
8. "Same length"
9. Transverse structure unique to muscle cells (two words)

Down

1. Motor neuron plus the muscle fibers (two words)
2. Junction between nerve endings and muscle fibers
3. Plasma membrane of striated muscle fiber
5. Principle that states a muscle fiber will contract fully or not at all (three words)
6. "Same tension"
7. Fine subunit of muscle fiber

APPLYING WHAT YOU KNOW

47. Throughout Linda's life, she wanted to be a star in the 100-meter dash. However, no matter how hard she trained, she could never excel in this sport. On the other hand, she *did* achieve great success in much longer track events, especially the 10-kilometer race. Explain Linda's situation from the aspect of which skeletal muscle fiber type she may possess disproportionately by virtue of her genetics.

48. John is working in a hospital while he is studying to become a physician. One of his duties is to transport recently deceased patients to the morgue. While moving the patients onto the gurney, he is surprised to discover how stiff the bodies can be. Which physiological phenomenon is responsible for this stiffness? Exactly why is it that these muscles can temporarily display stiffness?

Student Name _____

DID YOU KNOW?

- The simple act of walking requires the use of 200 muscles in the human body.
- People who are on bed rest or totally inactive lose approximately 1% muscle strength per day.

ONE LAST QUICK CHECK ✔

Multiple Choice—select the best answer.

49. When a muscle does not shorten and no movement results, the contraction is:
    - a. isometric.
    - b. isotonic.
    - c. twitch.
    - d. tetanic.

50. Pushing against a wall is an example of which type of contraction?
    - a. isotonic
    - b. isometric
    - c. twitch
    - d. tetanic

51. Prolonged inactivity causes muscles to shrink in mass, a condition called:
    - a. hypertrophy.
    - b. disuse atrophy.
    - c. paralysis.
    - d. muscle fatigue.

52. Which of the following statements about a motor unit is true?
    - a. It consists of a muscle cell group and motor neuron.
    - b. The point of contact between the nerve ending and the muscle fiber is called the *neuromuscular junction.*
    - c. Chemicals generate events within the muscle cell that result in contraction of the muscle cell.
    - d. All of the above.

53. What happens if a given muscle cell is stimulated by a threshold stimulus?
    - a. It shows an "all or none" response.
    - b. It shows a tetanus response.
    - c. It shows a subminimal response.
    - d. All of the above.

54. What is a quick, jerky response of a given muscle to a single stimulus called?
    - a. isometric
    - b. lockjaw
    - c. tetanus
    - d. twitch

True or false

55. ___F___ The point of contact between the nerve ending and the muscle fiber is called a *motor neuron.*

56. ___T___ A motor neuron together with the cells it innervates is called a *motor unit.*

57. ___T___ If muscle cells are stimulated repeatedly without adequate periods of rest, the strength of the muscle contraction will decrease, resulting in fatigue.

58. ___T___ The minimal level of stimulation required to cause a fiber to contract is called the *threshold stimulus.*

59. _____T_____   Weakness of abdominal muscles can lead to a hernia.

60. _____T_____   There are two types of smooth muscle: visceral and multiunit.

61. _____T_____   Cardiac muscle is also known as *striated involuntary*.

62. _____T_____   The length/tension relationship states that the maximal strength a muscle can develop is related to the length of the fibers.

63. _____F_____   Skeletal muscles have little effect on body temperature.

CHAPTER 12

NERVOUS SYSTEM CELLS

The nervous system organizes and coordinates the millions of impulses received each day to make communication with and enjoyment of our environment possible. The functioning unit of the nervous system is the neuron. Three types of neurons exist—sensory, motor, and interneurons—which are classified according to the direction in which they transmit impulses. Nerve impulses travel over routes made up of neurons and provide the rapid communication necessary for maintaining life.

Your study of the nervous system begins with the simplest concept of impulse conduction known as the *reflex arc*. It then progresses to the more complex pathways such as divergence/convergence. An understanding of the anatomy and physiology of the nervous system cells is necessary before you progress to the complexity of this system and its multiple divisions.

I   ORGANIZATION OF THE NERVOUS SYSTEM

Matching—identify each part of the nervous system with its definition.

1. ____C____ consists of the brain and spinal cord

2. ____f____ composed of nerves arising from brain and spinal cord

3. ____a____ PNS subdivision that transmits incoming information from the sensory organs to CNS

4. ____h____ produces the "fight or flight" response

5. ____g____ subdivision that carries information from the CNS to skeletal muscle

6. ____b____ subdivision of efferent division that transmits information to smooth muscle, cardiac muscle, and glands

7. ____d____ consists of all outgoing motor pathways

8. ____e____ coordinates the body's normal resting activities

a. afferent division
b. autonomic nervous system
c. central nervous system
d. efferent nervous system
e. parasympathetic division
f. peripheral nervous system
g. somatic nervous system
h. sympathetic division

******If you had difficulty with this section, review pages **342-344**

II   CELLS OF THE NERVOUS SYSTEM

Matching—identify each type of cell with its characteristics.

9. ____b____ has the ability of phagocytosis

10. ____a____ helps to form the blood-brain barrier

11. ____d____ produces fatty myelin sheath in PNS

12. ____a____ largest and most numerous of the neuroglial cells

13. ____c____ produces myelin sheath in CNS

14. ____d____ type of neuroglia that forms the neurilemma

15. ____a____ "star-cell"

16. ____c____ disorder of this cell associated with multiple sclerosis

a.   astrocyte
b.   microglia
c.   oligodendrocyte
d.   Schwann cell

Multiple Choice—select the best answer.

17. Which of the following are classified as nerve fibers?
    a.   axon
    b.   dendrites
    c.   both a and c
    d.   none of the above

18. Which of the following conduct impulses towards the cell body?
    a.   axons
    b.   dendrites
    c.   Nissl bodies
    d.   none of the above

19. A neuron with one axon and several dendrites is a:
    a.   multipolar neuron.
    b.   unipolar neuron.
    c.   bipolar neuron.
    d.   none of the above.

20. Which type of neuron lies entirely within the CNS?
    a.   afferent
    b.   efferent
    c.   interneuron
    d.   none of the above

21. Which sequence best represents the course of an impulse over a reflex arc?
    a.   receptor, synapse, sensory neuron, motor neuron, effector
    b.   effector, sensory neuron, synapse, motor neuron, receptor
    c.   receptor, motor neuron, synapse, sensory neuron, effector
    d.   receptor, sensory neuron, interneuron, motor neuron, effector

Student Name _____

Labeling—label the following illustration showing the structure of a typical neuron.

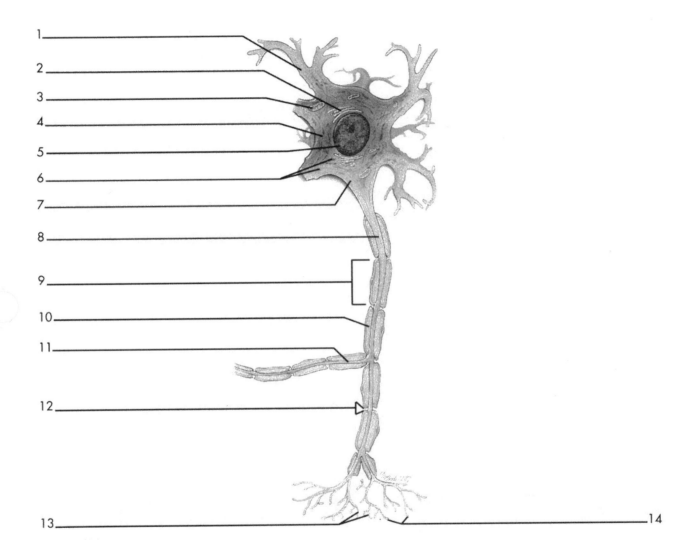

1 _____

2 _____

3 _____

4 _____

5 _____

6 _____

7 _____

8 _____

9 _____

10 _____

11 _____

12 _____

13 _____   14

Labeling—using the terms provided, label the following illustration of a myelinated axon.

neurilemma (sheath of Schwann cell)   myelin sheath
plasma membrane of axon   node of Ranvier
nucleus of Shwann cell   neurofibrils

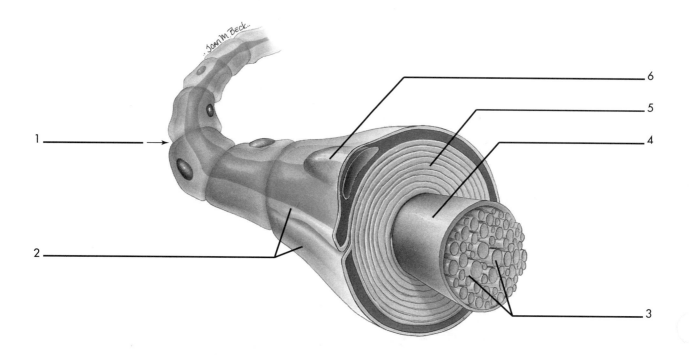

Labeling—identify the classification of each type of neuron in the following illustrations.

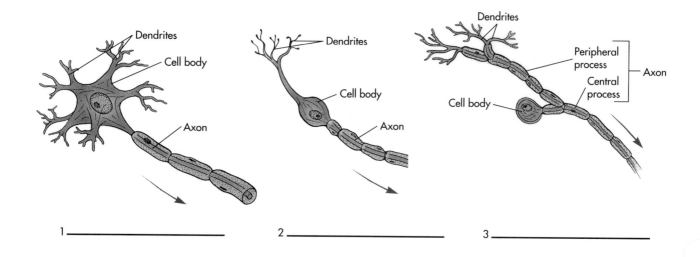

1 _____   2 _____   3 _____

Student Name _____

Labeling—using the terms provided, label the following illustration of a reflex arc.

gray matter   cell body   white matter
interneuron   spinal nerve   synapse
sensory neuron axon   motor neuron axon   dendrite

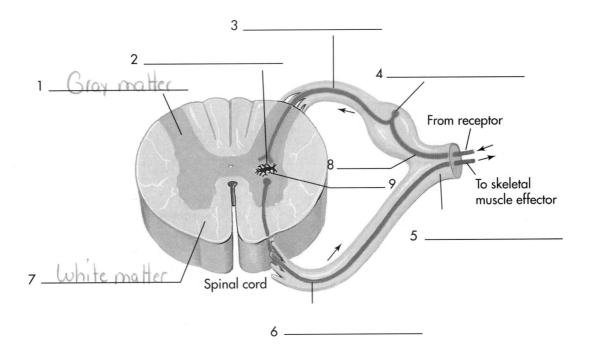

1 _____ Gray matter _____

2 _____

3 _____

4 _____

From receptor

8 _____

9 _____

To skeletal
muscle effector

5 _____

7 _____ White matter _____

Spinal cord

6 _____

****** If you had difficulty with this section, review pages **344-351**

III NERVES AND TRACTS

Multiple Choice—select the best answer.

22. A complete nerve, consisting of numerous fascicles and their blood supply, is held together by a fibrous coat called the:
    a. endoneurium.   c. epineurium.
    b. perineurium.   d. fascicle.

23. Small, distinct regions of gray matter within the CNS are usually called:
    a. white matter.   c. ganglia.
    b. nuclei.   d. fascicle.

24. Nerves that contain mostly efferent fibers are called:
    a. sensory nerves.   c. mixed nerves.
    b. motor nerves.   d. Schwann nerves.

25. Gray matter in the CNS consists of:
    a. nerve fibers.   c. axons.
    b. neuroglia.   d. cell bodies.

26. Most nerves in the human nervous system are:
    a. sensory nerves.   c. mixed nerves.
    b. motor nerves.   d. reflex nerves.

****** If you had difficulty with this section, review pages **350-352**

IV   REPAIR OF NERVE FIBERS

True or false

27. _____   Neurons have a vast ability to repair themselves.

28. _____   Regeneration of nerve fibers will occur if the cell body is intact and the fibers have a neurilemma.

29. _____   There are no differences between the CNS and PNS concerning the repair of damaged fibers.

******If you had difficulty with this section, review pages **352-353**

V   NERVE IMPULSES

Multiple Choice—select the best answer.

30. Compared with the inside of the cell, the outside of most cell membranes is:
    a.   positive.
    b.   negative.
    c.   equal.
    d.   none of the above.

31. The difference in electrical charge across a plasma membrane is called:
    a.   depolarization.
    b.   membrane potential.
    c.   both a and b.
    d.   none of the above.

32. A neuron's resting membrane potential is:
    a.   70 mV.   c.   30 mV.
    b.   −70 mV.   d.   −30 mV.

33. Which of the following statements is true concerning the sodium-potassium pump?
    a.   Three sodium ions are pumped out of the neuron for every two potassium ions pumped into the neuron.
    b.   Two sodium ions are pumped out of the neuron for every three potassium ions pumped into the neuron.
    c.   Three sodium ions are pumped out of the neuron for every three chloride ions pumped into the neuron.
    d.   Three sodium ions are pumped out of the neuron for every three potassium ions pumped into the neuron.

True or false

34. _____   A membrane that exhibits a membrane potential is said to be *polarized.*

35. _____   A slight shift away from the resting membrane potential in a specific region of the plasma membrane is often called a *stimulus-gated channel.*

36. _____   Chlorine ions (Cl-) are the dominant extracellular cations.

******If you had difficulty with this section, review pages **353-355**

Student Name_____

VI   ACTION POTENTIAL

Multiple Choice—select the best answer.

37.   During a relative refractory period:
    a.   an action potential is impossible.
    b.   an action potential is possible only in response to a very strong stimuli.
    c.   an action potential is occurring.
    d.   none of the above.

38.   Voltage-gated channels are:
    a.   membrane channels that close during voltage fluctuations.
    b.   membrane channels that open in response to voltage fluctuations.
    c.   membrane channels that are altered from an extremely high stimulus.
    d.   none of the above.

39.   When current leaps across an insulating myelin sheath from node of Ranvier to node of Ranvier, the type of impulse conduction is:
    a.   repolarization.
    b.   refraction.
    c.   saltatory conduction.
    d.   diffusion.

40.   The larger the diameter of a nerve fiber:
    a.   the slower the speed of conduction.
    b.   the faster the speed of conduction.
    c.   Fiber diameter does not influence speed of conduction.
    d.   the more the speed fluctuates.

True or false

41.   _____   *Action potential* and *nerve impulse* are synonymous.

42.   _____   When repolarization has occurred, an impulse cannot be conducted.

43.   _____   The action potential is an all-or-none response.

44.   _____   Many anesthetics function by inhibiting the opening of sodium channels and thus blocking the initiation and conduction of nerve impulses.

******If you had difficulty with this section, review pages **355-359**

VII   SYNAPTIC TRANSMISSION

Multiple Choice—select the best answer.

45.   Which of the following structures is *NOT* a component of a chemical synapse?
    a.   synaptic knob
    b.   synaptic cleft
    c.   neurotransmitter
    d.   plasma membrane of postsynaptic neuron

46.   A synaptic knob is located on the:
    a.   synaptic cleft.   c.   dendrite.
    b.   axon.   d.   cell body.

47.   Which of the following is true of spatial summation?
    a.   Neurotransmitters released simultaneously from several presynaptic knobs converge on one postsynaptic neuron.
    b.   Simultaneous stimulation of more than one postsynaptic neuron occurs.
    c.   Impulses are fired in a rapid succession by the same neuron.
    d.   Speed of impulse transmission is increased when several neurotransmitters are released.

True or false

48. _____   In an adult, the nervous system is replete with both electrical synapses and chemical synapses.

49. _____   Rapid succession stimulation of a postsynaptic neuron by a synaptic knob can have a cumulative effect over time that can result in an action potential.

50. _____ Ca^{++} ions cause the release of neurotransmitters across the synaptic cleft.

Labeling—using the terms provided, label the following illustration of a chemical synapse.

synaptic knob
stimulus-gated Na^+ channels
presynaptic cell
synaptic cleft

postsynaptic cell action potential
voltage-gated K^+ channels
voltage-gated Ca^{++} channels

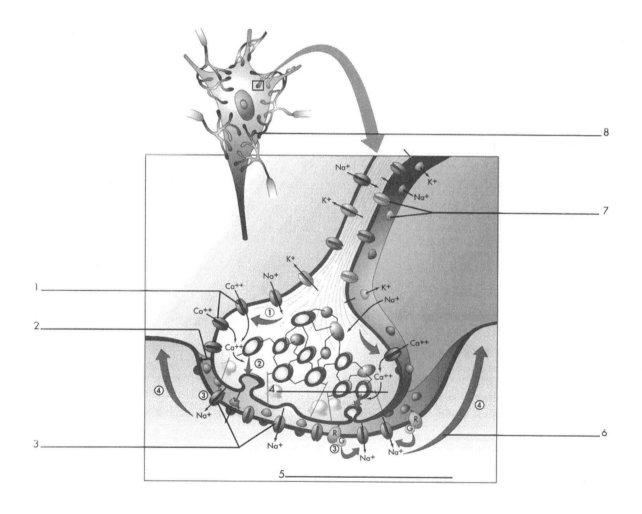

******If you had difficulty with this section, review pages **359-362**

Student Name _____

VII NEUROTRANSMITTERS

Multiple Choice—select the best answer.

51. Neurotransmitters are released in a synapse and bind to:
    a. presynaptic terminals.
    b. the synaptic cleft.
    c. the base of the axon.
    d. receptors on the postsynaptic terminal.

52. The main chemical classes of neurotransmitters include all of the following *EXCEPT*:
    a. acetylcholine.
    b. norepinephrine.
    c. amino acids.
    d. neuropeptides.

53. Which of the following is *NOT* an example of an amine neurotransmitter?
    a. serotonin
    b. histamine
    c. glycine
    d. dopamine

54. Severe depression can be caused by a deficit in which of the following neurotransmitters?
    a. acetylcholine
    b. amino acids
    c. amines
    d. neuropeptides

55. Which of the following is *NOT* a catecholamine?
    a. epinephrine
    b. norepinephrine
    c. dopamine
    d. serotonin

True or false

56. _____ Many biologists now believe that neuropeptides are the most common neurotransmitters in the CNS.

57. _____ Cocaine produces a temporary feeling of well-being by blocking the uptake of dopamine.

******If you had difficulty with this section, review pages **363-367**

VIII MECHANISMS OF DISEASE

Fill in the blanks.

58. _____ _____ is a disorder of the nervous system that involves the glia rather than neurons.

59. _____ is a common type of brain tumor that is usually benign but may still be life-threatening.

60. A highly malignant form of astrocytic tumor is known as _____ _____.

61. Joseph Merrick, the so-called Elephant Man, suffered from _____ _____.

62. Most disorders of the nervous system cells involve _____ rather than neurons.

******If you had difficulty with this section, review page **368**

Crossword Puzzle

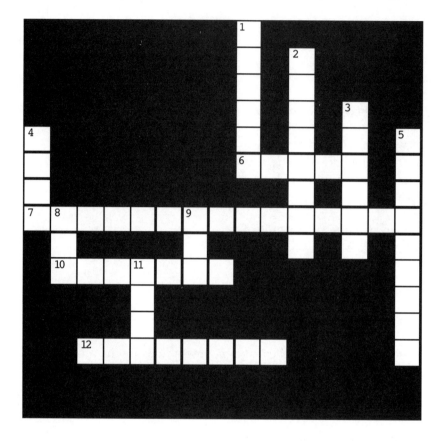

Across

6. Bundle of peripheral nerve fibers
7. Membrane potential of an active neuron (two words)
10. Place where signals are transmitted from one to another neuron
12. Transmits impulses toward the cell body

Down

1. Consists of a cell body, an axon, and one or more dendrites
2. _____ potential or difference in electrical charge across the plasma membrane
3. White, fatty substance
4. Supporting cell of the nervous system
5. Signal conduction route to and from the CNS (two words)
8. Center of entire nervous system (abbrev.)
9. Nerves that lie in the "periphery" (abbrev.)
11. Transmits impulses away from the cell body

APPLYING WHAT YOU KNOW

63. Jim is experiencing muscular weakness, loss of coordination, visual impairment, and speech disturbances. Which disease of the CNS could he be experiencing? Which nervous tissue cells are most likely involved? What specifically occurs to both the neurons and neuroglia of the CNS? What are the possible treatments and what are the theories as to the cause of this disease?

64. John is a professional football player who, upon a severe compressing blow to the head, lost the ability to move his lower body. He was rushed to the hospital where the doctors suspected crushing and bruising to the spinal cord. What are the chances of the damaged nervous tissue repairing itself?

DID YOU KNOW?

- In the adult human body, there are 46 miles of nerves.

ONE LAST QUICK CHECK

Circle the correct answer.

65. A synaptic knob is a tiny bulge at the end of the (presynaptic or postsynaptic) neuron's axon.

66. Acetylcholine is an example of a (neurotransmitter or protein molecule receptor).

67. Neurotransmitters are chemicals that allow neurons to (communicate or reproduce) with one another.

68. Neurotransmitters are distributed (randomly or specifically) into groups of neurons.

69. Endorphins and enkephalins are neurotransmitters that inhibit conduction of (fear or pain).

70. Unipolar neurons are always (sensory or motor) neurons.

71. In the peripheral nervous system, small regions of gray matter are known as (nuclei or ganglion).

72. The distal tips of axons form branches called (telodendria or axon hillock).

Matching—select the best choice for the following words and insert the correct letter in the blanks.

73. _____ axon

74. _____ supporting cells

75. _____ astrocytes

76. _____ sensory

77. _____ conduct impulses

78. _____ forms the myelin sheath
                 around central nerve fibers

79. _____ phagocytosis

80. _____ efferent

81. _____ multiple sclerosis

82. _____ multipolar

a.   neurons
b.   neuroglia

CHAPTER 13

CENTRAL NERVOUS SYSTEM

Approximately one hundred billion neurons make up the brain. Everything we are and everything we hope to become are centered in this structure which is about the size of a small bowling ball. Our personality, communication skills, memory, and sensations depend upon the successful functioning of the brain. We are still in the infancy of our knowledge of this unique organ as it still holds many mysteries for scientists to yet uncover. We are fascinated by the fact that although all pain is felt and interpreted in the brain, the brain itself has no pain sensation—even when cut! This simple example illustrates the complexity of the brain and some of the challenges ahead in identifying and understanding its capabilities for our body.

The central nervous system (CNS) is made up of the spinal cord and brain. The spinal cord provides access to and from the brain by means of ascending and descending tracts. In addition, the spinal cord functions as the primary reflex center of the body. The brain consists of the brain stem, cerebellum, diencephalon, and cerebrum. These areas provide the extraordinary network necessary to receive, interpret, and respond to most of our impulses. Your study of the CNS will give you an appreciation of the complex mechanisms necessary to perform your daily tasks.

I   COVERINGS OF THE BRAIN AND SPINAL CORD

Multiple Choice—select the best answer.

1. From superficial to deep, which is the correct order of location of the meninges?
    a. dura mater, arachnoid membrane, pia mater
    b. pia mater, arachnoid membrane, dura mater
    c. arachnoid, pia mater, dura mater
    d. dura mater, pia mater, arachnoid membrane

2. The falx cerebri separates the:
    a. two hemispheres of the cerebellum.
    b. cerebellum from the cerebrum.
    c. two hemispheres of the cerebrum.
    d. dura mater from the arachnoid.

3. The cerebrospinal fluid resides in the:
    a. epidural space.
    b. subarachnoid space.
    c. subdural space.
    d. piarachnoid space.

4. The layer of the meninges that serves as the inner periosteum of the cranial bones is the:
    a. pia mater.
    b. arachnoid membrane.
    c. dura mater.

Labeling—label the coverings of the brain on the following diagram.

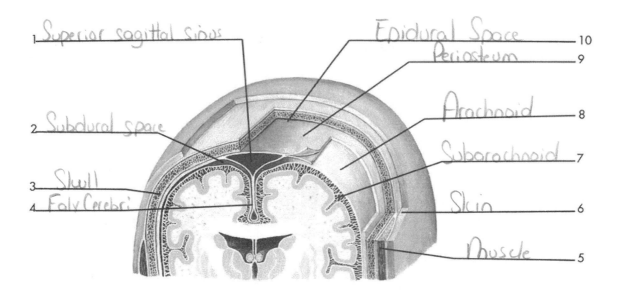

1. Superior sagittal sinus
2. Subdural space
3. Skull
4. Falx Cerebri

10. Epidural Space
9. Periosteum
8. Arachnoid
7. Subarachnoid
6. Skin
5. Muscle

******If you had difficulty with this section, review pages **374-376**

II CEREBROSPINAL FLUID

Multiple Choice—select the best answer.

5. Formation of the cerebrospinal fluid occurs mainly in the:
    a. cerebral aqueduct.
    b. superior sagittal sinus.
    c. choroid plexuses.
    d. median foramen.

6. The lateral ventricles are located within the:
    a. cerebrum.
    b. cerebellum.
    c. spinal cord.
    d. none of the above.

7. CSF is absorbed into the venous blood via the:
    a. cisterna magna.   c. falx cerebri.
    b. choroid plexus.   d. arachnoid villus.

8. Cerebrospinal fluid is *NOT* found in the:
    a. central canal.
    b. subarachnoid space.
    c. third ventricle.
    d. subdural space.

True or false

9. _____ The four large, fluid-filled spaces within the brain are called *ventricles.*

10. _____ Interference of the CSF circulation, causing the fluid to accumulate in the subarachnoid space, is referred to as *external hydrocephalus.*

Student Name_____

Labeling—label the following illustration of the fluid spaces of the brain.

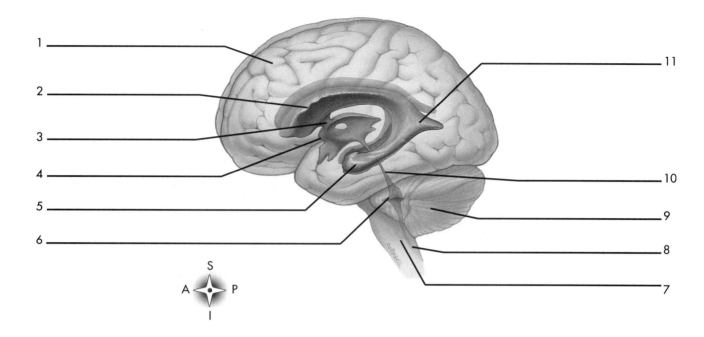

Labeling—label the following illustrations depicting the flow of cerebrospinal fluid and the layers of the brain.

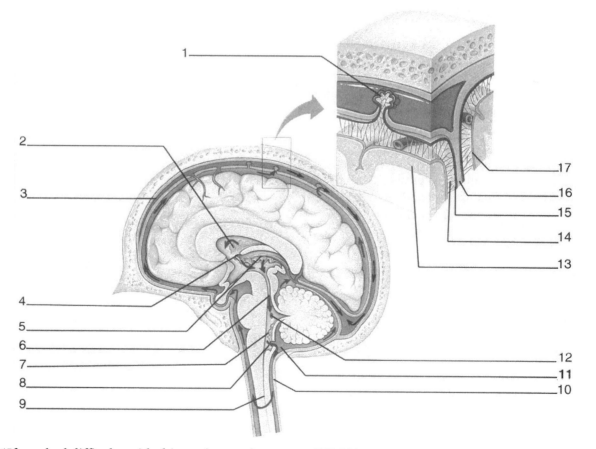

******If you had difficulty with this section, review pages **377-380**

III   THE SPINAL CORD

Matching—identify each ascending, or sensory, tract with its corresponding function.

11. _____   transmits impulses of crude touch and pressure

12. _____   transmits impulses of subconscious kinesthesia

13. _____   transmits impulses of crude touch, pain, and temperature cuneatus

14. _____   transmits impulses of discriminating touch and kinesthesia

a.   lateral spinothalamic tract
b.   anterior spinothalamic tract
c.   fasciculi gracilis and cuneatus
d.   spinocerebellar tract

Matching—identify each descending, or motor, tract with its corresponding function.

15. _____   transmits impulses that control voluntary movement of muscles on the same side of the body

16. _____   transmits inhibitory impulses to skeletal muscles

17. _____   transmits facilitory impulses to skeletal muscles

18. _____   transmits impulses that control voluntary movement of muscles on the opposite side of the body

19. _____   transmits impulses that coordinate body movements and maintenance of posture

a.   lateral corticospinal tract
b.   anterior corticospinal tract
c.   lateral reticulospinal tract
d.   medial reticulospinal tract
e.   rubrospinal tract

Student Name _____

Labeling—match each spinal cord term with its corresponding number in the following illustration.

_____ white matter

_____ anterior median fissure

_____ cauda equina

_____ spinal nerve

_____ posterior column

_____ gray matter

_____ lumbar enlargement

_____ cervical enlargement

_____ end of spinal cord

_____ anterior column

_____ central canal

_____ dorsal nerve root

_____ filum terminale

_____ lateral column

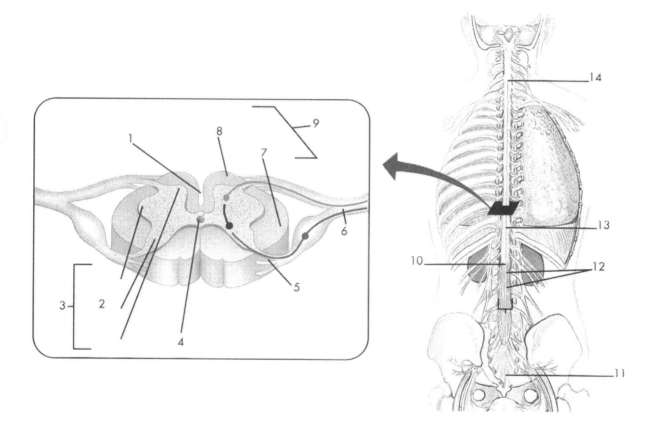

Labeling—using the terms provided, label the major tracts of the spinal cord on the following diagram.

fasciculus gracilis   rubrospinal   anterior spinocerebellar
anterior spinothalamic   reticulospinal   spinotectal
lateral spinothalamic   fasciculus cuneatus   vestibulospinal
lateral corticospinal   posterior spinocerebellar   tectospinal
anterior corticospinal

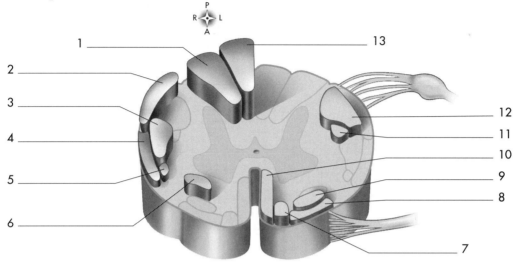

******If you had difficulty with this section, review pages **380-383**

IV   THE BRAIN

Multiple Choice—select the best answer.

20. Which of the following is *NOT* a part of the brainstem?
     a.   medulla oblongata
     b.   hypothalamus
     c.   pons
     d.   midbrain

21. Which of the following is *NOT* a component of the midbrain?
     a.   cerebral peduncles
     b.   corpora quadrigemina
     c.   superior colliculi
     d.   all of the above are part of the midbrain

22. The internal white matter of the cerebellum is the:
     a.   arbor vitae.
     b.   vermis.
     c.   peduncle.
     d.   none of the above.

23. The part of the brain that secretes releasing hormones is the:
     a.   thalamus.   c.   medulla.
     b.   hypothalamus.   d.   pons.

24. Regulation of the body's biological clock and production of melatonin is performed by the:
     a.   pons.   c.   cerebellum.
     b.   thalamus.   d.   pineal body.

25. The central sulcus divides the:
     a.   temporal lobe and parietal lobe.
     b.   cerebrum into two hemispheres.
     c.   frontal lobe and parietal lobe.
     d.   occipital lobe and parietal lobe.

26. The part of the cerebrum integral to consciousness is:
     a.   Broca's area.
     b.   the reticular activating system.
     c.   the limbic system.
     d.   the insula.

Student Name_____

27. The two cerebral hemispheres are connected by the:
   a. corpus callosum.
   b. mammillary body.
   c. hippocampus.
   d. central sulcus.

28. Emotions involve the functioning of the cerebrum's:
   a. Broca's area.
   b. limbic system.
   c. reticular activating system.
   d. caudate nucleus.

29. The type of brain wave associated with deep sleep is:
   a. delta.   c. alpha.
   b. beta.   d. theta.

True or false

30. _____ The cerebellum is the second largest portion of the brain.

31. _____ Functions of the cerebellum include language, memory, and emotions.

32. _____ The vomiting reflex is mediated by the cerebellum.

33. _____ The shallow grooves of the cerebrum are called *sulci*.

34. _____ The islands of gray matter inside the hemispheres of the cerebrum are called the *basal ganglia*.

Labeling—label the following illustration of the left hemisphere of the cerebrum.

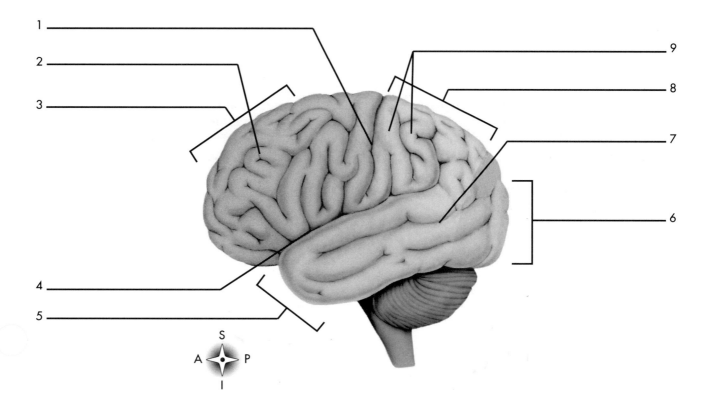

Labeling—label the functional areas of the cerebral cortex on the following illustration.

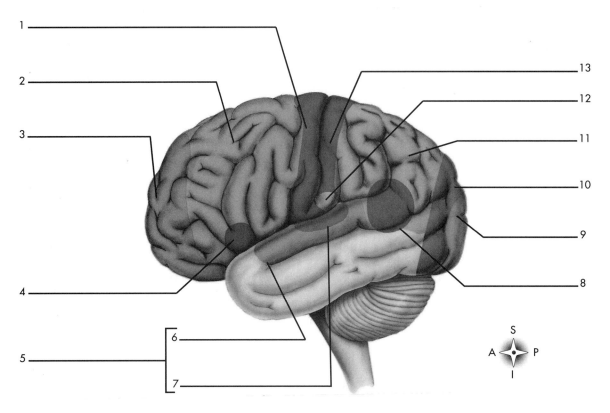

******If you had difficulty with this section, review pages **383-397**

IV   SOMATIC SENSORY AND MOTOR PATHWAYS

Multiple Choice—select the best answer.

35. Which of the following is *NOT* a pathway that
     produces sensations to touch and pressure?
     a.   medial lemniscal system
     b.   spinothalamic pathway
     c.   rubrospinal tract

36. Axons from the anterior gray horn of the
     spinal cord terminate in:
     a.   cerebral cortex.
     b.   sensory receptors.
     c.   skeletal muscle.
     d.   none of the above.

37. Absence of reflexes is indicative of injury to:
     a.   lower motor neurons.
     b.   upper motor neurons.
     c.   lower sensory neurons.
     d.   upper sensory neurons.

Student Name _____

True or false

38. _____ Poliomyelitis results in flaccid paralysis via destruction of anterior horn neurons.

39. _____ Ascending tracts carry only motor information, whereas descending pathways carry only sensory information.

******If you had difficulty with this section, review pages **381** and **400-403**

VI MECHANISMS OF DISEASE

Matching—identify each disorder with its corresponding definition.

40. _____ an inherited form of dementia in which the symptoms first appear between 30 and 40 years of age

    a.   Alzheimer's disease
    b.   cerebrovascular accident
    c.   epilepsy
    d.   Huntington's disease

41. _____ a hemorrhage from or cessation of blood flow to the cerebral vessels, which destroys neurons

42. _____ a degenerative disease that affects memory, generally developing during the middle to late adult years and causing characteristic lesions in the cortex

43. _____ recurring or chronic seizure episodes involving sudden bursts of abnormal neuron activity

******If you had difficulty with this section, review pages **404-405**

Crossword Puzzle

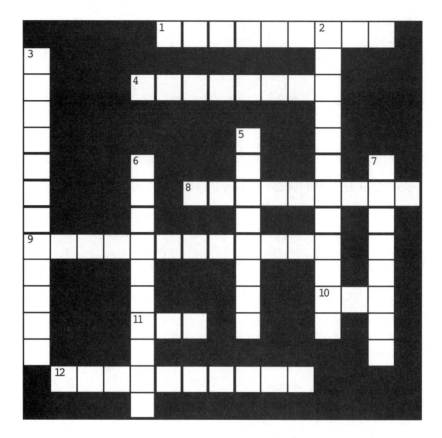

Across

1. _____ formation consisting of gray and white matter located in medulla
4. Largest division of the brain
8. Contains midbrain, pons, and medulla
9. Helps maintain normal body temperature
10. Electroencephalogram (abbrev.)
11. Cerebrospinal fluid (abbrev.)
12. Second largest part of the brain

Down

2. "Emotional brain" (two words)
3. "Between brain"
5. Part of diencephalon
6. Large, fluid-filled spaces within the brain
7. Membranous coverings of brain

APPLYING WHAT YOU KNOW

44. Baby Dania was born with an excessive accumulation of cerebrospinal fluid in the ventricles. A catheter was placed in the ventricle and the fluid was drained by means of a shunt into the circulating bloodstream. What condition does this medical history describe?

45. Julius is exhibiting loss of memory, increasingly limited attention span, deteriorating motor control, and changes in his personality. What is the general term that can be used to describe his condition? What specific condition may he be suffering from?

Student Name_____

DID YOU KNOW?

- The short-term memory capacity for most people is between five and nine items or digits. This is one reason that phone numbers were kept to seven digits (not including the area code).
- The soft mass of the adult brain is motionless. Though it consumes up to 24% of the blood's oxygen supply, it does not grow, divide, or contract.

ONE LAST QUICK CHECK ✓

Matching—select the best choice and insert the correct letter in the answer blank.

46. _____ stroke

47. _____ paralysis

48. _____ a crippling disease that in-volves permanent, nonprogressive damage to motor control areas of the brain

49. _____ an imaging technique for the brain that involves scanning the head with a revolving x-ray generator

50. _____ a scanning method that determines the functional characteristics of the brain by introducing a radioactive substance into the blood supply of the brain

51. _____ used to visualize blood flow in the brain

52. _____ a scanning method that uses a magnetic field to induce brain tissues to emit radio waves

53. _____ measurement of electrical activity of the brain

54. _____ characteristic of Alzheimer's disease

55. _____ caused by the HIV virus

a. SPECT
b. MRI
c. CT
d. hemiplegia
e. cerebral palsy
f. EEG
g. AIDS
h. CVA
i. dementia
j. PET

Multiple Choice—select the best answer.

56. The portion of the brain stem that joins the spinal cord to the brain is the:
    a. pons.
    b. cerebellum.
    c. diencephalon.
    d. hypothalamus.
    e. medulla.

57. Which one of the following is *NOT* a function of the brain stem?
    a. conducts sensory impulses from the spinal cord to the higher centers of the brain
    b. conducts motor impulses from the cerebrum to the spinal cord
    c. conducts heartbeat, respiration, and blood vessel diameter
    d. contains centers for speech and memory

58. Which one of the following is *NOT* part of the diencephalon?
    a. cerebrum
    b. thalamus
    c. pituitary gland
    d. third ventricle gray matter

59. Which one of the following parts of the brain helps in the association of sensations with emotions, as well as aiding in the arousal or alerting mechanism?
    a. pons
    b. hypothalamus
    c. cerebellum
    d. thalamus
    e. none of the above is correct

60. Which one of the following is *NOT* a function of the cerebrum?
    a. language
    b. consciousness
    c. memory
    d. conscious awareness of sensations
    e. all of the above are functions of the cerebrum

61. The area of the cerebrum responsible for the perception of sound lies in the _____ lobe.
    a. frontal
    b. temporal
    c. occipital
    d. parietal

62. Visual perception is located in the _____ lobe.
    a. frontal
    b. temporal
    c. occipital
    d. parietal

63. Which one of the following is *NOT* a function of the cerebellum?
    a. maintains equilibrium
    b. helps produce smooth, coordinated movements
    c. helps maintain normal posture
    d. associates sensations with emotions

64. The largest section of the brain is the:
    a. cerebellum.
    b. pons.
    c. cerebrum.
    d. midbrain.

65. Which statement is false?
    a. The spinal cord performs two general functions.
    b. A lumbar puncture is performed to withdraw cerebrospinal fluid.
    c. The cardiac, vasomotor, and respiratory control centers are called the *vital centers*.
    d. REM sleep is almost always a dreamless sleep.

66. Parkinson's disease is a disease of the:
    a. myelin.
    b. axons.
    c. neuroglia.
    d. cerebral nuclei.

CHAPTER 14

PERIPHERAL NERVOUS SYSTEM

While you concentrate on this chapter, your body is performing a multitude of functions. Fortunately for us, the beating of the heart, digestion of food, breathing, and most of our day-to-day processes do not require our supervision or thought. They function automatically, and the division of the nervous system that regulates these functions is known as the *autonomic nervous system*.

The autonomic nervous system is a division of the peripheral nervous system (PNS). There are two functional divisions of the PNS—the afferent (sensory) division and the efferent (motor) division. The efferent division is divided into the somatic nervous system which is responsible for voluntary motor responses and the autonomic nervous system which is responsible for involuntary motor responses. The autonomic nervous system consists of two divisions called the *sympathetic system* and the *parasympathetic system*. The sympathetic system functions as an emergency system and prepares us for "fight or flight." The parasympathetic system dominates control of many visceral effectors under normal everyday conditions. Together, these two divisions regulate the body's automatic functions in an effort to assist with the maintenance of homeostasis. Your understanding of this chapter will alert you to the functions and complexity of the peripheral nervous system and the "automatic pilot" of your body—the autonomic system.

I   SPINAL NERVES

Multiple Choice—select the best answer.

1. Which of the following is an *incorrect* statement?
    a. There are 7 cervical nerve pairs.
    b. There are 12 thoracic nerve pairs.
    c. There are 5 lumbar nerve pairs
    d. All of the above are correct statements.

2. The spinal root that has a noticeable swelling is the:
    a. ventral root.
    b. anterior root.
    c. dorsal root.
    d. none of the above.

3. The dorsal root ganglion contains:
    a. sensory neuron cell bodies.
    b. motor neuron cell bodies.
    c. both sensory neuron and motor neuron cell bodies.
    d. motor neuron fibers.

4. The phrenic nerve innervates the:
    a. spleen.
    b. diaphragm.
    c. chest muscles.
    d. none of the above.

5. The femoral nerve arises from the:
    a. lumbar plexus.   c. coccygeal plexus.
    b. sacral plexus.   d. brachial plexus.

True or false

6. _____   The lower end of the spinal cord is called the *cauda equina.*

7. _____   There are 31 pairs of spinal nerves, all of which are composed of both motor and sensory fibers.

8. _____   Herpes zoster is a unique bacterial infection that almost always affects the skin of a single dermatome.

9. _____   *Dermatome* is a term referring to a skeletal muscle group innervated by motor neuron axons from a given spinal nerve.

10. _____   The brachial plexus is found deep within the shoulder.

Labeling—using the terms provided, label the spinal nerves on the following illustration.

cervical plexus	cervical vertebrae	thoracic nerves
brachial plexus	sacral nerves	lumbar nerves
thoracic vertebrae	lumbar vertebrae	sacrum
coccyx	cervical nerves	dura mater
coccygeal nerve	cauda equina	

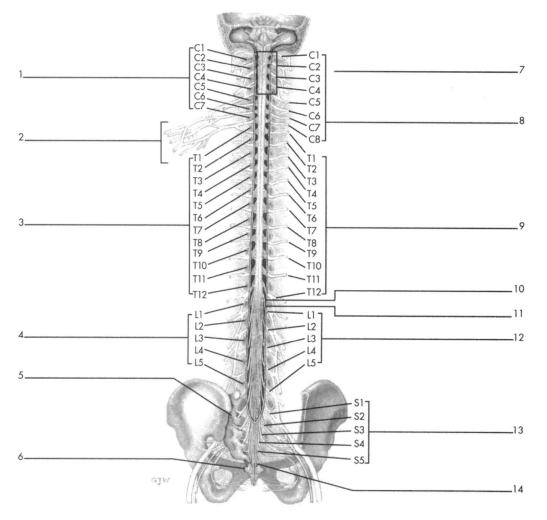

****** If you had difficulty with this section, review pages **413-421**

Student Name _____

II CRANIAL NERVES

Matching—identify each cranial nerve with its corresponding function.

11. ___g___ facial expressions

12. ___a___ sense of smell

13. ___j___ peristalsis

14. ___h___ hearing and balance

15. ___b___ vision

16. ___e___ chewing

17. ___i___ swallowing

18. ___c___ regulation of pupil size

19. ___d___ innervation of the superior oblique muscle of the eye

20. ___f___ abduction of the eye

21. ___l___ tongue movements

22. ___k___ shoulder movements

a. olfactory
b. optic
c. oculomotor
d. trochlear
e. trigeminal
f. abducens
g. facial
h. vestibulocochlear
i. glossopharyngeal
j. vagus
k. accessory
l. hypoglossal

Labeling—identify the cranial nerves by matching each term with its corresponding number in the following illustration.

_____ glossopharyngeal nerve (IX)

_____ olfactory nerve (I)

_____ abducens nerve (VI)

_____ vestibulocochlear nerve (VIII)

_____ vagus nerve (X)

_____ hypoglossal nerve (XII)

_____ trigeminal nerve (V)

_____ oculomotor nerve (III)

_____ facial nerve (VII)

_____ trochlear nerve (IV)

_____ accessory nerve (XI)

_____ optic nerve (II)

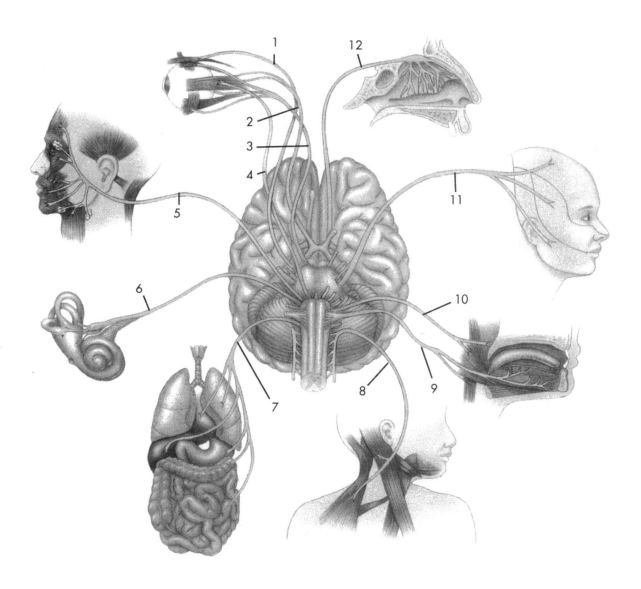

******If you had difficulty with this section, review pages **421-429**

Student Name_____

III SOMATIC MOTOR NERVOUS SYSTEM

Multiple Choice—select the best answer.

23. Somatic effectors are:
     a. smooth muscle. c. cardiac muscle.
     b. skeletal muscle. d. gland.

24. When stimulating the outer sole of the foot, a normal infant will extend the great toe. This is called the:
     a. Babinski reflex. c. tendon reflex.
     b. plantar reflex. d. corneal reflex.

25. Which is the neurotransmitter in a somatic motor pathway?
     a. acetylcholine c. amino acids
     b. amines d. neuropeptides

Labeling—label the neural pathway involved in the patellar reflex on the following illustration.

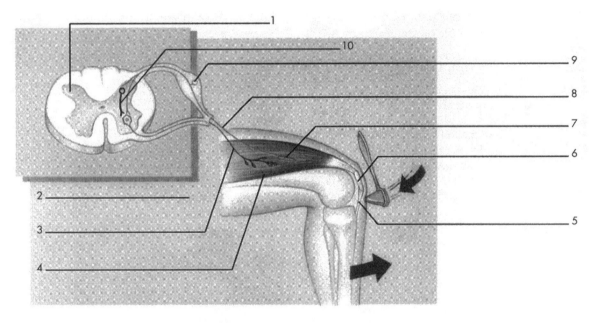

******If you had difficulty with this section, review pages **429-431**

IV AUTONOMIC NERVOUS SYSTEM

Multiple Choice—select the best answer.

26. Somatic motor and autonomic pathways share all of the following *EXCEPT:*
     a. direction of impulse conduction.
     b. effectors located outside the CNS.
     c. number of neurons between CNS and effector.
     d. acetylcholine as a possible neurotransmitter.

27. Within the sympathetic chain ganglion, the preganglionic fiber may:
     a. synapse with a sympathetic postganglionic neuron.
     b. send an ascending branch through the sympathetic trunk.
     c. pass through chain and synapse in a collateral ganglion.
     d. all of the above.

28. Beta receptors bind with:
    a. acetylcholine.
    b. norepinephrine.
    c. toxin muscarine.
    d. none of the above.

29. Which of the following is *NOT* an example of sympathetic stimulation?
    a. constriction of the bronchioles
    b. decreased secretion of the pancreas
    c. constriction of the urinary sphincters
    d. dilation of skeletal muscle blood vessels

30. "Fight or flight" physiological changes include all of the following *EXCEPT*:
    a. increased conversion of glycogen to glucose.
    b. constriction of respiratory airways.
    c. increased perspiration.
    d. dilation of blood vessels in skeletal muscles.

True or false

31. _____ Conduction of autonomic effectors requires only one efferent neuron.

32. _____ Each spinal nerve branches into three rami: a ventral branch, a dorsal branch, and an autonomic or visceral branch.

33. _____ The sympathetic division is also called the *thoracolumbar division*.

34. _____ The sympathetic division is the dominant controller of the body at rest.

35. _____ Sympathetic responses are usually widespread, involving many organ systems at once.

Labeling—using the terms provided, label the following diagram of autonomic conduction paths.

sympathetic ganglion
postganglionic neuron axon
sympathetic trunk
sympathetic rami

collateral ganglion
preganglionic sympathetic neuron axon
somatic motor neuron axon

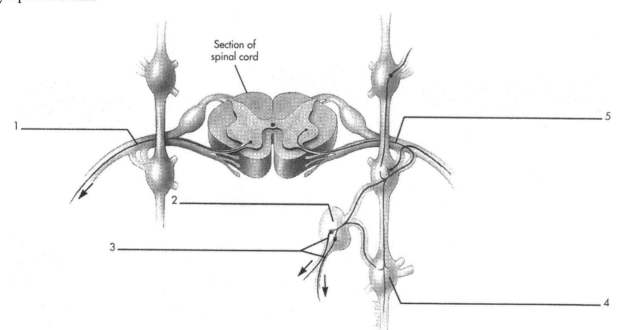

Section of spinal cord

******If you had difficulty with this section, review pages **431-441**

Student Name _____

Crossword Puzzle

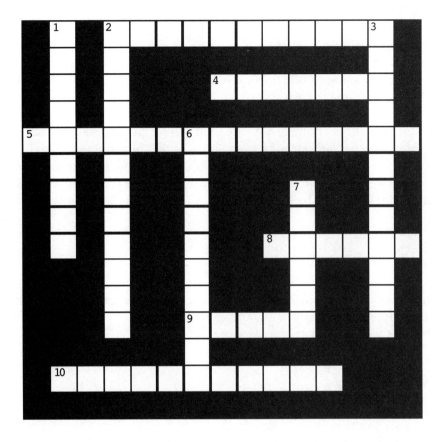

Across

2. Division that serves as the "fight-or-flight" reaction
4. Along with autonomic nerve and plexuses, makes up efferent autonomic pathway
5. Division that controls most autonomic effectors most of the time
8. Action that results from a nerve impulse passing over a reflex arc
9. Large branches of spinal nerve
10. "Horse's tail" (two words)

Down

1. "Skin section"
2. 31 pairs (two words)
3. Trochlear is an example (two words)
6. A spinal nerve may also be called this (two words)
7. Complex network formed by ventral rami of most spinal nerves

APPLYING WHAT YOU KNOW

36.   Cara experiences great anxiety prior to her college final exams. As the professor distributes the exam, she experiences a classic "fight or flight" reaction. Which division of the autonomic nervous system is responsible for this phenomenon? Which body systems are affected and how do they respond? What is Cara's risk of chronic exposure to such stress?

37.   Greg is under great stress from trying to advance in his career, pursue graduate school, and raise two small children. After a particularly stressful event, he noticed a burning sensation in his axillary and pectoral regions. Days later he experienced an eruption of red swollen plaques in the same area. What condition is he experiencing? What is the name of the responsible pathogen? Why did he experience the symptoms that he did? What may be the reason that the pathogen was capable of breaching his immune system?

DID YOU KNOW?

- The human brain continues sending out electrical wave signals for up to 37 hours after death.
- The brain begins to lose cells at a rate of 50,000 per day by age 30.
- Eighty percent of the average human brain is water.

ONE LAST QUICK CHECK ✔

Matching—identify the term on the left with the proper selection on the right.

38.   _____ autonomic nervous system

39.   _____ autonomic neurons

40.   _____ preganglionic neurons

41.   _____ visceral effectors

42.   _____ sympathetic system

43.   _____ somatic nervous system

a.   division of ANS
b.   tissues to which autonomic neurons conduct impulses
c.   voluntary actions
d.   regulates body's involuntary effectors
e.   efferent neurons that make up the ANS
f.   conduct impulses between the spinal cord and a ganglion

Multiple Choice—select the best answer.

44.   Dendrites and cell bodies of sympathetic preganglionic neurons are located in the:
a.   brain stem and sacral portion of the spinal cord.
b.   sympathetic ganglia.
c.   gray matter of the thoracic and upper lumbar segments of the spinal cord.
d.   ganglia close to effectors.

45.   Which of the following is *NOT* correct?
a.   Sympathetic preganglionic neurons have their cell bodies located in the lateral gray column of certain parts of the spinal cord.
b.   Sympathetic preganglionic axons pass along the dorsal root of certain spinal nerves.
c.   There are synapses within sympathetic ganglia.
d.   Sympathetic responses are usually widespread, involving many organs.

Student Name_____

46. Another name for the parasympathetic nervous system is:
    a. thoracolumbar. d. ANS.
    b. craniosacral.   e. cholinergic.
    c. visceral.

47. Which statement is *NOT* correct?
    a. Sympathetic postganglionic neurons have their dendrites and cell bodies in sympathetic ganglion or collateral ganglia.
    b. Sympathetic ganglions are located in front of and at each side of the spinal column.
    c. Separate autonomic nerves distribute many sympathetic postganglionic axons to various internal organs.
    d. Very few sympathetic preganglionic axons synapse with postganglionic neurons.

Matching—select the correct response and insert the letter in the answer blank.

48. _____ constricts pupils

49. _____ "goose pimples"

50. _____ increases sweat secretion

51. _____ increases secretion of digestive juices and insulin

52. _____ constricts blood vessels

53. _____ slows heartbeat

54. _____ relaxes bladder

55. _____ increases epinephrine secretion

56. _____ increases peristalsis

57. _____ stimulates lens for near vision

a. sympathetic control
b. parasympathetic control

Matching—select the best choice for the following words and insert the correct letter in the answer blank.

58. _____ 12 pairs

59. _____ dermatome

60. _____ vagus

61. _____ shingles

62. _____ 31 pairs

63. _____ optic

64. _____ C1

65. _____ plexus

a. cranial nerves
b. spinal nerves

CHAPTER 15

SENSE ORGANS

Consider this scene for a moment. You are walking along a beautiful beach watching the sunset. You notice the various hues and are amazed at the multitude of shades that cover the sky. The waves are melodious as they splash along the shore and you wiggle your feet with delight as you sense the warm, soft sand trickling between your toes. You sip on a soda and then inhale the fresh salt air as you continue your stroll along the shore. It is a memorable scene, but one that would not be possible without the assistance of your sense organs. The sense organs pick up messages that are sent over nerve pathways to specialized areas in the brain for interpretation. They make communication with and enjoyment of the environment possible. The visual, auditory, tactile, olfactory, and gustatory sense organs not only protect us from danger but also add an important dimension to our daily pleasures of life. Your study of this chapter will give you an understanding of another one of the systems necessary for homeostasis and survival.

I   SENSORY RECEPTORS

Multiple Choice—select the best answer.

1. Which of the following is *NOT* a general sense?
    a. touch
    b. taste
    c. temperature
    d. pain

2. Which of the following is *NOT* a true statement?
    a. Mechanoreceptors are activated by stimuli that "deform" the receptor.
    b. Taste and smell are examples of chemoreceptors.
    c. Photoreceptors respond to light stimuli.
    d. Thermoreceptors are activated by pressure.

3. Which of the following structures is a disc-shaped nerve ending that is responsible for discerning light touch?
    a. Merkel discs
    b. pacinian corpuscles
    c. nociceptors
    d. Golgi tendon receptors

4. Which of the following is *NOT* a propriocep-tor?
    a. muscle spindle
    b. root hair plexus
    c. Golgi tendon receptor
    d. all of the above are proprioceptors

5. Proprioceptors:
    a. function in relation to movements and body position.
    b. are superficial.
    c. are receptors for touch, pain, heat, and cold.
    d. are widely distributed throughout the skin.

True or false

6. _____ Mechanoreceptors are activated by a change in temperature.

7. _____ Free nerve endings are the simplest, most common, and most widely distributed sensory receptors.

8. _____ Somatic sense receptors located in muscles and joints are called *visceroreceptors*.

9. _____ Golgi tendon receptors are stimulated by excessive muscle contraction.

10. _____ Exteroceptors are often called *cutaneous receptors* because of their placement in the skin.

******If you had difficulty with this section, review pages **448-453**

II THE SENSE OF SMELL AND THE SENSE OF TASTE

Multiple Choice—select the best answer.

11. Olfactory receptors and taste buds are:
    a. thermoreceptors.
    b. chemoreceptors.
    c. nociceptors.
    d. mechanoreceptors.

12. The number of pure, or "primary," olfactory scents is approximately:
    a. 4.   c. 30.
    b. 15.   d. 100.

13. All of the following are primary taste sensations *EXCEPT*:
    a. sweet.   c. spicy.
    b. sour.   d. bitter.

14. Nerve impulses responsible for the sensation of taste are carried in all of the following cranial nerves *EXCEPT*:
    a. VII.   c. IX.
    b. VIII.   d. X.

True or false

15. _____ Olfaction requires the chemical response of a dissolved substance for a stimulus.

16. _____ The olfactory receptor cells lie in an excellent position functionally to smell delicate odors.

17. _____ The transmission pathway for olfactory sensations is as follows: olfactory cilia, olfactory bulb, olfactory tract, thalamic, and olfactory centers of the brain.

18. _____ The tip of the tongue reacts best to bitter taste.

Student Name_____

Labeling—label the midsagittal section of the nasal area on the following illustration.

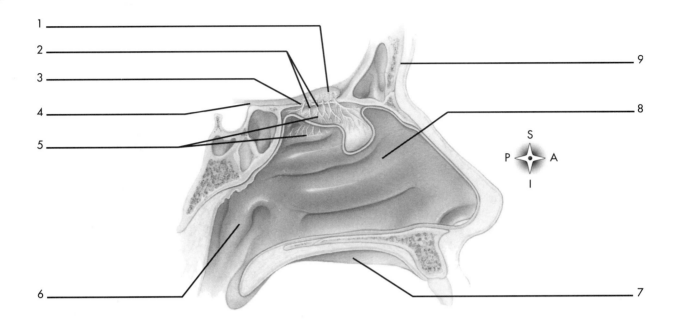

1 _____

2 _____

3 _____

4 _____

5 _____

6 _____

9 _____

8 _____

7 _____

******If you had difficulty with this section, review pages **453-456**

III   SENSE OF HEARING AND BALANCE: THE EAR

Multiple Choice—select the best answer.

19. Which of the following is a structure of the middle ear?
    a. incus
    b. oval window
    c. cranial nerve VII
    d. vestibule

20. The auditory tube connects the:
    a. inner ear and cranial nerve VIII.
    b. middle ear and the auditory ossicles.
    c. middle ear and the nasopharynx.
    d. oval window and the round window.

21. The only structure of the inner ear concerned with hearing is the:
    a. utricle.
    b. saccule.
    c. semicircular canals.
    d. cochlear duct.

22. The sense organ(s) responsible for the sense of balance is/are located in the:
    a. vestibule.
    b. cochlea.
    c. semicircular canals.
    d. both a and c.

23. Dynamic equilibrium depends upon the functioning of the:
    a. organ of Corti.
    b. crista ampullaris.
    c. both a and c.
    d. none of the above.

24. The neuronal pathway of hearing begins at the:
    a. vestibular nerve.
    b. cochlear nerve.
    c. vestibulocochlear nerve.
    d. cranial nerve VII.

25. The passageway leading to the tympanic membrane is the:
    a. external auditory canal.
    b. auditory tube.
    c. Eustachian tube.
    d. oval window.

True or false

26. _____   The membranous labyrinth is filled with endolymph.

27. _____   The correct order of the auditory ossicles from deep to the tympanic membrane is incus, malleus, and stapes.

28. _____   If the hairs of the organ of Corti are damaged, nerve deafness results—even if the vestibulocochlear nerve is healthy.

29. _____   Movement of the tympanic membrane from sound waves initiates vibration of the auditory ossicles.

30. _____   *Vertigo* essentially means "fear of heights."

Labeling—identify the structures of the ear by matching each term with its corresponding number on the following illustration.

_____ auditory tube   _____ malleus   _____ incus

_____ stapes   _____ round window   _____ vestibule

_____ cochlea   _____ auricle   _____ temporal bone

_____ semicircular canals   _____ vestibular nerve _____ cochlear nerve

_____ facial nerve   _____ oval window   _____ tympanic membrane

_____ external auditory meatus

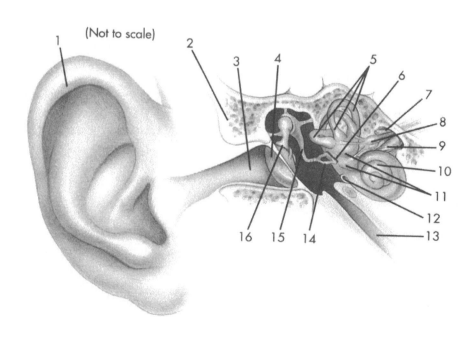

(Not to scale)

******If you had difficulty with this section, review pages **456-464**

Student Name_____

IV VISION: THE EYE

Multiple Choice—select the best answer.

31. From superficial to deep, the three layers of tissue that compose the eyeball are:
    a. sclera, retina, choroid.
    b. choroid, sclera, retina.
    c. sclera, choroid, retina.
    d. retina, choroid, sclera.

32. The anterior portion of the sclera is called the:
    a. cornea.   c. lens.
    b. iris.   d. conjunctiva.

33. The neurons of the retina—in the order in which they conduct impulses—are:
    a. photoreceptor neurons, bipolar neurons, ganglion neurons.
    b. photoreceptor neurons, ganglion neurons, bipolar neurons.
    c. bipolar neurons, photoreceptor neurons, ganglion neurons.
    d. bipolar neurons, ganglion neurons, photoreceptor neurons.

34. All of the axons of ganglion neurons extend back to an area of the posterior eyeball called the:
    a. fovea centralis.
    b. macula lutea.
    c. canal of Schlemm.
    d. optic disc.

35. Which of the following spaces contains vitreous humor?
    a. anterior chamber
    b. posterior chamber
    c. anterior cavity
    d. posterior cavity

36. The white of the eye is called the:
    a. sclera.   c. retina.
    b. choroid.   d. cornea.

37. The function of the lacrimal gland is to:
    a. secrete aqueous humor.
    b. secrete vitreous humor.
    c. secrete tears.
    d. none of the above.

38. Accommodation of the lens for near vision necessitates:
    a. increased curvature of the lens.
    b. relaxation of the ciliary muscle.
    c. contraction of the suspensory ligament.
    d. dilation of the pupil.

39. People whose acuity is worse than 20-200 after correction are considered to be:
    a. nearsighted.
    b. farsighted.
    c. legally blind.
    d. none of the above.

40. An intrinsic eye muscle is the:
    a. iris.   c. sclera.
    b. pupil.   d. retina.

True or false

41. _____ The canal of Schlemm drains the vitreous humor from the anterior chamber.

42. _____ All the muscles associated with the eye are smooth or involuntary.

43. _____ Conjunctivitis is a highly contagious infection.

44. _____ The correct order of flow of tears is as follows: lacrimal gland, lacrimal duct, punctum, lacrimal canal, lacrimal sac, and nasolacrimal duct.

45. _____ Deficiency of the blue-sensitive photopigments is the most common form of color blindness.

46. _____ The opening and separation of opsin and retina in the presence of light is called *bleaching*.

47. _____ The retina is the incomplete innermost coat of the eyeball in that it has no anterior portion.

48. _____ *Refraction* means "the deflection or bending of light rays."

49. _____ A person with a 20-100 vision can see objects at 100 feet that a person with normal vision can see at 20 feet.

50. _____ Detached retinas are more common in myopic eyes because of the elongated shape.

Labeling—label the horizontal section through the eyeball on the following illustration.

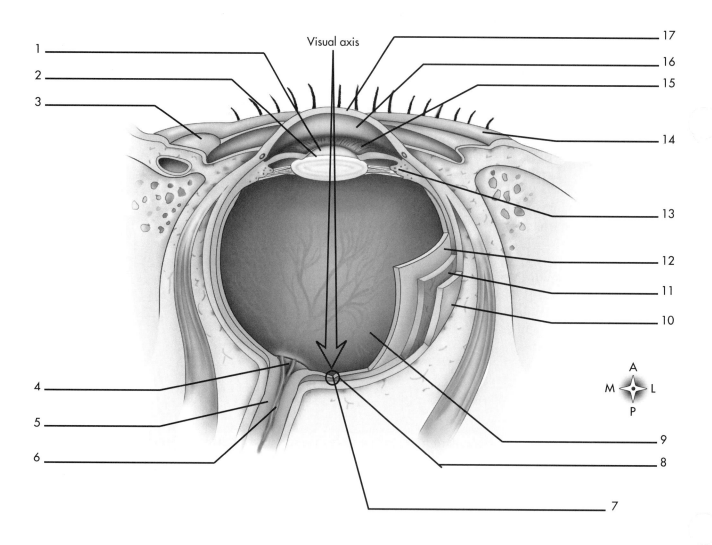

Student Name _____

Labeling—label the extrinsic muscles of the right eye on the following illustration.

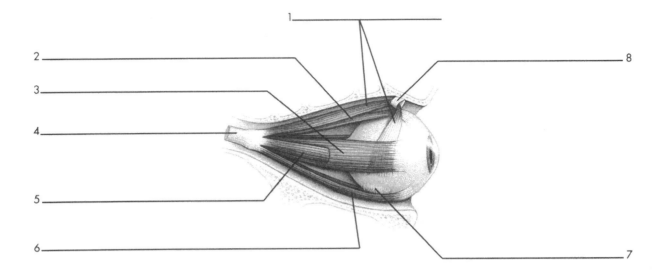

Labeling—label the structures of the lacrimal apparatus on the following illustration.

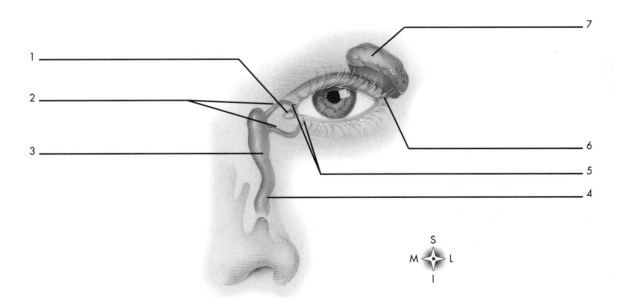

******If you had difficulty with this section, review pages **464-473**

V   MECHANISMS OF DISEASE

Matching—identify the best answer from the choices given and insert the letter in the answer blank.

51. _____ inherited bone disorder that impairs conduction by causing structural irregularities in the stapes

52. _____ "ringing in the ear"

53. _____ middle ear infection

54. _____ sensation of spinning

55. _____ progressive hearing loss associated with aging

56. _____ chronic inner ear disease characterized by progressive nerve deafness and vertigo

a. tinnitus
b. presbycusis
c. otosclerosis
d. otitis media
e. vertigo
f. Meniere's disease

Matching—select the best answer from the choices given and insert the letter in the answer blank.

57. _____ nearsightedness

58. _____ an irregularity in the cornea

59. _____ "pink-eye"

60. _____ Chlamydial conjunctivitis

61. _____ cloudy spots in the eye's lens

62. _____ often caused by diabetes mellitus

63. _____ farsightedness

64. _____ "night blindness"

65. _____ loss of only the center of the visual field

66. _____ excessive intraocular pressure caused by abnormal accumulation of aqueous humor

a. trachoma
b. retinopathy
c. myopia
d. glaucoma
e. astigmatism
f. conjunctivitis
g. nyctalopia
h. hyperopia
i. scotoma
j. cataracts

******If you had difficulty with this section, review pages **473-476**

Student Name_____

Crossword Puzzle

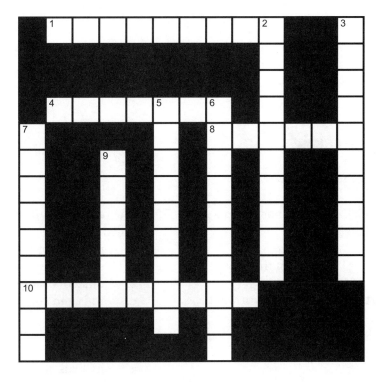

Across

1. Photopigment in rods
4. "Snail"
8. Provides information related to head position or acceleration
10. Smell

Down

2. Pain receptor
3. Deflection of light rays
5. Inner ear
6. Crista _____; dynamic equilibrium
7. Taste
9. Innermost coat of eyeball

APPLYING WHAT YOU KNOW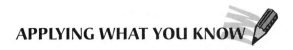

67. Kim became ill repeatedly with throat infections during her first few years of school. Lately, however, she has noticed that whenever she has a throat infection, her ears become very sore also. What might be the cause of this additional problem?

68. Deb is a woman with unusually poor vision. Without glasses, she needs to stand 20 feet away from an object to see it, whereas a person with normal vision could see that same object from 400 feet. How would you quantify her visual acuity? What must she score in a visual acuity exam after correction with glasses to avoid being designated as legally blind? With which type of refraction disorder is she afflicted? What shape lenses would be required to focus a clear image on her retina?

DID YOU KNOW?

- Synesthesia is a rare condition in which the senses are combined. Synesthetes see words, taste colors and shapes, and feel flavors.
- A human can taste one gram of salt in 500 liters of water (0.0001M).

ONE LAST QUICK CHECK ✔

Multiple Choice—select the best answer.

69. Where are the specialized mechanoreceptors of hearing and balance located?
    a.   inner ear
    b.   malleus
    c.   helix
    d.   all of the above

70. The organ of Corti is the sense organ of what sense?
    a.   sight
    b.   hearing
    c.   pressure
    d.   taste

71. Where are taste sensations interpreted?
    a.   cerebral cortex
    b.   nasal cavity
    c.   area of stimulation
    d.   none of the above

72. An eye physician is a/an:
    a.   oculist.
    b.   optometrist.
    c.   ophthalmologist.
    d.   none of the above.

73. Which of the following statements about the sclera is true?
    a.   It is a mucous membrane.
    b.   It is called the *white of the eye*.
    c.   It lies behind the iris.
    d.   All of the above

74. Which of the following are encapsulated nerve endings?
    a.   gustatory receptors
    b.   pacinian corpuscles
    c.   olfactory receptors
    d.   all of the above

75. The retina contains microscopic receptor cells called:
    a.   mechanoreceptors.
    b.   chemoreceptors.
    c.   olfactory receptors.
    d.   rods and cones.

76. Which two involuntary muscles make up the front part of the eye?
    a.   malleus and incus
    b.   iris and ciliary muscle
    c.   retina and pacinian muscle
    d.   sclera and iris

77. Which of the following statements about gustatory sense organs is true?
    a.   They are called *taste buds*.
    b.   The are innervated by cranial nerves VII and IX.
    c.   They work together with the olfactory senses.
    d.   All of the above

78. The external ear consists of the:
    a.   auricle and auditory canal.
    b.   labyrinth.
    c.   organ of Corti and cochlea.
    d.   none of the above.

Student Name_____

True or false

79. _____ The tympanic membrane separates the middle ear from the external ear.

80. _____ Glaucoma may result from a blockage of flow of vitreous humor.

81. _____ With the condition of presbyopia the eye lens loses its elasticity.

82. _____ The crista ampullaris is located in the nasal cavity.

83. _____ Myopia occurs when images are focused in front of the retina rather than on it.

84. _____ Light enters through the pupil and the size of the pupil is regulated by the iris.

85. _____ The retina is the innermost layer of the eye and contains structures called *rods*.

86. _____ The olfactory receptors are chemical receptors.

87. _____ Meissner's corpuscle is a tactile corpuscle.

88. _____ The macula provides information related to head position or acceleration.

CHAPTER 16

ENDOCRINE SYSTEM

The endocrine system has often been compared to a fine concert symphony. When all instruments are playing properly, the sound is melodious. If one instrument plays too loud or too soft, however, it affects the overall quality of the entire performance.

The endocrine system is a ductless system that releases hormones into the bloodstream to help regulate body functions. The pituitary gland may be considered the conductor of the orchestra, because it stimulates many of the endocrine glands to secrete their powerful hormones. All hormones, whether stimulated in this manner or by other control mechanisms, are interdependent. A change in the level of one hormone may affect the level of many other hormones.

In addition to the endocrine glands, prostaglandins, or "tissue hormones," are powerful substances similar to hormones that have been found in a variety of body tissues. These hormones are often produced in a tissue and diffuse only a short distance to act on cells within that area. Prostaglandins influence respiration, blood pressure, gastrointestinal secretions, and the reproductive system and may some day play an important role in the treatment of diseases such as hypertension, asthma, and ulcers.

The endocrine system is a system of communication and control. It differs from the nervous system in that hormones provide a slower, longer-lasting effect than do nerve stimuli and responses. Your understanding of the "system of hormones" will alert you to the mechanism of our emotions, response to stress, growth, chemical balances, and many other body functions.

I   THE ENDOCRINE SYSTEM AND HORMONES

Multiple Choice—select the best answer.

1. The chemical messengers of the endocrine system are:
    a.   hormones.
    b.   neurotransmitters.
    c.   target tissues.
    d.   target organs.

2. Which of the following statements is true of the endocrine system?
    a.   The cells secreting the chemical messengers are called *neurons.*
    b.   The distance traveled by the chemical messengers is short (across a microscopic synapse).
    c.   Its effects are slow to appear, yet long-lasting.
    d.   None of the above.

3. Which of the following is *NOT* an endocrine gland?
    a.   pineal gland
    b.   placenta
    c.   parathyroid gland
    d.   intestines

4. The neuroendocrine system performs all of the following *EXCEPT*:
    a.   communication.
    b.   control.
    c.   conduction.
    d.   integration.

5. The many hormones secreted by endocrine tissues can be classified simply as:
    a. steroid or nonsteroid hormones.
    b. anabolic or catabolic hormones.
    c. sex or nonsex hormones.
    d. tropic or hypotropic hormones.

6. Nonsteroid hormones include:
    a. proteins.   c. glycoproteins.
    b. peptides.   d. all of the above.

7. Anabolic hormones:
    a. target other endocrine glands and stimulate their growth and secretion.
    b. target reproductive tissue.
    c. stimulate anabolism in their target cells.
    d. stimulate catabolism in their target cells.

8. The second messenger most often involved in nonsteroid hormone action is:
    a. cAMP.   c. ATP.
    b. mRNA.   d. GTP.

9. The control of hormone secretion is:
    a. usually part of a negative feedback loop.
    b. rarely part of a positive feedback loop.
    c. both a and b.
    d. none of the above.

10. When a small amount of hormone allows a second hormone to have its full effect on a target cell, the phenomenon is called:
    a. synergism.   c. antagonism.
    b. permissiveness.   d. combination.

True or false

11. _____ The nervous system functions at a much greater speed than the endocrine system.

12. _____ The most widely used method of hormone classification is by chemical structure.

13. _____ Steroid hormone receptors are usually attached in the plasma membrane of a target cell.

14. _____ Production of too much hormone of a diseased gland is termed *hyposecretion.*

15. _____ Input from the nervous system influences secretions of hormones.

Student Name_____

Labeling—label the locations of the major endocrine glands on the following illustration.

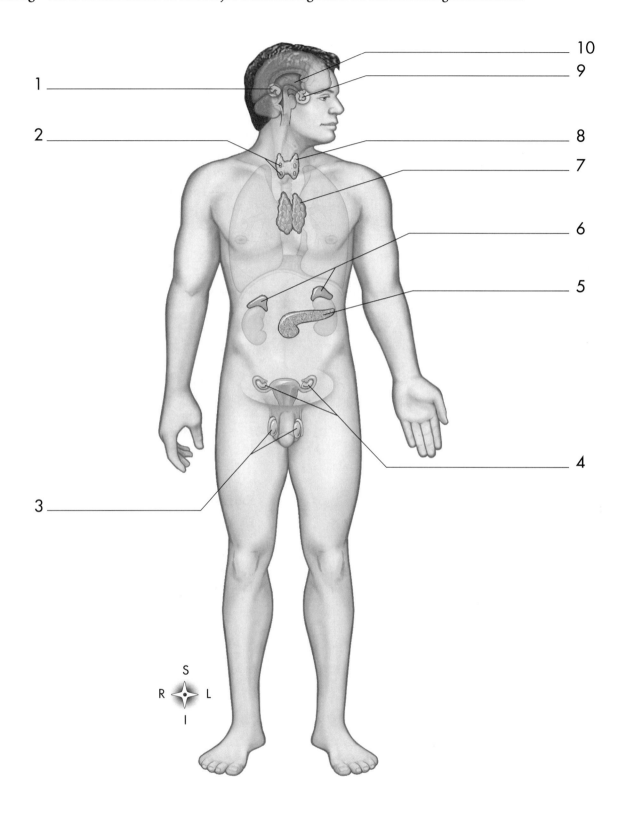

1 _____

2 _____

3 _____

10 _____

9 _____

8 _____

7 _____

6 _____

5 _____

4 _____

******If you had difficulty with this section, review pages **484-493**

II PROSTAGLANDINS

Multiple Choice—select the best answer.

16. Prostaglandins are referred to as:
  a.   growth hormones.
  b.   tissue hormones.
  c.   target cells.
  d.   thyroxins.

17. Which of the following is *FALSE*?
  a.   Prostaglandins tend to integrate activities of neighboring cells.
  b.   The first prostaglandin was discovered in semen.
  c.   Aspirin produces some of its effects by increasing PGE synthesis.
  d.   PGFs have been used to induce labor and accelerate delivery of a baby.

******If you had difficulty with this section, review pages **494-495**

III PITUITARY GLAND

Multiple Choice—select the best answer.

18. The pituitary is attached to the hypothalamus by a stalk called the:
  a.   physis.
  b.   infundibulum.
  c.   pars intermedia.
  d.   none of the above.

19. The vascular link between the hypothalamus and the adenohypophysis is called the:
  a.   hypophyseal portal system.
  b.   hepatic portal system.
  c.   releasing hormone portal system.
  d.   both a and c.

20. Which of the following organs links the nervous system with the endocrine system?
  a.   pituitary   c.   thalamus
  b.   pineal gland   d.   hypothalamus

21. Hypersecretion of prolactin can cause:
  a.   insufficient milk production in nursing women.
  b.   atrophy of breast tissue in nonnursing women.
  c.   impotence in men.
  d.   both a and b.

22. Psychosomatic relationships between human body systems and the brain:
  a.   are not believed to exist.
  b.   are a real phenomenon.
  c.   have a minimal effect on human physiology.
  d.   none of the above.

Student Name_____

Matching—identify each hormone with its corresponding function or description.

23. _____ promotes development and secretion in the adrenal cortex

24. _____ promotes growth by stimulating protein anabolism and fat mobilization

25. _____ promotes development of ovarian follicles in females and sperm in males

26. _____ triggers ovulation in females and production of testosterone in males

27. _____ promotes milk secretion

28. _____ stimulates uterine contractions and milk ejection into mammary ducts

29. _____ may affect skin pigmentation

30. _____ stimulates development and secretion in the thyroid gland

31. _____ promotes water retention in kidney tubules

a. adrenocorticotropic hormone (ACTH)
b. antidiuretic hormone (ADH)
c. follicle-stimulating hormone (FSH)
d. growth hormone (GH)
e. luteinizing hormone (LH)
f. melanocyte-stimulating hormone (MSH)
g. oxytocin (OT)
h. prolactin (PRL)
i. thyroid-stimulating hormone (TSH)

Labeling—label the location and structure of the pituitary gland on the following illustration.

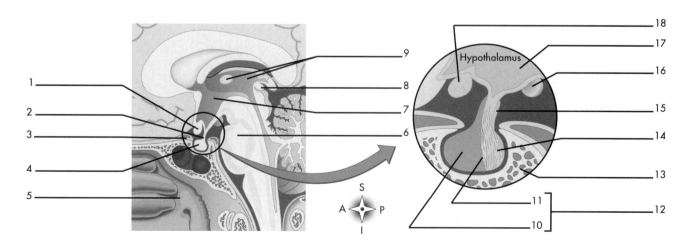

******If you had difficulty with this section, review pages **495-502**

IV PINEAL, THYROID, AND PARATHYROID GLANDS

Multiple Choice—select the best answer.

32. Which thyroid hormone is released in greatest quantity?
    a. T_3
    b. T_4
    c. triiodothyronine
    d. calcitonin

33. The principal thyroid hormone is:
    a. thyroxine.
    b. triiodothyronine.
    c. T_4.
    d. both a and c.

34. The two lobes of the thyroid are connected by the:
    a. infundibulum.
    b. isthmus.
    c. peninsula.
    d. islet.

35. High blood calcium levels can cause all of the following *EXCEPT*:
    a. constipation.
    b. muscle spasms.
    c. lethargy.
    d. coma.

36. PTH increases calcium absorption in the intestines by activating:
    a. vitamin A.
    b. vitamin C.
    c. vitamin D.
    d. iron.

True or false

37. _____ Calcitonin acts to lower blood calcium levels.

38. _____ The parathyroid glands are located on the anterior surface of the thyroid gland.

39. _____ Hypersecretion of thyroid hormone can cause Graves' disease.

40. _____ The pineal gland functions to support the body's biological clock.

41. _____ The structural units of thyroid tissue are called *colloids*.

Labeling—label the following illustration showing the structure of the thyroid and parathyroid glands.

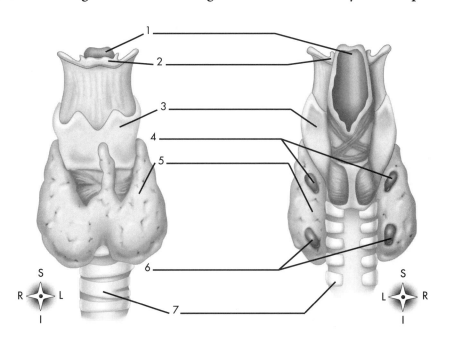

******If you had difficulty with this section, review pages **502-506**

Student Name _____

V ADRENAL GLANDS

Multiple Choice—select the best answer.

42. Which of the following hormones is *NOT* secreted by the adrenal cortex?
    a. aldosterone
    b. epinephrine
    c. adrenal androgens
    d. adrenal estrogens

43. Which of the following hormones is *NOT* secreted by the adrenal medulla?
    a. epinephrine
    b. norepinephrine
    c. adrenaline
    d. all of the above are secreted by adrenal medulla

44. The most physiologically important mineralo-corticoid is:
    a. aldosterone.   c. renin.
    b. angiotension II.   d. angiotension I.

True or false

45. _____ The outer portion of an adrenal gland is called the *adrenal cortex*.

46. _____ Hypersecretion of cortisol from the adrenal cortex produces a collection of symptoms called Addison's disease.

47. _____ The renin-angiotensin mechanism is a negative feedback mechanism that helps maintain homeostasis of blood pressure.

******If you had difficulty with this section, review pages **506-510**

VI PANCREATIC ISLETS

Multiple Choice—select the best answer.

48. Glucagon functions to:
    a. promote the entry of glucose into cells.
    b. convert glucose into glycogen.
    c. increase blood glucose concentration.
    d. decrease blood glucose concentration.

49. Insulin functions to:
    a. decrease blood concentration of glucose, amino acids, and fatty acids.
    b. increase blood concentration of glucose, amino acids, and fatty acids.
    c. inhibit the secretion of growth hormone.
    d. both a and c.

True or false

50. _____ Somatostatin has the primary role of inhibiting the secretion of the other pancreatic hormone.

51. _____ Pancreatic polypeptide is the dominant pancreatic hormone in the regulation of blood glucose homeostasis.

Matching—identify each pancreatic islet cell type with its appropriate hormone secretion.

52. _____   insulin

53. _____   somatostatin

54. _____   glucagon

55. _____   pancreatic polypeptide

a.   alpha cells
b.   beta cells
c.   delta cells
d.   pancreatic polypeptide cells

******If you had difficulty with this section, review pages **510-512**

VII   OTHER ENDOCRINE GLANDS AND TISSUES

Multiple Choice—select the best answer.

56. The major hormone produced by the corpus luteum is:
    a.   progesterone.
    b.   estrogen.
    c.   chorionic gonadotropin.
    d.   none of the above.

57. Testosterone is produced by:
    a.   seminiferous tubules.
    b.   interstitial cells.
    c.   LH.
    d.   the scrotum.

58. The hormone that can be detected during the early part of a woman's pregnancy with an over-the-counter kit is:
    a.   LH.   c.   hCG.
    b.   estrogen.   d.   ANH.

True or false

59. _____   Thymosin is a major digestive hormone.

60. _____   Atrial natriuretic hormone aids in the homeostasis of blood volume and blood pressure.

61. _____   Secretin plays a major regulatory role in the digestive process.

******If you had difficulty with this section, review pages **513-514**

Student Name _____

VIII   MECHANISMS OF DISEASE

Matching—identify the disease with its appropriate description.

62. _____ acromegaly

63. _____ Addison's disease

64. _____ Cushing's syndrome

65. _____ Graves' disease

66. _____ myxedema

67. _____ osteoporosis

68. _____ goiter

69. _____ winter depression

a. hypersecretion of ACTH
b. lack of iodine
c. hypersecretion of thyroid hormone
d. hypersecretion of melatonin
e. hypersecretion of GH (adults)
f. extreme hyposecretion of thyroid (adult)
g. hyposecretion of estrogen in postmenopausal women
h. hyposecretion of adrenal cortex

******If you had difficulty with this section, review pages **518-520**

Crossword Puzzle

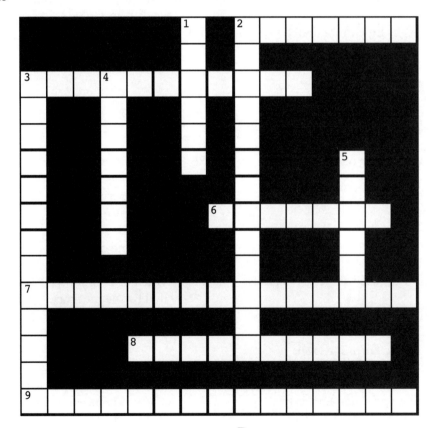

Across

2. Secretes thyroxin
3. Secretes parathormone
6. Secreted by endocrine system
7. Anterior pituitary
8. A cell with one or more receptors for a particular hormone (two words)
9. Posterior pituitary gland

Down

1. Located in the mediastinum beneath sternum
2. Hormones that target other endocrine glands (two words)
3. Tissue hormone
4. Secretes aldosterone
5. Primary sex organs

APPLYING WHAT YOU KNOW

70.   After a visit with the doctor, Amanda and Bill were elated to learn of the high levels of human chorionic gonadotropin in Amanda's urine. Why would this couple be so delighted? Which organ produced this hormone in her body and what is its function?

71.   Dania has been experiencing excessive thirst, hunger, and copious urination. Which endocrine system syndrome may she be experiencing? What are the actual physiological mechanisms that are causing her symptoms? How is she most likely to be treated?

72.   Mrs. Hart was pregnant and was 2 weeks past her due date. Her doctor suggested that she enter the hospital and he would induce labor. What hormone will he give Mrs. Hart?

DID YOU KNOW?

- Midgets and dwarfs almost always have normal-sized children, even if both parents are midgets or dwarfs.
- The pituitary weighs little more than a small paper clip.

ONE LAST QUICK CHECK ✔

Multiple Choice—select the best answer.

73.   What does the outer zone of the adrenal cortex secrete?
   a.   mineralocorticoids
   b.   sex hormones
   c.   glucocorticoids
   d.   epinephrine

74.   From what condition does diabetes insipidus result?
   a.   low insulin levels
   b.   high glucagon levels
   c.   low antidiuretic hormone levels
   d.   high steroid levels

75.   Which of the following statements is true regarding a young child whose growth is stunted, metabolism is low, sexual development is delayed, and mental development is retarded?
   a.   The child suffers from cretinism.
   b.   The child has an underactive thyroid.
   c.   The child could suffer from a pituitary disorder.
   d.   All of the above.

76.   What can result when too much growth hormone is produced by the pituitary gland?
   a.   hyperglycemia
   b.   a pituitary giant
   c.   both a and b
   d.   none of the above

77.   Which of the following glands is *NOT* regulated by the pituitary?
   a.   thyroid   c.   adrenals
   b.   ovaries   d.   thymus

78.   Which of the following statements about the antidiuretic hormone is true?
   a.   It is released by the posterior lobe of the pituitary.
   b.   It causes diabetes insipidus when produced in insufficient amounts.
   c.   It decreases urine volume.
   d.   All of the above.

79. What controls the development of the body's immune system?
    a. pituitary
    c. pineal body
    b. thymus
    d. thyroid

80. Administration of which of the following would best treat a person suffering from rheumatoid arthritis?
    a. gonadocorticoids
    b. glucagon
    c. mineralocorticoids
    d. glucocorticoids

81. Which endocrine gland is composed of cell clusters called the islets of Langerhans?
    a. adrenals
    c. pituitary
    b. thyroid
    d. pancreas

82. Which of the following statements concerning prostaglandins is true?
    a. They control activities of widely separated organs.
    b. They can be called *tissue hormones.*
    c. They diffuse over long distances to act on cells.
    d. All of the above.

Matching—select the most correct answer from the column on the right for each item in the column on the left (only one answer is correct).

83. _____ goiter

84. _____ ovulation

85. _____ diabetes mellitus

86. _____ lactation

87. _____ diabetes insipidus

88. _____ chorionic gonadotropins

89. _____ Cushing's syndrome

90. _____ labor

91. _____ acromegaly

92. _____ aldosterone

a. glucocorticoid hormones
b. antidiuretic hormone
c. mineralocorticoid
d. oxytocin
e. growth hormone
f. placenta
g. luteinizing hormone
h. insulin
i. prolactin
j. thyroid hormones

CHAPTER 17

BLOOD

Blood, the river of life, is the body's primary means of transportation. Although it is the respiratory system that provides oxygen for the body, the digestive system that provides nutrients, and the urinary system that eliminates wastes, none of these functions could be provided for the individual cells without the blood. In less than one minute, a drop of blood will complete a trip through the entire body, distributing nutrients and collecting the wastes of metabolism.

Blood is divided into plasma (the liquid portion of blood) and the formed elements (the blood cells). There are three types of blood cells: red blood cells, white blood cells, and platelets. Together these cells and plasma provide a means of transportation that delivers the body's daily necessities.

Although all of us have red blood cells that are similar in shape, we have different blood types. Blood types are identified by the presence of certain antigens in the red blood cells. Every person's blood belongs to one of four main blood groups: Type A, B, AB, or O. Any one of the four groups or "types" may or may not have the Rh factor present in the red blood cells. If an individual has a specific antigen called the *Rh factor* present in his or her blood, the blood is Rh positive. If this factor is missing, the blood is Rh negative. Approximately 85% of the population have the Rh factor (Rh positive) while 15% do not have the Rh factor (Rh negative).

Your understanding of this chapter is necessary to prepare a proper foundation for the study of the circulatory system.

I   COMPOSITION OF BLOOD AND RED BLOOD CELLS

Multiple Choice—select the best answer.

1.   The composition of blood is:
   a.   55% plasma, 45% formed elements.
   b.   45% plasma, 55% formed elements.
   c.   50% plasma, 50% formed elements.
   d.   none of the above.

2.   A hematocrit of 45% means that in every 100 ml of whole blood:
   a.   there are 45 ml of red blood cells and 55 ml of plasma.
   b.   there are 45 ml of plasma and 55 ml of red blood cells.
   c.   45% of the formed elements are red blood cells.
   d.   plasma is 45% of the circulating whole blood.

3.   Reduced red blood cell numbers cause:
   a.   polycythemia.   c.   anemia.
   b.   buffy coat.   d.   both a and c.

4.   Which of the following formed elements carry oxygen?
   a.   leukocytes   c.   thrombocytes
   b.   erythrocytes   d.   monocytes

5.   All formed elements arise from which stem cell?
   a.   proerythroblast   c.   lymphoblast
   b.   megakaryoblast   d.   hemocytoblast

True or false

6. _____   *Hematocrit* and *packed cell volume (PCV)* are synonymous terms.

7. _____   A reticulocyte count can indicate to a physician the rate of leukocyte formation.

8. _____   Oxygen deficiency increases RBC numbers by increasing the secretion of erythropoietin by the kidneys.

9. _____   The life span of circulating RBCs is about 10 to 12 days.

10. _____   Heme is broken down into iron and amino acids for use in the synthesis of new RBCs.

Labeling—label the different types of leukocytes on the following illustration.

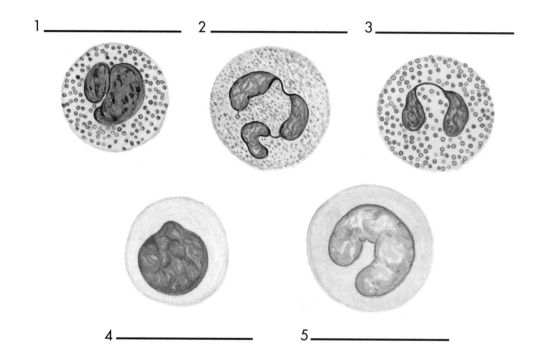

1 _____   2 _____   3 _____

4 _____   5 _____

******If you had difficulty with this section, review pages **530-538**

Student Name _____

II WHITE BLOOD CELLS AND PLATELETS

Matching—identify each term with its corresponding description.

11. _____ classification of leukocytes that contain cytoplasmic granules

12. _____ most numerous leukocytes

13. _____ granulocytes that release heparin and histamine

14. _____ granulocytes that protect against infections from parasitic worms and allergic reactions

15. _____ agranulocytes that produce antibodies

16. _____ agranulocytes that enter tissue spaces as macrophages

17. _____ cell fragments that function in blood clotting and hemostasis

18. _____ cells from which platelets are formed

19. _____ classification of leukocytes without cytoplasmic granules

20. _____ classification of formed elements that are nucleated cells lacking hemoglobin

a. agranulocytes
b. basophils
c. eosinophils
d. granulocytes
e. leukocytes
f. lymphocytes
g. megakaryocytes
h. monocytes
i. neutrophils
j. platelets

III BLOOD TYPES

Multiple Choice—select the best answer.

21. A person with antibody A in his or her plasma would have which blood type?
    a. type A   c. type AB
    b. type B   d. type O

22. People with type O blood are considered to be universal donors because their blood contains:
    a. neither A nor B antigens on their RBCs.
    b. both A and B antigens in their blood plasma.
    c. the Rh antigen on their RBCs.
    d. none of the above.

23. Blood transfusions are safer than ever due to:
    a. screening procedures such as the nucleic acid test.
    b. new freezing techniques.
    c. new phlebotomy techniques.
    d. all of the above.

True or false

24. _____   Type AB blood is considered to be the universal recipient.

25. _____   Type AB blood contains both the A and B antibodies in its plasma.

26. _____   Most blood contains the anti-Rh antibodies.

******If you had difficulty with this section, review pages **538-545**

IV   BLOOD PLASMA

True or false

27. _____   Plasma is a pale yellow fluid that accounts for more than half the blood volume.

28. _____   Serum is whole blood minus the clotting elements.

29. _____   Synthesis of plasma proteins occurs in the spleen.

******If you had difficulty with this section, review page **545**

V   BLOOD CLOTTING

Multiple Choice—select the best answer.

30. Which of the following is *NOT* a critical component of coagulation?
    a.   thrombin
    b.   fibrinolysis
    c.   fibrinogen
    d.   fibrin

31. For prothrombin to be synthesized by the liver, adequate amounts of which vitamin is required?
    a.   vitamin A
    b.   vitamin C
    c.   vitamin D
    d.   vitamin K

32. Which of the following does *NOT* hasten clotting?
    a.   rough spot in the endothelium
    b.   abnormally slow blood flow
    c.   heparin
    d.   all of the above hasten clotting

******If you had difficulty with this section, review pages **545-549**

Student Name_____

VI   MECHANISMS OF DISEASE

Fill in the blanks.

33.   _____ is an excess of RBCs.

34.   _____ _____ often results from the destruction of bone marrow by

drugs, toxic chemicals, or radiation.

35.   An anemia resulting from a dietary deficiency of vitamin B_{12} is _____

_____.

36.   A type of hemolytic anemia common to African Americans is _____

_____ _____.

37.   _____ refers to an abnormally low WBC count.

38.   A _____ is a stationary clot.

39.   A circulating clot is a(n) _____.

40.   _____ is a type of X-linked inherited disorder that results from a failure to

form blood-clotting factor VIII, IX, or XI.

******If you had difficulty with this section, review pages **549-551**

Crossword Puzzle

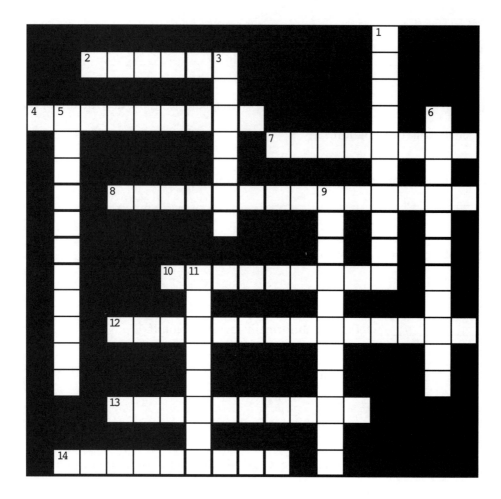

Across

2. Liquid portion of blood
4. WBC
7. Thrombocyte
8. Blood cells (two words)
10. Least numerous of the WBCs
12. RBC formation
13. Oxygen-carrying mechanism of blood
14. Largest of the leukocytes

Down

1. Movement of formed elements through vessel wall
3. Agglutinogen
5. RBC
6. 65% of WBCs
9. 2-5% of circulating WBCs
11. Agglutinin

Student Name_____

APPLYING WHAT YOU KNOW

41. Pepper is an elite competitive cyclist who wanted to gain a physiological advantage over his competitors. He decided to have his own blood drawn and stored so that it could be infused into him prior to competition. What is the theory behind this practice? How effective is this procedure?

42. Mrs. Payne's blood type is O positive. Her husband's type is O negative. Her newborn baby's blood type is O negative. Is there any need for concern with this combination?

43. After Mrs. Wiedeke's baby was born, the doctor applied a gauze dressing for a short time on the umbilical cord. He also gave the baby a dose of vitamin K. Why did the doctor perform these two procedures?

DID YOU KNOW?

- In the second it takes to turn the page of a book, you will lose about 3 million red blood cells. During that same second, your bone marrow will have produced the same number of new ones.
- There is enough iron in a human to make a small nail.

ONE LAST QUICK CHECK ✔

Multiple Choice—select the best answer.

44. Which of the following statements is false?
    a. Sickle cell anemia is caused by a genetic defect.
    b. Leukemia is characterized by a low number of WBCs.
    c. Polycythemia is characterized by an abnormally high number of erythrocytes.
    d. Pernicious anemia is caused by a lack of vitamin B_{12}.

45. Deficiency in the number or function of erythrocytes is called:
    a. leukemia.
    b. anemia.
    c. polycythemia.
    d. leukopenia.

46. Which of the following statements does *NOT* describe a characteristic of leukocytes?
    a. They are disc-shaped cells that do not contain a nucleus.
    b. They have the ability to fight infection.
    c. They provide defense against certain parasites.
    d. They provide immune defense.

47. Which of the following substances is *NOT* found in serum?
    a. clotting factors
    b. water
    c. hormones
    d. all of the above are found in serum

48. Which of the following substances is *NOT* found in blood plasma?
    a. water
    b. oxygen
    c. hormones
    d. none of the above

49. An allergic reaction may increase the number of:
    a. eosinophils.
    b. neutrophils.
    c. lymphocytes.
    d. monocytes.

50. What is a blood clot that is moving through the body called?
    a. embolism
    b. fibrosis
    c. heparin
    d. thrombosis

51. When could difficulty with the Rh blood factor arise?
    a. Rh-negative man and woman produce a child
    b. Rh-positive man and woman produce a child
    c. Rh-positive woman and an Rh-negative man produce a child
    d. Rh-negative woman and an Rh-positive man produce a child

52. What is the primary function of hemoglobin?
    a. fight infection
    b. produce blood clots
    c. carry oxygen
    d. transport hormones

53. Are any of the following steps *NOT* involved in blood clot formation?
    a. A blood vessel is injured and platelet factors are formed.
    b. Thrombin is converted into prothrombin.
    c. Fibrinogen is converted into fibrin.
    d. All of the above are involved in blood clot formation.

Matching—select the most correct answer for each item on the left.

54. _____ lymphocytes

55. _____ erythrocytes

56. _____ type AB

57. _____ basophils

58. _____ leukemia

59. _____ platelets

60. _____ type O

61. _____ Rh factor

62. _____ autologous transfusion

63. _____ neutrophils

a. heparin
b. contains anti-A and anti-B antibodies
c. clotting
d. immunity
e. erythroblastosis fetalis
f. anemia
g. cancer
h. contains A and B antigens
i. reinfusion into self
j. phagocytosis

CHAPTER 18

ANATOMY OF THE CARDIOVASCULAR SYSTEM

The heart is actually two pumps—one moves blood to the lungs, the other pushes it out into the body. These two functions seem rather elementary in comparison to the complex and numerous functions performed by most of the other body organs, and yet if this pump stops, within a few short minutes all life ceases.

The heart is divided into two upper compartments called *atria*, or receiving chambers, and two lower compartments, or discharging chambers, called *ventricles*. By age 45, approximately 300,000 tons of blood will have passed through these chambers to be circulated to the blood vessels. This closed system of circulation provides distribution of blood to the entire body (systemic circulation) and to specific regions, such as the pulmonary circulation or coronary circulation.

One hundred thousand miles of blood vessels make up the elaborate transportation system that circulates materials for energy, growth, and repair, and eliminates wastes from your body. These vessels, called *arteries, veins,* and *capillaries,* are exchange vessels, or connecting links, between the arteries and veins. The pumping action of the heart keeps blood moving through the closed system of vessels. This closed system of circulation provides distribution of blood to the entire body and to specific regions such as the pulmonary circulation or hepatic portal circulation. Your review of the anatomy of this system will provide you with an understanding of the complex transportation mechanism necessary to provide oxygen and nutrients to our tissues.

I HEART

Multiple Choice—select the best answer.

1. The visceral pericardium is found:
   a. inside the fibrous pericardium.
   b. adhering to the surface of the heart.
   c. lining the inside of the chambers of the heart.
   d. comprising the bulk of the heart tissue.

2. The correct layers of the heart, from superficial to deep, are:
   a. myocardium, pericardium, endocardium.
   b. epicardium, myocardium, pericardium.
   c. epicardium, myocardium, endocardium.
   d. endocardium, myocardium, epicardium.

3. The atrioventricular valves are also called:
   a. cuspid valves.
   b. semilunar valves.
   c. aortic valves.
   d. pulmonary valves.

4. Respectively, the right and left atrioventricular valves are also referred to as:
   a. tricuspid, mitral.
   b. bicuspid, tricuspid.
   c. mitral, bicuspid.
   d. bicuspid, mitral.

5. Semilunar valves prevent backflow of blood into the:
   a. atria.
   b. lungs.
   c. vena cava.
   d. ventricles.

183

6. The most abundant blood supply goes to the:
   a. right atrium.   c. left atrium.
   b. right ventricle.   d. left ventricle.

7. Branching of an artery as it progresses from proximal to distal is called:
   a. ischemia.   c. anastomosis.
   b. infarction.   d. both a and c.

8. The cavity of the heart that normally has the thickest wall is the:
   a. right atrium.   c. left atrium.
   b. right ventricle.   d. left ventricle.

9. Which of the following is a semilunar valve?
   a. aortic   c. mitral
   b. pulmonary   d. both a and b

10. The pacemaker of the heart is/are the:
    a. AV bundle.   c. AV node.
    b. SA node.   d. Purkinje fibers.

Labeling

11. Trace the blood flow through the heart by numbering the following structures in the correct sequence. Start with number 1 for the vena cava and proceed until you have numbered all the structures.

_____ tricuspid

_____ pulmonary arteries

_____ bicuspid valve

_____ vena cava

_____ right ventricle

_____ aorta

_____ pulmonary veins

_____ pulmonary semilunar valve

_____ left ventricle

_____ right atrium

_____ left atrium

_____ aortic semilunar valve

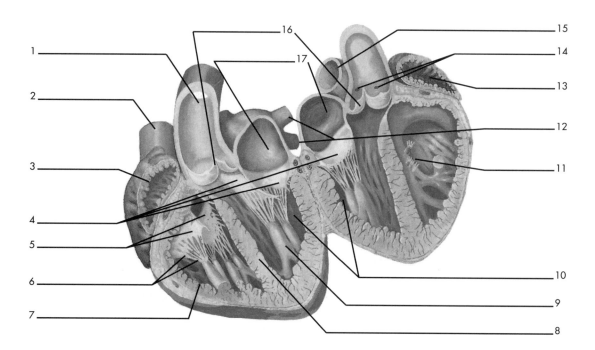

******If you had difficulty with this section, review pages **556-565**

Student Name_____

Fill in the blanks.

12. A noninvasive technique for evaluating the internal structures and motions of the heart and great
    vessels is known as _____.

13. Increased serum levels in the blood are often indicative of a recent myocardial infarction. These levels
    are monitored by blood tests known as _____ _____ _____.

14. A safe, noninvasive method of evaluating blood flow in coronary arteries or to evaluate ventricular
    function is _____ _____ _____.

15. Rhythmic compressions of the heart combined with effective artificial respiration in cases of cardiac
    arrest is known as _____ _____.

******If you had difficulty with this section, review pages **557-565**

II BLOOD VESSELS

Match the term on the left with the proper selection on the right.

16.	_____ arteries	a.	smooth muscle cells that guard the entrance to capillaries
17.	_____ capillaries	b.	carry blood to the heart
		c.	carry blood into the venules
18.	_____ tunica adventitia	d.	carry blood away from the heart
19.	_____ tunica intima	e.	outermost layers of arteries and veins
		f.	large venous spaces
20.	_____ sinuses	g.	endothelium
21.	_____ veins		
22.	_____ precapillary sphincters		

True or false

23. _____ Veins are the only blood vessels to contain semilunar valves.

24. _____ The walls of veins are much thicker than arteries.

25. _____ The flow of blood through the capillary bed is referred to as *microcirculation.*

26. _____ Arteries are often referred to as *capacitance vessels.*

Labeling—label the structure of blood vessels depicted in the following diagrams.

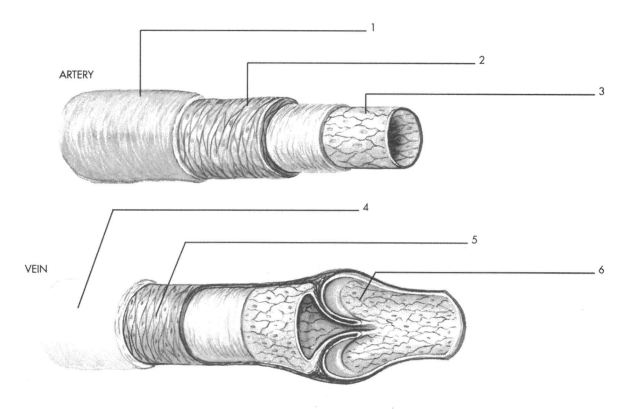

******If you had difficulty with this section, review pages **566-569**

III   MAJOR BLOOD VESSELS

Multiple Choice—select the best answer.

27. The aorta carries blood out of the:
   a.   right atrium.   c.   left atrium.
   b.   right ventricle.   d.   left ventricle.

28. The superior vena cava returns blood to the:
   a.   left atrium.   c.   right atrium.
   b.   left ventricle.   d.   right ventricle.

29. Blood returns from the lungs during pulmonary circulation via the:
   a.   pulmonary artery.
   b.   pulmonary veins.
   c.   aorta.
   d.   inferior vena cava.

30. The hepatic portal circulation serves the body by:
   a.   removing excess glucose and storing it in the liver as glycogen.
   b.   detoxifying blood.
   c.   assisting the body to maintain proper blood glucose.
   d.   all of the above.

31. The structure used to bypass the liver in the fetal circulation is the:
   a.   foramen ovale.
   b.   ductus venosus.
   c.   ductus arteriosus.
   d.   umbilical vein.

Student Name_____

32. The foramen ovale serves the fetal circulation by:
    a. connecting the aorta and the pulmonary artery.
    b. shunting blood from the right atrium directly into the left atrium.
    c. bypassing the liver.
    d. bypassing the lungs.

33. The structure used to connect the aorta and pulmonary artery in the fetal circulation is the:
    a. ductus arteriosus.
    b. ductus venosus.
    c. aorta.
    d. foramen ovale.

34. Which of the following is *NOT* an artery?
    a. femoral   c. coronary
    b. popliteal   d. inferior vena cava

Fill in the blanks.

35. Blood flow from the heart to all parts of the body and back again is known as _____

    _____.

36. Small vessels join the anterior and posterior arteries to form an arterial circle at the base of the brain

    known as the _____ _____ _____.

37. _____ are the ultimate extensions of capillaries.

38. When blood is in the capillaries of abdominal digestive organs, it must flow through the

    _____ _____ _____.

39. If either hepatic portal circulation or venous return from the liver is interfered with, a condition known

    as _____ may occur.

40. Two _____ _____ carry circulation to the placenta and one

    _____ _____ returns blood from the placenta.

41. Many arteries have corresponding _____ with the same name.

Labeling—label the principal veins of the body on the following illustration.

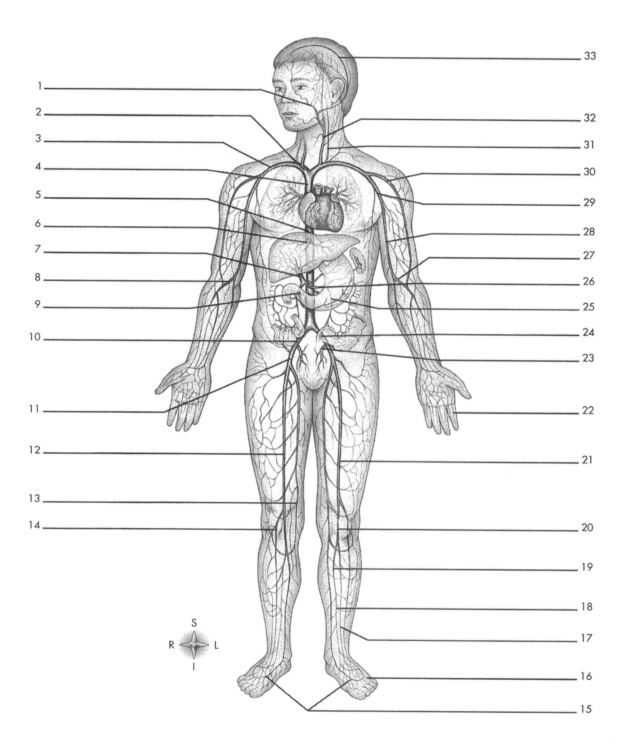

Student Name_____

Labeling—label the principal arteries of the body on the following illustration.

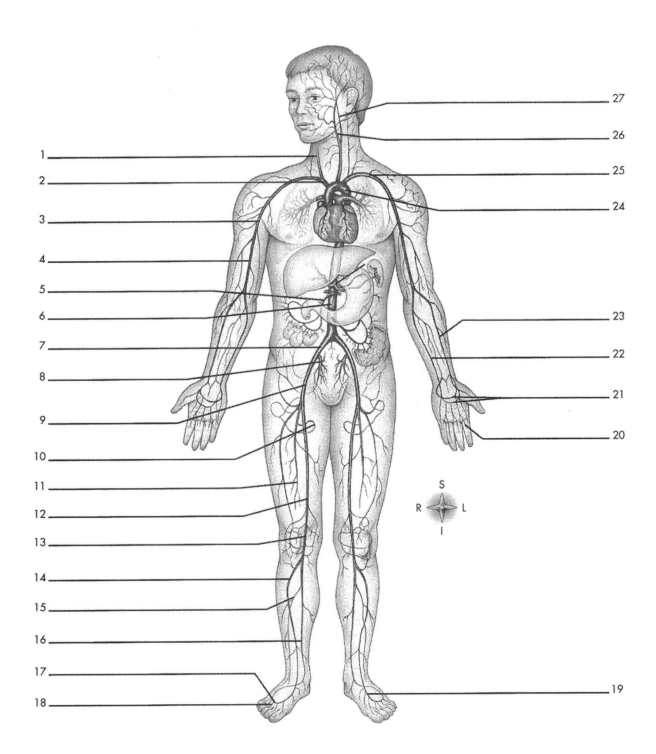

1 _____
2 _____
3 _____
4 _____
5 _____
6 _____
7 _____
8 _____
9 _____
10 _____
11 _____
12 _____
13 _____
14 _____
15 _____
16 _____
17 _____
18 _____

27
26
25
24
23
22
21
20
19

Labeling—label the following depiction of fetal circulation.

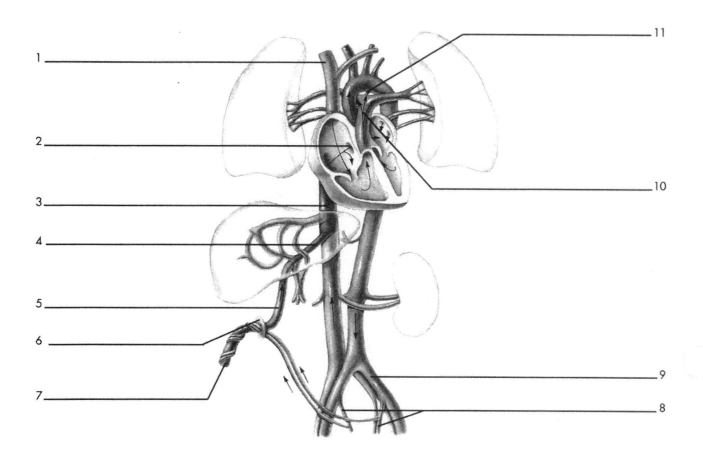

1 _____

2 _____

3 _____

4 _____

5 _____

6 _____

7 _____

11 _____

10 _____

9 _____

8 _____

******If you had difficulty with this section, review pages **569-584**

Student Name_____

IV MECHANISMS OF DISEASE

Match the term on the left with the proper selection on the right.

42. _____ heart attack

43. _____ decreased blood supply to a tissue

44. _____ tissue death

45. _____ necrosis that has progressed to decay

46. _____ a type of arteriosclerosis caused by lipids

47. _____ a section of an artery that has become abnormally widened

48. _____ varicose veins in the rectum

49. _____ vein inflammation

50. _____ clot formation

51. _____ cerebral vascular accident

52. _____ leaking of bicuspid valve

53. _____ narrower-than-normal valve

a. atherosclerosis
b. ischemia
c. aneurysm
d. necrosis
e. gangrene
f. hemorrhoids
g. phlebitis
h. stroke
i. myocardial infarction
j. thrombus
k. stenosed valves
l. MVP

******If you had difficulty with this section, review pages **584-588**

Crossword Puzzle

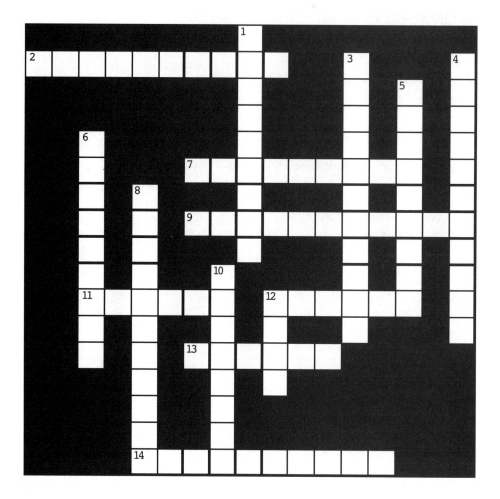

Across

2. Visceral layer of the serous pericardium
7. "Pumping chamber" of the heart
9. Membrane that surrounds the heart
11. Carries blood away from the heart
12. Small vein
13. "Receiving chamber" of the heart
14. Muscle of the heart

Down

1. _____ circulation (blood flow to lungs and back)
3. Delicate interior layer of the heart
4. Provides collateral circulation to a part
5. Small artery
6. Connects arterioles to venules
8. Cells that line the circulatory system
10. _____ circulation (blood flow throughout the system)
12. Vessel that returns blood to the heart

Student Name _____

APPLYING WHAT YOU KNOW

54. Mr. Shearer was admitted to the emergency room with severe swelling in his extremities, difficulty in breathing, and an elevated blood pressure. His doctor advised him that he had "left-sided heart failure." What is the other name for this condition and could you elaborate on the possible serious outcome of this diagnosis if Mr. Shearer does not respond to this treatment?

55. Else was experiencing angina pectoris. Her doctor suggested a surgical procedure that would require the removal of a vein from another region of her body. What is the name of this surgical procedure?

56. Mr. Wertz called his doctor and informed him that during the night he had experienced some "heart-burn" and "night sweats." His wife had insisted that he call the doctor even though he felt better. Mr. Wertz's doctor ordered blood work to be done and was not surprised when the serum levels of CPK, AST, and LDH came back elevated. How would you explain this elevation in blood serum levels?

DID YOU KNOW

- Your heart pumps more than 5 quarts of blood every minute… that's 2,000 gallons a day!

ONE LAST QUICK CHECK

Multiple Choice—select the best answer.

57. The superior vena cava carries blood to the:
    a. left ventricle.
    b. coronary arteries.
    c. right atrium.
    d. pulmonary veins.

58. Which of the following statements is *NOT* true regarding pericarditis?
    a. It may be caused by infection or trauma.
    b. It often causes severe chest pain.
    c. It may result in impairment of the pumping action of the heart.
    d. All of the above statements are true.

59. The outside covering that surrounds and protects the heart is called the:
    a. endocardium.
    b. myocardium.
    c. pericardium.
    d. ectocardium.

60. A valve that permits blood to flow from the right ventricle into the pulmonary artery is called:
    a. tricuspid.
    b. mitral.
    c. aortic semilunar.
    d. pulmonary semilunar.

61. Hemorrhoids can best be described as:
    a. varicose veins.
    b. varicose veins in the rectum.
    c. thrombophlebitis of the rectum.
    d. clot formation in the rectum.

62. A common type of vascular disease that occludes arteries by lipids and other substances is:
    a. an aneurysm.
    b. atherosclerosis.
    c. varicose veins.
    d. thrombophlebitis.

Matching—select the most appropriate answer for each item on the left (there is only one correct answer for each item).

63. _____ largest artery

64. _____ decreased blood supply

65. _____ leg vein

66. _____ fetal circulation

67. _____ arterial procedure

68. _____ vein inflammation

69. _____ lung circulation

70. _____ weakened artery

71. _____ largest vein

72. _____ myocardial infarction

a. ischemia
b. phlebitis
c. foramen ovale
d. aneurysm
e. vena cava
f. angioplasty
g. aorta
h. pulmonary
i. great saphenous vein
j. heart attack

CHAPTER 19

PHYSIOLOGY OF THE CARDIOVASCULAR SYSTEM

The beating of the heart must be coordinated in a rhythmic manner if the heart is to pump effectively. That is achieved by electrical impulses that are stimulated by specialized structures embedded in the walls of the heart. The sinoatrial node, atrioventricular node, bundle of His, and Purkinje fibers combine efforts to produce the tiny electrical currents necessary to contract the heart. A healthy heart is necessary to pump blood throughout the body to nourish and oxygenate cells continuously. Any interruption or failure of this system may result in serious pathology.

Blood pressure is the force of blood in the vessels. This force is highest in the arteries and lowest in the veins. Normal blood pressure varies among individuals and depends upon the volume of blood in the arteries. The larger the volume of blood in the arteries, the more pressure is exerted on the walls of the arteries and the higher the arterial pressure. Conversely, the less blood in the arteries, the lower the blood pressure.

A functional cardiovascular system is vital for survival because without circulation, tissues would lack a supply of oxygen and nutrients. Waste products would begin to accumulate and could become toxic. Your review of this system will provide you with an understanding of the complex transportation mechanism of the body necessary for survival.

1. Under resting conditions, the SA node fires at an intrinsic rhythmical rate of:
   a. 65 to 70 beats per minute.
   b. 70 to 75 beats per minute.
   c. 75 to 80 beats per minute.
   d. 80 to 85 beats per minute.

2. The normal pattern of impulse conduction through the heart is:
   a. AV node, SA node, AV bundle, Purkinje fibers.
   b. SA node, AV node, AV bundle, Purkinje fibers.
   c. AV bundle, AV node, SA node, Purkinje fibers.
   d. AV node, SA node, Purkinje fibers, AV bundle.

3. An ECG P wave represents:
   a. depolarization of the atria.
   b. repolarization of the atria.
   c. depolarization of the ventricles
   d. repolarization of the ventricles.

4. Repolarization of the atria is:
   a. clearly depicted by the QRS complex.
   b. masked by the massive ventricular depolarization.
   c. masked by the massive ventricular repolarization.
   d. none of the above.

5. Contraction of the ventricles produces:
   a. the first heart sound (lub).
   b. the second heart sound (dupp).
   c. both of these.
   d. none of these.

True or false

6.   _____   The contraction phase of the cardiac cycle is referred to as *systole.*

7.   _____   *Tachycardia* refers to a heartbeat under 50 beats per minute.

8.   _____   The term *dysrhythmia* refers to abnormal heart sounds.

9.   _____   PVC is an acronym for *premature ventricular contraction.*

10.   _____   Isovolumetric ventricular contraction occurs between the start of ventricular systole and the opening of the semilunar valves.

Labeling—label the following ECG deflection waves.

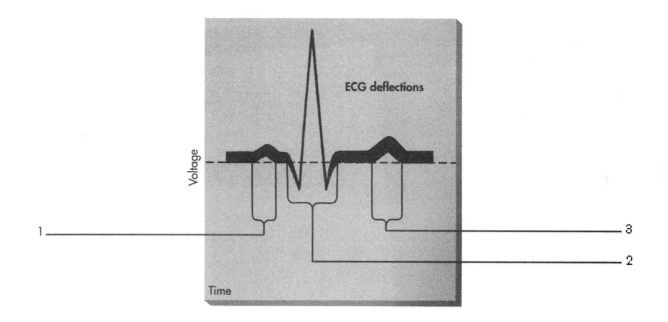

******If you had difficulty with this section, review pages **593-604**

II   CIRCULATION AND BLOOD PRESSURE

Multiple Choice—select the best answer.

11.   Blood pressure at the venae cavae and right atrium is:
a.   120 mm Hg.   c.   80 mm Hg.
b.   100 mm Hg.   d.   0 mm Hg.

12.   Starling's law of the heart states that:
a.   blood flows from areas of high pressure to areas of low pressure.
b.   the volume of blood ejected from the ventricle is constant.
c.   the more stretched the heart fibers are at the beginning of a contraction, the stronger is their contraction.
d.   average heart rate is 72 beats per minute.

Student Name_____

13. Parasympathetic control of the heart involves the:
    a. glossopharyngeal nerve (cranial nerve IX).
    b. vagus nerve (cranial nerve X).
    c. carotid sinus.
    d. aortic sinus.

14. The vagus nerve is said to act as a(n) _____ on the heart.
    a. temperature monitor
    b. positive feedback loop
    c. ejection mechanism
    d. brake

15. Under normal conditions, blood viscosity changes:
    a. frequently.
    b. during hemorrhage only.
    c. under stress.
    d. very little.

16. A dominance of sympathetic impulses increases heart rate and stroke volume and constricts reservoir vessels in response to:
    a. decreased O_2, increased CO_2 and/or decreased pH.
    b. increased O_2, increased CO_2 and/or decreased pH.
    c. decreased O_2, decreased CO_2 and/or decreased pH.
    d. decreased O_2, increased CO_2 and/or increased pH.

17. The difference between systolic and diastolic pressure is called:
    a. bruit pressure.
    b. pulse pressure.
    c. laminar pressure.
    d. none of the above.

18. The popliteal pulse point is found:
    a. at the bend of the elbow.
    b. on the dorsum of the foot.
    c. behind the knee.
    d. behind the medial malleolus.

19. Peripheral resistance is primarily affected by:
    a. the length of myocardial fibers.
    b. blood viscosity and the diameter of arterioles.
    c. the capacity of the blood reservoirs.
    d. the elasticity of the heart.

20. At rest, most of the body's blood supply resides in the:
    a. pulmonary loop.
    b. systemic arteries and arterioles.
    c. capillaries.
    d. systemic veins and venules.

True or false

21. _____ Stroke volume is determined by multiplying cardiac output and heart rate.

22. _____ A slow and weakly beating heart tends to have a decreased cardiac output.

23. _____ Starling's law operates in humans as a major regulator of stroke volume under ordinary conditions.

24. _____ Cardiac output can increase from 5 to 6 L/min during strenuous exercise.

25. _____ Skeletal muscle is of minor consequence in venous blood return to the heart.

26. _____ 100% of the fluid that leaves the capillaries at the arterial end is recovered by the venous end of the capillary.

27. _____ Systolic blood pressure is the force with which the blood is pushing against the artery wall when the ventricles are contracting.

28. _____   Velocity of blood decreases as blood flows from the aorta toward the capillaries.

29. _____   The axillary artery is one of the six arteries identified to stop arterial bleeding.

30. _____   Hypoxic conditions act as a major stimulant to chemoreceptors.

******If you had difficulty with this section, review pages **604-622**

III   MECHANISMS OF DISEASE

Fill in the blanks.

31.   Complications of septicemia may result in _____ _____.

32.   _____ _____ results from any type of heart failure.

33.   An acute type of allergic reaction called _____ results in _____ _____.

34.   _____ _____ results from widespread dilation of blood vessels caused by an imbalance in autonomic stimulation of smooth muscles in vessel walls.

35.   Hypovolemia means_____ _____ _____.

36.   A type of septic shock that results from staphylococcal infections that begin in the vagina of menstruating women and spread to the blood is _____ _____ _____.

******If you had difficulty with this section, review pages **622-624**

Student Name_____

Crossword Puzzle

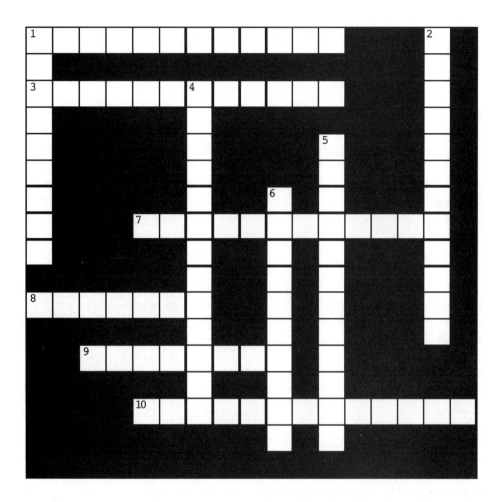

Across

1. Sensitive to pressure
3. Complete heartbeat (two words)
7. Volume pumped per heartbeat (two words)
8. Heart contracting
9. Heart at rest
10. Determined by stroke volume and heart rate (two words)

Down

1. SA node
2. Amount of blood returned to the heart by veins
4. Reflex that functions in hypoxia or hypercapnia emergencies
5. Increase in diameter of blood vessel
6. Resistance that helps determine arterial blood pressure

APPLYING WHAT YOU KNOW

37. Kim received a gunshot wound to her leg during a robbery attempt. She experienced severe hemorrhaging that significantly decreased her blood volume. Which kind of shock is she at risk for? Name the physiological mechanisms that her body has initiated to attempt to maintain circulatory homeostasis.

38. Upon examination with electrocardiogram, John was diagnosed with a cardiac dysrhythmia that displayed very slow ventricular contractions and large intervals between the P wave and the R peak of the QRS complex. What is the physiological explanation for his symptoms? What can physicians do to restore his heart's conduction system?

DID YOU KNOW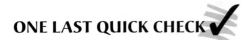

- Every pound of excess fat contains 200 miles of additional capillaries.
- If laid out in a straight line, the average adult's circulatory system would be nearly 60,000 miles long—enough to circle the Earth 2.5 times.

ONE LAST QUICK CHECK ✔

Multiple Choice—select the best answer.

39. The medical term for high blood pressure is:
    a. arteriosclerosis.
    b. cyanosis.
    c. hypertension.
    d. central venous pressure.

40. Septic shock is caused by:
    a. complications of toxins in the blood.
    b. a nerve condition.
    c. a drop in blood pressure.
    d. blood vessel dilation.

41. Hypovolemic shock is caused by:
    a. heart failure.
    b. dilated blood vessels.
    c. a drop in blood pressure.
    d. a severe allergic reaction.

42. Which vessels collect blood from the capillaries and return it to the heart?
    a. arteries   c. veins
    b. sinuses   d. arterioles

43. Which of the following events, if any, would *NOT* cause the blood pressure to increase?
    a. hemorrhaging
    b. increasing the viscosity of the blood
    c. increasing the strength of the heartbeat
    d. all of the above

Matching—identify the most appropriate answer for each item on the left.

44. _____ influences circulation of blood
45. _____ SA node
46. _____ depolarization of atria
47. _____ dysrhythmia
48. _____ bradycardia
49. _____ heart at rest
50. _____ blood remaining in ventricles
51. _____ pressoreflexes
52. _____ hypercapnia
53. _____ ischemia
54. _____ bruits
55. _____ pulse point

a. P wave
b. abnormal heart rate
c. below 50 beats per minute
d. baroreflexes
e. hemodynamics
f. inadequate blood supply
g. diastole
h. excess carbon dioxide
i. residual volume
j. occur in carotid arteries
k. pacemaker
l. dorsalis pedis

CHAPTER 20

LYMPHATIC SYSTEM

The lymphatic system is a system similar to the circulatory system. Lymph, like blood, flows through an elaborate route of vessels. In addition to lymphatic vessels, the lymphatic system consists of lymph nodes, lymph, and the spleen. Unlike the circulatory system, the lymphatic vessels do not form a closed circuit. Lymph flows only once through the vessels before draining into the general blood circulation. This system is a filtering mechanism for microorganisms and serves as a protective device against foreign invaders, such as cancer.

As your text suggests, this system can also be likened to the wastewater system of our communities. Lymph circulates to bring contaminants to the system that are harmful to the bodies. Toxins are filtered and the fluid returned cleansed, just as our wastewater systems remove harmful substances and return it cleansed for our eventual use. Your knowledge of this system is necessary to understand the function of the lymphatic system in maintaining fluid balance in the tissues and the role that plays in the body's immune system.

I   LYMPHATIC VESSELS, LYMPH, AND CIRCULATION OF LYMPH

Multiple Choice—select the best answer.

1. The most important function(s) of the lymphatic system is/are:
   a. fluid balance of the internal environment.
   b. immunity.
   c. both a and b.
   d. none of the above.

2. Lymphatic capillaries that operate in the villi of the small intestine are called:
   a. lymphatics.   c. Peyer's patches.
   b. lacteals.   d. lymph nodes.

3. Lymph from the entire body drains into the thoracic duct, *EXCEPT* lymph from the:
   a. upper right quadrant.
   b. upper left quadrant.
   c. lower limbs.
   d. entire head and neck.

4. Which of the following is *NOT* a difference between lymphatics and veins?
   a. Lymphatics have thinner walls.
   b. Lymphatics contain more valves.
   c. Lymphatics contain lymph nodes.
   d. Lymphatics endure greater pressure.

5. If lymphatic return is blocked, which of the following will *NOT* occur?
   a. Blood protein concentration will fall.
   b. Blood osmotic pressure will fall.
   c. CO_2 levels in the blood will rise.
   d. Tissue edema will occur.

6. Lymphatic circulation is maintained by all of the following *EXCEPT*:
   a. breathing movements.
   b. heart.
   c. skeletal muscle contractions.
   d. valves.

7. Lymphatic circulation begins with:
   a. lymphatic capillaries.
   b. lymphatic veins.
   c. lymphatic venules.
   d. lymphatic arterioles.

True or false

8. _____ The lymphatic system could be referred to as a specialized component of the circulatory system.

9. _____ Lymphatic vessels, like vessels in the blood vascular system, form a closed loop of circulation.

10. _____ Both lymph and interstitial fluid closely resemble blood plasma in composition.

11. _____ Lymph has a clotting ability similar to that of blood.

12. _____ The milky lymph found in lacteals after digestion is called *chyle.*

13. _____ Breathing movements and skeletal muscle actions establish the lymph pressure gradient necessary for the circulation of lymph.

14. _____ Activities that result in central movement, or flow, of lymph are called *lymphokinetic actions.*

******If you had difficulty with this section, review pages **629-632**

II   LYMPH NODES

Multiple Choice—select the best answer.

15. The small depression of a lymph node from which the efferent lymph vessel arises is termed the:
    a.   sinus.
    b.   hilus.
    c.   capsule.
    d.   nodule

16. The lymph nodes located in front of the ear are called the:
    a.   submaxillary groups.
    b.   inguinal lymph nodes.
    c.   cervical lymph nodes.
    d.   none of the above.

17. An infection of a lymph node is called:
    a.   adenitis.
    b.   noditis.
    c.   lymphitis.
    d.   lysis.

18. The lymphatic tissue of lymph nodes serves as the final maturation site for:
    a.   monocytes.
    b.   lymphocytes.
    c.   both a and b.
    d.   none of the above.

True or false

19. _____ Even though some lymph nodes occur in clusters, most occur as single nodes.

20. _____ Cortical nodules are composed of packed lymphocytes that surround an area called the *germinal center.*

Student Name_____

Labeling—label the principal organs of the lymphatic system on the following illustration.

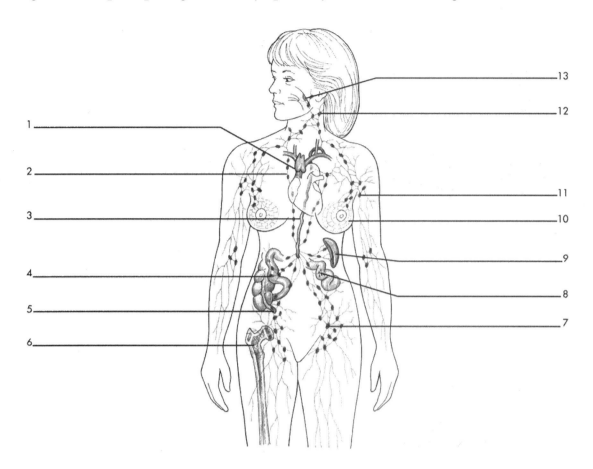

Labeling—label the structure of a lymph node on the following diagram.

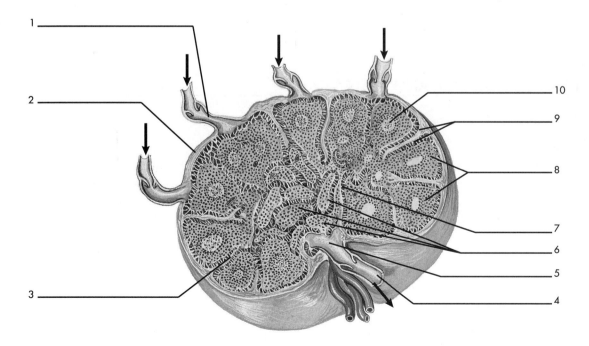

******If you had difficulty with this section, review pages **632-634**

III   LYMPHATIC DRAINAGE OF THE BREAST

Multiple Choice—select the best answer.

21.   Over 85% of the lymph from the breast enters
       lymph nodes of the:
       a.   axillary region.
       b.   supraclavicular region.
       c.   brachial region.
       d.   subscapular region.

22.   The breast—mammary gland and surround-
       ing tissue—is drained by:
       a.   lymphatics that originate in and drain
             the skin over the breast, with exception
             of the areola and nipple.
       b.   lymphatics that originate in and drain
             the substance of the breast itself, includ-
             ing the skin of the areola and nipple.
       c.   both a and b.
       d.   none of the above.

Labeling—label the lymphatic drainage of the breast on the following illustration.

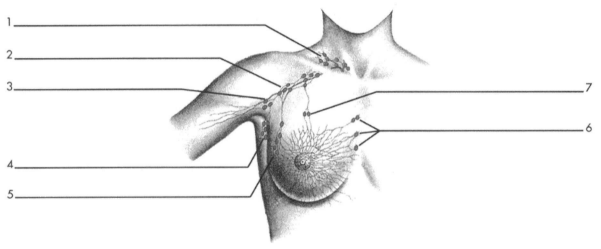

******If you had difficulty with this section, review pages **634-636**

IV   TONSILS, THYMUS, AND SPLEEN

Multiple Choice—select the best answer.

23.   Adenoids are swollen:
       a.   pharyngeal tonsils.
       c.   lingual tonsils.
       b.   palatine tonsils.
       d.   none of the above.

24.   The thymus secretes:
       a.   T$_3$.   c.   thymosin.
       b.   T$_4$.   d.   both a and c

25.   The thymus is located:
       a.   deep to the thyroid.
       b.   in the axillary region.
       c.   in the mediastinum.
       d.   none of the above.

Student Name _____

True or false

26. _____ As a person ages, the thymus increases in size; this process is called *involution*.

27. _____ The spleen functions solely in the defense from foreign microorganisms.

28. _____ The spleen removes imperfect platelets from the blood.

******If you had difficulty with this section, review pages **636-639**

V   MECHANISMS OF DISEASE

Fill in the blanks.

29. _____ is a term that refers to a tumor of the cells of lymphoid tissue.

30. A middle ear infection is known as_____ _____ _____.

31. Septicemia is also known as _____ _____.

32. Adenoids cause _____ obstruction.

33. Two principal categories of lymphomas are _____ and _____ lymphoma.

******If you had difficulty with this section, review pages **639-640**

Crossword Puzzle

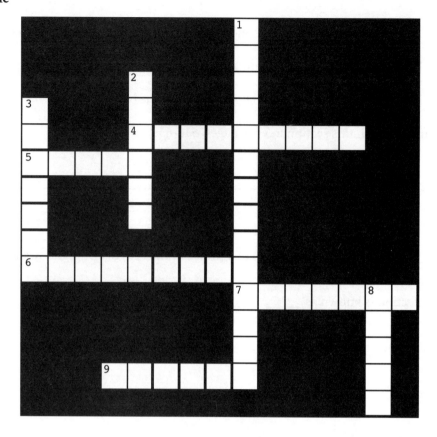

Across

4. Vessels that originate as lacteals in villi
5. Found in lacteals after digestion
6. Functions in defense and hematopoiesis (two words)
7. Palatine are an example
9. Active in production of T cells

Down

1. Activities that result in lymph flow
2. Destroys red blood cells
3. Located in villi
8. Fluid found in lymphatic vessels

APPLYING WHAT YOU KNOW

34. Nancy was diagnosed with hemolytic anemia. Is a splenectomy a viable option? Can she live without her spleen? Why is removal of the spleen considered a treatment of choice?

35. Baby Wilson was born without a thymus gland. Immediate plans were made for a transplant to be performed. In the meantime, baby Wilson was placed in strict isolation. For what reason was he placed in isolation?

DID YOU KNOW?

- According to the Centers for Disease Control and Prevention (CDC), 18 million courses of antibiotics are prescribed for the common cold in the United States per year. Research shows that colds are caused by viruses. Fifty million unnecessary antibiotics are prescribed for viral respiratory infections.

Student Name_____

ONE LAST QUICK CHECK ✔

Matching—select the best response

36. _____ palatine, pharyngeal, and lingual are examples

37. _____ hematopoiesis

38. _____ destroys worn-out red blood cells

39. _____ located in mediastinum

40. _____ serves as a reservoir for blood

41. _____ T-lymphocytes

42. _____ largest at puberty

a. thymus
b. tonsils
c. spleen

True or false

43. _____ The cisterna chyli is a dilated structure on the thoracic duct that serves as a storage area for lymph moving into the venous system.

44. _____ Healthy capillaries "leak" proteins.

45. _____ Thoracic duct lymph is "pumped" into the venous system during inspiration.

46. _____ Lymph nodes have several afferent and efferent vessels.

47. _____ Lymphedema is swelling due to an accumulation of lymph.

48. _____ An anastomosis is the removal of a part.

49. _____ The spleen is located below the diaphragm, above the right kidney and descending colon.

50. _____ Splenomegaly is removal of the spleen.

CHAPTER 21

IMMUNE SYSTEM

The immune system is the armed forces division of the body. Ready to attack at a moment's notice, the immune system defends us against the major enemies of the body: microorganisms, foreign transplanted tissue cells, and our own cells that have turned malignant.

The most numerous cells of the immune system are the lymphocytes. These cells circulate in the body's fluids seeking invading organisms and destroying them with powerful lymphotoxins, lymphokines, or antibodies.

Phagocytes, another large group of immune system cells, assist with the destruction of foreign invaders by a process known as *phagocytosis.* Neutrophils and macrophages ingest and digest the invaders, rendering them harmless to the body.

Another weapon that the immune system possesses is complement. Normally a group of inactive enzymes present in the blood, complement can be activated to kill invading cells by drilling holes in their cytoplasmic membranes, which allows fluid to enter the cell until it bursts. Your review of this chapter will give you an understanding of how the body defends itself from the daily invasion of destructive substances.

I   NONSPECIFIC IMMUNITY

Multiple Choice—select the best answer.

1. Which of the following cells is *NOT* involved with nonspecific immunity?
    a. natural killer cells
    b. neutrophils
    c. monocytes
    d. lymphocytes

2. The "first line of defense" in nonspecific immunity is:
    a. inflammation.
    b. phagocytosis.
    c. mechanical and chemical barriers.
    d. complement.

3. About 15% of the total number of lymphocyte cells are:
    a. natural killer (NK) cells.
    b. macrophages.
    c. neutrophils.
    d. interferon.

4. The most numerous type of phagocyte is the:
    a. neutrophil.   c. histocyte.
    b. macrophage.   d. Kupffer cell.

5. Which of the following is a phagocytic monocyte that migrates out of the bloodstream?
    a. neutrophil
    b. macrophage
    c. phagosome
    d. none of the above

True or false

6. _____ The immune mechanism that provides a general defense by acting against anything recognized as nonself is termed *specific immunity.*

7. _____ Species resistance is the genetic characteristics of the human species that protect the body from certain pathogens.

8. _____ Interferon has been proven effective as a treatment against cancer.

9. _____ The complement cascade causes phagocytosis of the foreign cell that triggered it.

10. _____ Natural killer cells are a group of lymphocytes that kill many types of tumor cells and cells infected by different kinds of viruses.

******If you had difficulty with this section, review pages **644-649**

II SPECIFIC IMMUNITY

Multiple Choice—select the best answer.

11. B cells and T cells are examples of:
    a. monocytes.
    b. lymphocytes.
    c. neutrophils.
    d. macrophages.

12. Cell-mediated immunity involves:
    a. B cells.
    b. T cells.
    c. both a and b.
    d. neither a nor b.

13. The T cell subsets that are clinically important in diagnosing AIDS are:
    a. CD4.
    b. CD8.
    c. neither a nor b.
    d. both a and b.

14. An antibody consists of:
    a. two heavy and two light polypeptide chains.
    b. two heavy and one light polypeptide chains.
    c. one heavy and two light polypeptide chains.
    d. one heavy and one light polypeptide chains.

15. The amount of antibodies in a person's blood in response to exposure to a pathogen is called:
    a. toxoid.
    b. titer.
    c. both a and b.
    d. none of the above.

16. The most abundant circulating antibody is:
    a. IgM.
    b. IgG.
    c. IgA.
    d. IgE.

17. The specific cells that secrete antibodies are:
    a. B cells.
    b. T cells.
    c. plasma cells.
    d. none of the above.

18. T cells are sensitized by:
    a. direct exposure to an antigen.
    b. presentation of an antigen by a macrophage.
    c. antibodies produced by B cells.
    d. lymphokines.

19. *Complement* can best be described as:
    a. an antibody.
    b. an enzyme in the blood plasma.
    c. a hormone.
    d. a lymphokine.

20. The chemical messengers that T cells release into inflamed tissues are called:
    a. pathogens.
    b. lymphokines.
    c. lymphotoxins.
    d. suppressor cells.

Student Name_____

True or false

21. _____ Antibodies are proteins of the family called immunoglobulins.

22. _____ IgD is the most understood antibody.

23. _____ The first vaccination was against the cowpox virus.

24. _____ Toxoids and vaccines function similarly.

25. _____ Active immunity generally lasts longer than passive immunity.

26. _____ Abnormal antigens or "tumor markers" are present in the plasma membranes of some cancer cells in addition to self-antigens.

27. _____ PSA is elevated in both benign and malignant prostate disease.

28. _____ Sensitized T cells that release lymphotoxin are called "killer T cells."

29. _____ A fetus receives protection from the mother through active artificial immunity.

30. _____ A vaccination provides natural passive immunity.

******If you had difficulty with this section, review pages **649-661**

III   MECHANISMS OF DISEASE

True or false

31. _____ The human immunodeficiency virus has a profound impact on a person's number of CD12 subset of T cells.

32. _____ Once inside a cell, HIV uses its viral RNA to produce DNA; this process is called reverse transcription.

33. _____ A common autoimmune disease is SLE or "lupus."

34. _____ SCID is an immunosuppressive drug.

35. _____ Glomerulonephritis is an autoimmune disease of the neuromuscular junction.

******If you had difficulty with this section, review pages **661-664**

Crossword Puzzle

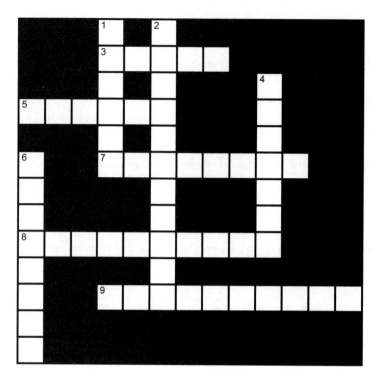

Across

3. Family of cells descended from one cell
5. Cell-mediated immunity (two words)
7. Immunity that recognizes specific threatening agents and responds to these only
8. Inhibits spread of a viral infection
9. Enlarged monocytes that are giant phagocytic cells

Down

1. Produce antibodies (two words)
2. Immunity that resists various threatening agents (general defense)
4. Foreign protein
6. Plasma protein (immunoglobulin)

APPLYING WHAT YOU KNOW

36. Trent, a newborn, received immune protection from his mother through the placenta and breast milk. Which specific type of immunity is this? His older sister, Carrie, also recently received immune protection from a host of illnesses; however, hers was achieved deliberately via immunization by her pediatrician. What specific types of immunity is she experiencing? How do her types of immunity differ from her brother's?

37. Marcia is a bisexual and an intravenous drug user. She has developed a type of skin cancer known as Kaposi's sarcoma. What, most likely, is Marcia's primary diagnosis? What are some of the medications that might be used to inhibit symptoms for a while?

DID YOU KNOW?

- The swine flu vaccine in 1976 caused more deaths and illness than the disease that it was intended to prevent.
- In the United States, the HIV infection rate is increasing four times faster in women than in men. Women tend to underestimate their risk.

Student Name _____

ONE LAST QUICK CHECK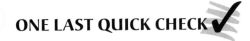

Multiple Choice—select the best answer.

38. T cells do which of the following?
    a. develop in the thymus
    b. form memory cells
    c. form plasma cells
    d. all of the above

39. Acquired immune deficiency syndrome is characterized by which of the following?
    a. caused by a retrovirus
    b. causes inadequate T cell formation
    c. can result in death from cancer
    d. all of the above

40. Interferon is:
    a. produced by B cells.
    b. a protein compound that protects other cells by interfering with the ability of a virus to reproduce.
    c. a group of inactive enzyme proteins normally present in blood.
    d. all of the above.

41. B cells do which of the following?
    a. develop into plasma cells and memory cells
    b. secrete antibodies
    c. develop from primitive cells in bone marrow called *stem cells*
    d. all of the above

42. Which of the following functions to kill invading cells by drilling a hole in their plasma membrane?
    a. interferon
    c. antibody
    b. complement
    d. memory cell

43. What is a rapidly growing population of identical cells that produce large quantities of specific antibodies called?
    a. complementary
    c. chemotactic
    b. lymphotoxic
    d. monoclonal

44. Which of the following is a form of passive natural immunity?
    a. A child develops measles and acquires immunity to subsequent exposure.
    b. Antibodies are injected into an infected individual.
    c. An infant receives protection through its mother's milk.
    d. Vaccinations are given against smallpox.

Matching—identify the term on the left with the proper selection on the right.

45. _____ nonspecific immunity

46. _____ inherited immunity

47. _____ acquired immunity

48. _____ immunization

a. inborn immunity
b. natural immunity
c. general protection
d. artificial exposure

CHAPTER 22

STRESS

Life without any stress would be very dull and boring. Often it is stress that stimulates us to achieve our dreams and experience success and happiness. Too much stress becomes unpleasant and tiring and can seriously interfere with our ability to function effectively. The challenge is to keep stress at a level that is healthy and enjoyable.

Although we react differently and in various degrees to stressors, we must acknowledge that in most individuals, stress leads to a physiological stress response. These responses may be as simple as an increase in heart rate or perspiration or as complex as a disease syndrome. And although we may not be aware of it on a day-to-day basis, stress can be cumulative and manifest itself long after apparent stressors have been resolved. Your study of this unit will alert you to the impact of stress on your body and the significant role it plays in homeostasis.

I SELYE'S CONCEPT OF STRESS

Multiple Choice—select the best answer.

1. The stages of general adaptation syndrome in the correct order are:
   a. alarm reaction, stage of exhaustion, stage of resistance.
   b. alarm reaction, stage of resistance, stage of exhaustion.
   c. stage of exhaustion, alarm reaction, stage of resistance.
   d. stage of exhaustion, stage of resistance, stage of alarm.

2. The "stress triad" refers to:
   a. alarm, exhaustion, resistance.
   b. hypertrophied adrenals, atrophied thymus and lymph nodes, and bleeding ulcers.
   c. stressor, stress, and response.
   d. health, stress, and disease.

3. Which of the following is *NOT* an alarm reaction response resulting from hypertrophy of the adrenal cortex?
   a. hyperglycemia
   b. decreased digestion
   c. decreased immunity
   d. decreased allergic responses

4. All of the following are true statements *EXCEPT*:
   a. stressors are extreme stimuli.
   b. stressors are always unpleasant, injurious, or painful.
   c. the emotions of fear, anxiety, and grief can act as stressors.
   d. stressors differ in individuals.

5. What determines which stimuli are stressors for each individual?
   a. past experience   c. heredity
   b. diet   d. all of the above

True or false

6. _____   Selye's stage of exhaustion is reached in each exposure to stressors.

7. _____   High-stress, hard-driving, competitive individuals who may be at greater risk of coronary heart disease are classified as "Type B."

8. _____   The state of resistance can be described as *adaptation*.

9. _____   Stressors are "bad" stimuli that should always be avoided.

10. _____   The stress response commonly referred to as "fight or flight" is evoked by increased sympathetic activity.

******If you had difficulty with this section, review pages **669-674**

II   SOME CURRENT CONCEPTS ABOUT STRESS

Multiple Choice—select the best answer.

11. CRH stimulates the anterior pituitary gland to secrete increased amounts of:
    a. glucocorticoids. c. ACTH.
    b. aldosterone.   d. ADH.

12. All of the following are effects of cortisol *EXCEPT*:
    a. increased protein catabolism.
    b. decreased immune responses.
    c. decreased allergic responses.
    d. fight or flight responses.

13. The dominant subjective reaction that occurs with psychological stress is:
    a. guilt.   c. depression.
    b. anxiety.   d. fear.

True or false

14. _____   The current definition of *stress* is "any stimulus that directly or indirectly stimulates neurons of the hypothalamus to release corticotropin-releasing hormone (CRH)."

15. _____   It is accepted among physiologists that a higher-than-normal blood level of corticoids results in a greater ability to resist stress.

16. _____   Physiological stress and psychological stress are clearly different phenomena.

17. _____   Hypervolemia and antidiuresis are common responses to stress.

18. _____   Stress is an issue only among adolescents and adults.

******If you had difficulty with this section, review pages **674-678**

Student Name _____

Crossword Puzzle

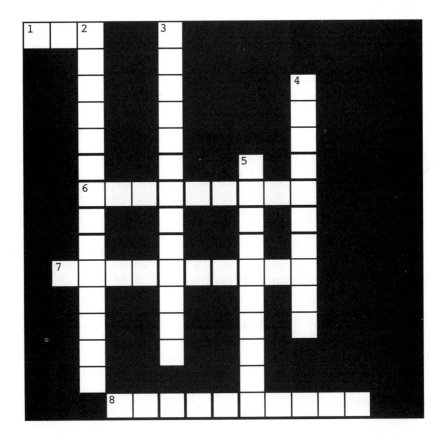

Across

1. General adaptation syndrome (abbrev.)
6. Agents that produce stress
7. Coping successfully with stress
8. GAS stage that develops only when stress is severe

Down

2. Also known as the stress response (two words)
3. Stage of GAS (two words)
4. GAS stage where sympathetic activity returns to normal
5. Hormones that increase during stress

APPLYING WHAT YOU KNOW

19. Merrilee has an adolescent crush on John. Whenever she is near him, she feels anxious, her pupils dilate, heart rate elevates, systolic blood pressure rises, blood glucose levels are above normal, and blood and urine levels of epinephrine and norepinephrine are elevated. What is the physiological term used to describe this syndrome? Beginning in the hypothalamus, trace the mechanisms that are causing this response. If this physiological scenario were extended and intense, what illnesses might Merrilee be at risk for?

20. Bill is going to his boss for his annual evaluation. He is planning to ask for a raise and hopes the evaluation will be good. Which subdivision of the autonomic nervous system will be active during this stressful conference? Should he have a large meal before his appointment? Support your answer with facts.

DID YOU KNOW?

- Laughing lowers levels of stress hormones and strengthens the immune system. Six-year-olds laugh an average of 300 times a day. Adults only laugh 15–100 times a day.
- A survey conducted at Iowa State College in 1969 suggests that a parent's stress at the time of conception plays a major role in determining a baby's sex. The child tends to be of the same sex as the parent who is under less stress.

ONE LAST QUICK CHECK ✔

Fill in the blanks.

21. _____ _____ _____ is the term for the group of changes that make the the presence of stress in the body known.

22. The stage of _____ develops only when stress is extremely severe or continues over a long period.

23. The hypothalamus releases _____ _____ _____ which acts as a trigger that initiates many diverse changes in the body.

24. The term that describes the stress responses that occur as a result of stimulation of the sympathetic centers is known as the _____ _____ _____

   _____.

25. _____ investigates physiological responses made by individuals to psychological stressors.

True or False

26. _____   Type B personalities are at greater risk of coronary disease than Type A personalities.

27. _____   Stress causes disruption in homeostasis.

28. _____   Smoking increases plasma adrenocorticoids by as much as 77%.

29. _____   Identical psychological stressors induce identical physiological responses in different individuals.

30. _____   Hans Selye identified a group of changes classic to stress and called them the *stress triad*.

CHAPTER 23

ANATOMY OF THE RESPIRATORY SYSTEM

As you sit reviewing this system your body needs 16 quarts of air per minute. Walking requires 24 quarts of air and running requires 50 quarts per minute. The respiratory system provides the air necessary for you to perform your daily activities and eliminates the waste gases from the air that you breathe. Take a deep breath and think of the air as entering some 250 million tiny air sacs similar in appearance to clusters of grapes. These microscopic air sacs expand to let air in and contract to force it out. These tiny sacs, or *alveoli*, are the functioning units of the respiratory system. They provide the necessary volume of oxygen and eliminate carbon dioxide 24 hours a day.

Air enters either through the mouth or the nasal cavity. Next it passes through the pharynx and past the epiglottis, through the glottis and the rest of the larynx. It then continues down the trachea, into the bronchi to the bronchioles, and finally through the alveoli. The reverse occurs for expelled air. Your review of this system is necessary to provide you with an understanding of this essential homeostatic mechanism—the breath of life.

I   UPPER RESPIRATORY TRACT

Multiple Choice—select the best answer.

1. Which of the following structures is *NOT* part of the upper respiratory tract?
    a.   trachea   c.   oropharynx
    b.   larynx   d.   nose

2. Which part of the respiratory system does *NOT* function as an air distributor?
    a.   trachea   c.   alveoli
    b.   bronchioles   d.   bronchi

3. Which sequence is the correct pathway for air movement through the nose and into the pharynx?
    a.   anterior nares, posterior nares, vestibule, nasal cavity meati
    b.   anterior nares, vestibule, posterior nares, nasal cavity meati
    c.   nasal cavity meati, anterior nares, vestibule, posterior nares
    d.   anterior nares, vestibule, nasal cavity meati, posterior nares

4. Which of the following is *NOT* a paranasal sinus?
    a.   frontal   c.   mandibular
    b.   maxillary   d.   sphenoid

5. The true vocal cords and the rima glottis are called the:
    a.   glottis.   c.   vestibular fold.
    b.   epiglottis.   d.   both a and b.

True or false

6. _____ Failure of the palatine bones to unite is called *cribriform palate*.

7. _____ The pharynx is a tubelike structure that opens only into the mouth and larynx.

8. _____ Enlarged pharyngeal tonsils are called *adenoids*.

9. _____ The more common name for the thyroid cartilage is *voice box*.

10. _____ The epiglottis moves up and down during swallowing to prevent food or liquids from entering the trachea.

Labeling—using the terms provided, label the following illustration of the respiratory system.

bronchioles	larynx	laryngopharynx
upper respiratory tract	primary bronchi	lower respiratory tract
nasopharynx	oropharynx	alveolar sac
nasal cavity	trachea	alveolar duct

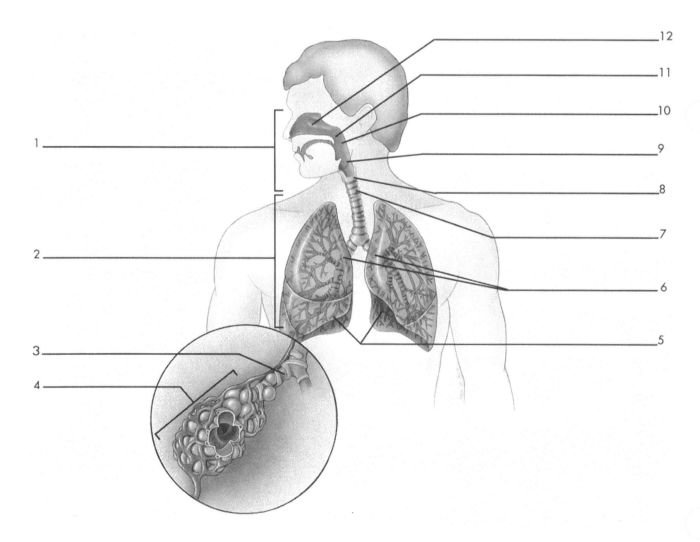

Student Name

Labeling—label the structures of the nasal cavity on the following illustration.

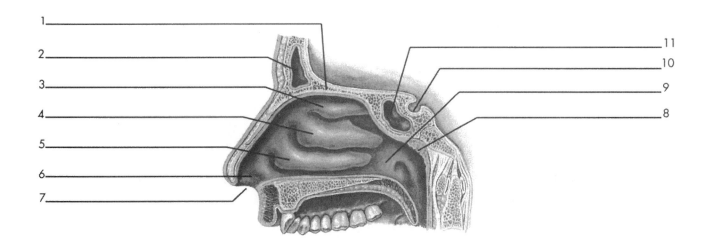

1. _____
2. _____
3. _____
4. _____
5. _____
6. _____
7. _____

11 _____
10 _____
9 _____
8 _____

Labeling—using the terms provided, label the three divisions of the pharynx and nearby structures on the following illustration.

opening of the eustachian tube
laryngopharynx
esophagus
oropharynx
vocal cords

pharyngeal tonsil
epiglottis
uvula
lingual tonsil
hyoid bone

trachea
nasopharynx
soft palate
palatine tonsil

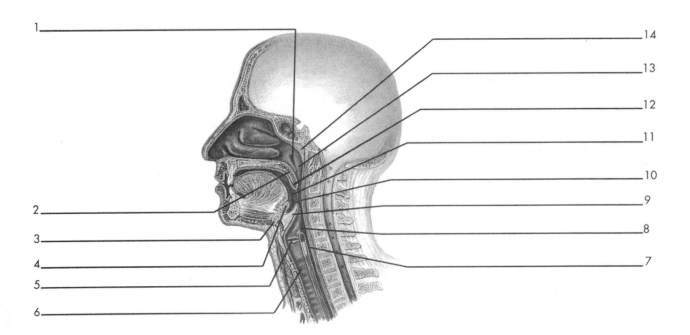

1. _____
2. _____
3. _____
4. _____
5. _____
6. _____

14 _____
13 _____
12 _____
11 _____
10 _____
9 _____
8 _____
7 _____

Labeling—label the structures related to the paranasal sinuses on the following illustration.

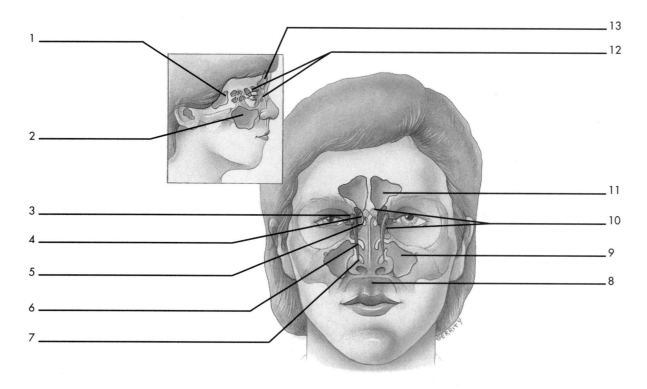

******If you had difficulty with this section, review pages **684-692**

II LOWER RESPIRATORY TRACT

Multiple Choice—select the best answer.

11. Aspirated objects tend to lodge in the:
    a. right bronchus.
    b. left bronchus.
    c. either right or left bronchus.
    d. none of the above.

12. The fluid coating the alveoli that reduces surface tension is called:
    a. bronchus.
    b. surfactant.
    c. alveolus.
    d. none of the above.

13. Which of the following is *NOT* a subdivision of the thoracic cavity?
    a. left pleural division
    b. right pleural division
    c. medial pleural division
    d. mediastinum

14. Which of the following is *NOT* a true statement?
    a. When the diaphragm relaxes, it returns to a domelike shape.
    b. When the diaphragm contracts, it pulls the floor of the thoracic cavity downward.
    c. Changes in thorax size bring about inspiration and expiration.
    d. Raising the ribs decreases the depth and width of the thorax.

Student Name_____

True or false

15. _____ The rings of cartilage that form the trachea are complete rings that prevent it from collapsing and shutting off the vital airway.

16. _____ The trachea divides into symmetrical primary bronchi.

17. _____ A tube is often placed in the trachea before a patient leaves the operating room, especially if he or she has had a muscle relaxant.

18. _____ The left lung is divided into three lobes by horizontal and oblique fissures.

19. _____ The apex of each lung is lateral and inferior.

20. _____ The exchange of gases between air and blood occurs in the alveoli.

Labeling—label the lobes and fissures of the lungs on the following illustration (anterior view).

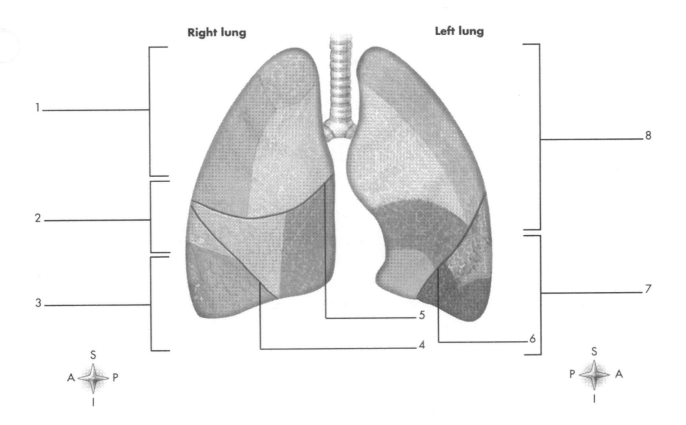

******If you had difficulty with this section, review pages **692-701**

III MECHANISMS OF DISEASE

Matching—identify each disorder with its corresponding description.

21. _____ malignancy of pulmonary tissue

22. _____ very serious, chronic, and highly infectious infection

23. _____ displacement of the nasal septum

24. _____ a common infection of the lower respiratory tract characterized by acute inflammation of the bronchial tree

25. _____ nosebleed

26. _____ an inflammation of the mucosa of the nasal cavity

27. _____ sore throat

28. _____ harsh, vibrating cough

a. acute bronchitis
b. deviated septum
c. epistaxis
d. lung cancer
e. pharyngitis
f. rhinitis
g. tuberculosis
h. croup

******If you had difficulty with this section, review pages **701-705**

Student Name _____

Crossword Puzzle

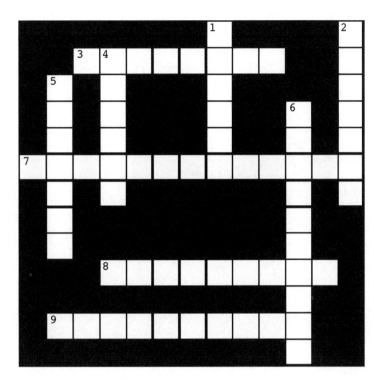

Across

3. "Gas exchanger"
7. Trachea, two primary bronchi, and their branches (two words)
8. There are four pairs of these sinuses
9. Small branch of bronchus

Down

1. Serous membrane in the thoracic cavity
2. "Windpipe"
4. "Voice box"
5. "Throat"
6. Conchae

APPLYING WHAT YOU KNOW

29. Mrs. Metheny's 6-year-old child had trouble swallowing. She had a high fever, appeared very anxious, and was drooling from her mouth. Mrs. Metheny called the EMS personnel who assessed the child, inserted an airway, and transported her immediately to the emergency room. What is a possible explanation for why her child is experiencing these symptoms? What is the causative agent for these symptoms? Is this a serious threat to her child?

30. Dr. Harry is a pediatrician who recently examined a 2-year-old boy who awakened in the middle of the night frightened and with the following symptoms: labored inspiration, harsh and vibrating cough, and a normal body temperature. What diagnosis might Dr. Harry give his patient? Is this life-threatening?

31. Mr. Gorski is a heavy smoker. Recently, he has noticed that when he gets up in the morning, he has a bothersome cough that brings up a large accumulation of mucus. This cough persists for several minutes and then leaves until the next morning. What is a possible explanation for this problem?

DID YOU KNOW?

- If the roof of your mouth is narrow, you are more likely to snore since you are not getting enough oxygen through your nose.
- Only about 10% of the air in the lungs is actually changed with each cycle of inhaling and exhaling when an at-rest person is breathing, but up to 80% can be exchanged during deep breathing or strenuous exercise.

ONE LAST QUICK CHECK ✔

Matching—choose the correct response.

32. _____	warms and humidifies air	a. nose
33. _____	air and food pass through here	b. pharynx
34. _____	sinuses	c. larynx
35. _____	conchae	
36. _____	septum	
37. _____	tonsils	
38. _____	middle ear infections	
39. _____	epiglottis	
40. _____	rhinitis	
41. _____	sore throat	
42. _____	epistaxis	

Fill in the blanks.

The organs of the respiratory system are designed to perform two basic functions. They serve as an (43)

_____ _____ and as a (44) _____ _____. In

addition to the above, the respiratory system (45) _____, (46) _____, and

(47) _____ the air we breathe. Respiratory organs include the (48) _____,

(49) _____, (50) _____, (51) _____, (52)

_____, and the (53) _____. The respiratory system ends in

millions of tiny, thin-walled sacs called (54) _____. (55) _____ of

gases takes place in these sacs. Two aspects of the structure of these sacs assist them in the exchange of gases.

First, an extremely thin membrane, the (56) _____ _____, allows for easy

exchange and second, the large number of air sacs makes an enormous (57) _____ area.

CHAPTER 24

PHYSIOLOGY OF THE RESPIRATORY SYSTEM

The respiratory system functions to diffuse gases into and out of the blood so that the organs of our body receive blood that is rich in oxygen and low in carbon dioxide. The exchange of gases that occurs within the body is a complex operation and each component of the pulmonary system contributes to successful ventilation. Air must enter the lungs (inspiration) from the external environment, an exchange must occur between the blood and the cells, and then air high in CO_2 is returned to the environment (expiration.)

Numerous anatomical and physiological mechanisms influence the successful exchange of gases throughout the process. The rate, depth, and pressure of pulmonary ventilation are dependent upon these structures to successfully perform their respiratory function. Your review of this system is necessary to provide you with an understanding of this essential homeostatic mechanism necessary for survival.

I PULMONARY VENTILATION

Multiple Choice—select the best answer.

1. Boyle's law states that:
   a. fluids move from areas of high pressure to low.
   b. the volume of a gas is inversely proportional to its pressure.
   c. the atmosphere exerts a pressure of 760 mm Hg.
   d. volume is directly proportional to temperature.

2. When the diaphragm contracts, the volume of the thorax increases, thoracic pressure:
   a. increases, and air is forced from the lungs.
   b. decreases, and air is forced from the lungs.
   c. decreases, and air rushes into the lungs.
   d. increases, and air rushes into the lungs.

3. Quiet inspiration is the function of:
   a. the diaphragm and internal intercostal.
   b. the diaphragm and external intercostal.
   c. the internal intercostal and external intercostal.
   d. none of the above.

4. During normal, quiet respiration, the amount of air exchanged between the lungs and atmosphere is called _____ and has a volume of _____ ml.
   a. tidal volume; 1200 ml
   b. vital capacity; 4500 ml
   c. tidal volume; 500 ml
   d. residual volume; 1200 ml

5. Functional residual capacity (FRC) equals:
   a. TV + IRV.
   b. TV + IRV + ERV + RV.
   c. TV + IRV + ERV.
   d. ERV + RV.

6. *Eupnea* is a term used to describe:
   a. rapid, deep respiration.
   b. cessation of respiration.
   c. slow, shallow respiration.
   d. normal breathing.

7. Under normal conditions, air in the atmosphere exerts a pressure of:
   a. 500 mm Hg.   c. 660 mm Hg.
   b. 560 mm Hg.   d. 760 mm Hg.

8.   Areas where gas exchange cannot take place are:
     a.   anatomical dead spaces.
     b.   nose, pharynx, larynx.
     c.   trachea and bronchi.
     d.   all of the above.

9.   All of the following are regulated processes associated with the functioning of the respiratory system *EXCEPT*:
     a.   control of cell metabolism rate.
     b.   gas exchange in lungs and tissue.
     c.   pulmonary ventilation.
     d.   transport of gases.

10. Dalton's law is also known as:
     a.   Henry's law.
     b.   Boyle's law.
     c.   Charles law.
     d.   the law of partial pressures.

True or false

11. _____   Temperature is the measurement of the motion of molecules.

12. _____   The largest amount of air that can enter and leave the lungs during respiration is termed *total lung capacity (TLC)*.

13. _____   Residual volume (RV) is the volume remaining in the respiratory tract after maximum expiration.

14. _____   The temporary cessation of breathing is termed *apnea*.

15. _____   It is not possible to exhale all of the air from your lungs.

Labeling—label the following diagram with the correct terminology for the lung volumes displayed.

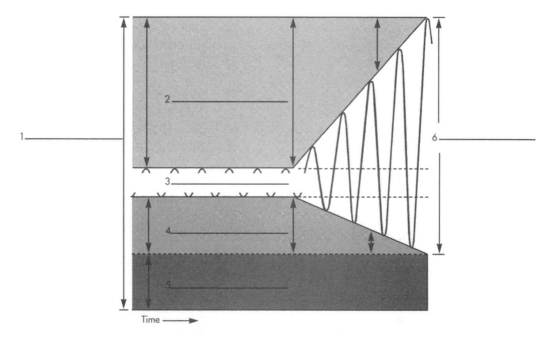

Time ⟶

******If you had difficulty with this section, review pages **708-717**

II PULMONARY GAS EXCHANGE

Multiple Choice—select the best answer.

16. If oxygen is 21% of the atmosphere, it will contribute _____ of the total atmospheric pressure.
    a. 21%
    c. 0.21%
    b. 79%
    d. .79%

17. If alveolar PO_2 equals 100 mm Hg and pulmonary capillary PO_2 equals 40 mm Hg, which of following will occur?
    a. O_2 will exit the alveoli and enter the capillary blood.
    b. Capillary O_2 will exit the alveoli at 100 mm Hg.
    c. PO_2 will equalize between the pulmonary capillary and alveoli.
    d. All of the above.

18. PO_2 at standard atmospheric pressure is approximately:
    a. 21 mm Hg.
    c. 160 mm Hg.
    b. 0.2 mm Hg.
    d. 760 mm Hg.

19. PCO_2 of systemic arterial blood is approximately:
    a. 40 mm Hg.
    c. 0.02 mm Hg.
    b. 46 mm Hg.
    d. 100 mm Hg.

True or false

20. _____ Air in the pleural space of the thoracic cavity is called a *pneumothorax*.

21. _____ *Partial pressure* and *tension* can be used interchangeably.

22. _____ The diameter of the pulmonary capillaries allows red blood cells to travel through at 10 abreast.

23. _____ Nitrogen is the gas of greatest concentration in atmospheric air.

******If you had difficulty with this section, review pages **716-720**

III BLOOD TRANSPORTATION OF GASES AND SYSTEMIC GAS EXCHANGE

Multiple Choice—select the best answer.

24. Oxygen is carried in blood:
    a. as oxyhemoglobin.
    b. dissolved in plasma.
    c. molecularly as HbO_2.
    d. all of the above.

25. Which of the following is *NOT* a manner in which CO_2 is transported in the blood?
    a. dissolved in plasma
    b. bound to the heme group of the hemoglobin molecule
    c. as bicarbonate ions
    d. bound to the polypeptide chains of hemoglobin

26. Increasing the carbon dioxide content of blood results in:
    a. increased H+ concentration of plasma.
    b. decreased blood pH.
    c. increased blood pH.
    d. both a and b.

27. Approximately 97% of oxygen is transported as _____, whereas the remaining 3% is transported dissolved in _____.
    a. plasma; hemoglobin
    b. oxyhemoglobin; bicarbonate ion
    c. oxyhemoglobin; plasma
    d. bicarbonate ion; carbonic acid

True or false

28. _____   The exact amount of oxygen in blood depends mainly upon the amount of hemoglobin present.

29. _____   As plasma PCO_2 increases, the CO_2 carrying capacity of blood decreases.

30. _____   Interstitial fluid PO_2 and intracellular fluid PO_2 are essentially the same.

31. _____   A right shift of the oxygen-hemoglobin dissociation curve due to increased PCO_2 is known as the *Bohr effect*.

******If you had difficulty with this section, review pages **720-727**

IV   REGULATION OF BREATHING

Multiple Choice—select the best answer.

32. The basic rhythm of the respiratory cycle seems to be generated by:
    a.   the medullary rhythmicity area.
    b.   the inspiratory center.
    c.   the expiratory center.
    d.   all of the above.

33. The diving reflex:
    a.   explains why some people can hold their breath for extended periods while under water.
    b.   is responsible for the astonishing recovery of near-drowning victims in cold water.
    c.   forces a submerged individual to exhale prior to surfacing.
    d.   both a and c.

True or false

34. _____   Input from the apneustic center in the pons inhibits the inspiratory center, causing a decrease in the length and depth of inspiration.

35. _____   Irritation of the phrenic nerve can cause extended periods of hiccups.

Student Name _____

Labeling—using the terms provided, label the respiratory centers of the brainstem on the following illustration.

medulla   respiratory centers   cortex
expiratory area   pons   limbic system
apneustic center   pneumotaxic center   respiratory muscles
inspiratory center

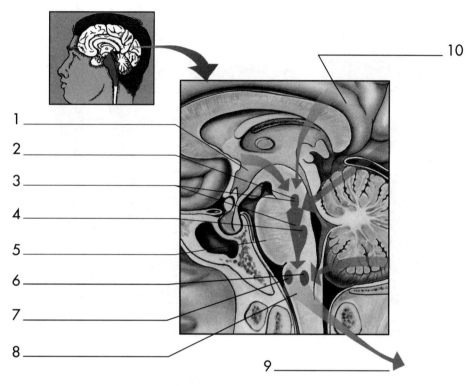

1 _____

2 _____

3 _____

4 _____

5 _____

6 _____

7 _____

8 _____

9 _____

10 _____

******If you had difficulty with this section, review pages **727-732**

V   MECHANISMS OF DISEASE

Fill in the blanks.

36. _____ or _____ _____ _____ _____ is a

    broad term used to describe conditions of progressive, irreversible obstruction of expiratory air flow.

37. _____ results from excessive tracheobronchial secretions that obstruct air flow.

38. _____ may result from the progression of chronic bronchitis or other conditions as

    air becomes trapped within alveoli causing them to enlarge and eventually rupture.

39. _____ is an obstructive disorder characterized by recurring spasms of the smooth

    muscle in the walls of the bronchial air passages.

******If you had difficulty with this section, review pages **732-735**

Crossword Puzzle

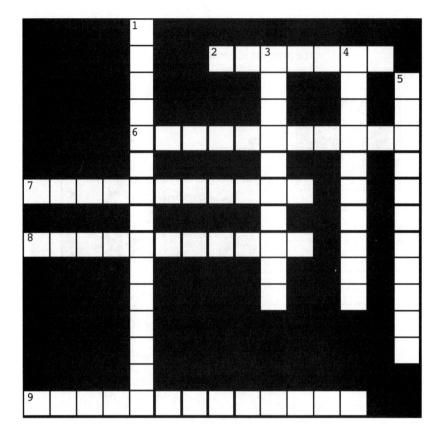

Across

2. Labored breathing
6. Inhaling
7. Volume of air exhaled after inspiration (two words)
8. Most carbon dioxide is carried in this form
9. Hemoglobin combined with oxygen

Down

1. "Tension" (two words)
3. Used to measure amount of air exchanged in breathing
4. Exhaling
5. Breathing

APPLYING WHAT YOU KNOW

40. Mr. Kehoe has smoked a considerable number of cigars and cigarettes during the last two decades. He is beginning to have difficulty breathing—especially upon exhalation. Which broad category of diseases may he be exhibiting symptoms of? What other diseases is he at risk for? What are the physiological mechanisms of these diseases?

41. While sledding on a frozen creek, Heather, a 12-year -old girl, fell through the ice. Her situation wasn't discovered for about half an hour. Upon rescue, she displayed fixed, dilated pupils; cyanosis; and no pulse. Miraculously, she recovered. Identify and explain the physiological phenomena that resulted in this astonishing recovery.

Student Name_____

DID YOU KNOW?

- Sinusitis affects 37 million Americans causing difficulty in breathing and chronic headaches.
- A person's nose and ears continue to grow throughout his or her life.

ONE LAST QUICK CHECK ✔

Multiple Choice—select the best answer.

42. The term that means the same thing as *breathing* is:
    a. gas exchange.
    b. respiration.
    c. inspiration.
    d. pulmonary ventilation.

43. Carbaminohemoglobin is formed when _____ bind(s) to hemoglobin.
    a. oxygen
    c. carbon dioxide
    b. amino acids
    d. nitrogen

44. Most of the oxygen transported by the blood is:
    a. dissolved to white blood cells.
    b. bound to white blood cells.
    c. bound to hemoglobin.
    d. bound to carbaminohemoglobin.

45. Which of the following does *NOT* occur during inspiration?
    a. elevation of the ribs
    b. elevation of the diaphragm
    c. contraction of the diaphragm
    d. chest cavity becomes longer from top to bottom

46. A young adult male would have a vital capacity of about _____ ml.
    a. 500
    c. 3300
    b. 1200
    d. 4800

47. The amount of air that can be forcibly exhaled after expiring the tidal volume is known as the:
    a. total lung capacity.
    b. vital capacity.
    c. inspiratory reserve volume.
    d. expiratory reserve volume.

48. Which one of the following is correct?
    a. VC = TV – IRV + ERV
    b. VC = TV + IRV – ERV
    c. VC = TV + IRV x ERV
    d. VC = TV + IRV + ERV

Matching—identify the term on the left with the proper selection on the right.

49. _____ tidal volume

50. _____ inspiratory reserve volume

51. _____ pneumothorax

52. _____ physiological dead space

53. _____ oxygen tension

54. _____ hemoglobin

55. _____ apneustic breathing

56. _____ chemoreceptors

57. _____ Hering-Breuer reflexes

58. _____ CO_2

a.   collapsed lung
b.   quaternary protein
c.   approximately 3300 ml
d. PO_2
e.   normal exhalation volume
f.   increased in emphysema
g.   helps control respirations
h.   respiratory stimulant
i.   long, deep inspiration
j.   sensitive to changes in arterial CO_2 and pH

CHAPTER 25

ANATOMY OF THE DIGESTIVE SYSTEM

Think of the last meal you ate. The different shapes, sizes, tastes, and textures that you so recently enjoyed. Think of those items circulating in your bloodstream in those same original shapes and sizes. Impossible? Of course. Because of this impossibility you can begin to understand and marvel at the close relationship of the digestive system to the circulatory system. It is the digestive system that changes our food, both mechanically and chemically, into a form that is acceptable to the blood and the body.

This change begins the moment you take the very first bite. Digestion starts in the mouth, where food is chewed and mixed with saliva. It then moves down the pharynx and esophagus by peristalsis and enters the stomach. In the stomach it is churned and mixed with gastric juices to continue the digestive process. As the food continues into the small intestine, it is further broken down chemically by intestinal fluids, bile, and pancreatic juice. These secretions prepare the food for absorption all along the course of the small intestine (duodenum, jejunum, and ileum). Products that are not absorbed pass on and enter the cecum of the large intestine and continue through the ascending colon, transverse colon, descending colon, sigmoid colon, into the rectum, and out the anus.

Products that are used in the cells undergo absorption. Absorption allows newly processed nutrients to pass through the walls of the digestive tract and into the bloodstream to be distributed to the cells. Your review of this system will help you understand the anatomy that provides the mechanical and chemical processes necessary to convert food into energy sources and compounds necessary for survival.

I   OVERVIEW OF THE DIGESTIVE SYSTEM

Multiple Choice—select the best answer.

1. Starting from the deepest layer and moving towards the most superficial, the layers of the wall of the GI tract are:
    a. mucosa, submucosa, serosa, muscularis.
    b. submucosa, mucosa, muscularis, serosa.
    c. mucosa, submucosa, muscularis, serosa.
    d. submucosa, serosa, muscularis, mucosa.

2. The serosa is actually:
    a. parietal peritoneum.
    b. visceral peritoneum.
    c. mesentery.
    d. none of the above.

True or false

3. ____T____   *Gastrointestinal tract* and *alimentary canal* are synonymous terms.

4. ____F____   The tissue layers of the GI tract are constant, with no variation in the different organs.

Matching—identify each digestive organ with its correct classification.

5.   _____A_____   mouth

6.   _____A_____   jejunum

7.   _____A_____   cecum

8.   _____B_____   pancreas

9.   _____B_____   teeth

10. _____B_____   liver

11. _____B_____   salivary glands

12. _____B_____   vermiform appendix

13. _____A_____   oropharynx

14. _____A_____   sigmoid colon

a.   GI tract segment
b.   accessory organ

Labeling—label the digestive organs on the following illustration.

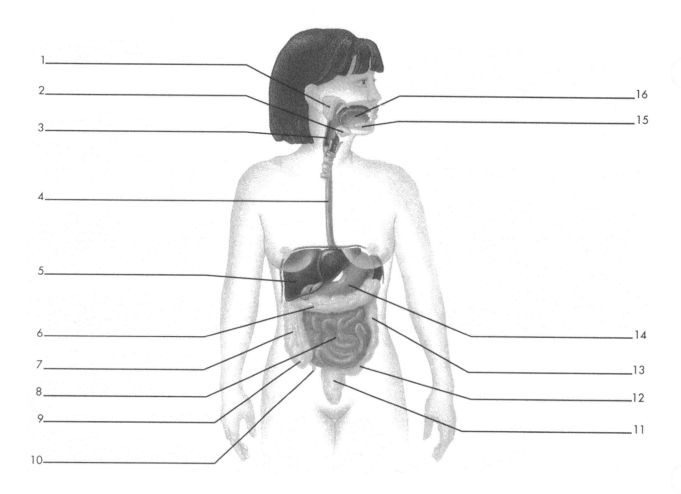

******If you had difficulty with this section, review pages **739-742**

Student Name_____

II   MOUTH AND PHARYNX

Multiple Choice—select the best answer.

15. The hard palate consists of portions of:
    a. three bones: two maxillae and one palatine.
    b. two bones: one maxillae and one palatine.
    c. three bones: one maxillae and two palatine.
    d. four bones: two maxillae and two palatine. *(circled)*

16. Which of the following is an accurate description of salivary glands?
    a. There are four pairs of salivary glands.
    b. They secrete about one liter of saliva per day. *(circled)*
    c. They are associated with buccal glands that secrete about 50% of the saliva.
    d. Both b and c are true.

17. The crown of a tooth is covered with:
    a. dentin.
    b. cementum.
    c. enamel. *(circled)*
    d. alveolar bone.

18. The type of teeth that do *NOT* appear as deciduous teeth are:
    a. incisors.
    b. canines.
    c. second molars.
    d. premolars. *(circled)*

19. The act of swallowing moves a mass of food called a _____ from the mouth to the stomach.
    a. dentin
    b. bolus *(circled)*
    c. fauces
    d. philtrum

True or false

20. ___T___ A typical tooth can be divided into three main parts: crown, neck, and root.

21. ___F___ The *philtrum* is a fold of mucous membrane that helps anchor the tongue to the floor of the mouth.

22. ___F___ There are 20 deciduous teeth and 30 permanent teeth.

23. ___T___ The act of swallowing is termed *deglutition.*

24. ___F___ The soft palate forms a partition between the mouth and oropharynx.

Labeling—label the structures of the tooth on the following illustration.

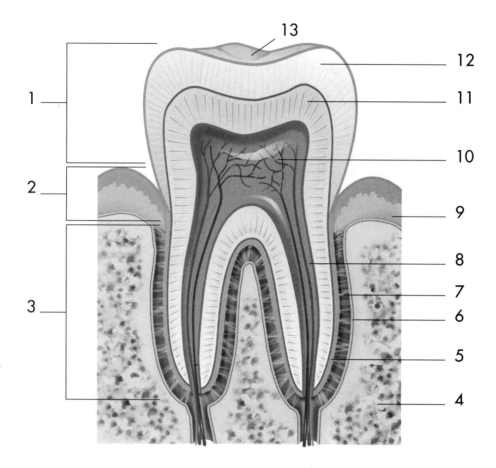

******If you had difficulty with this section, review pages **742-747**

III   ESOPHAGUS AND STOMACH

Multiple Choice—select the best answer.

25. Which of the following statements is *NOT* true of the esophagus?
     a.   It extends from the pharynx to the stomach.
     b.   It lies anterior to the trachea and posterior to the heart.
     c.   It resides in both the thoracic and abdominal cavities.
     d.   It pierces the diaphragm.

26. Which of the following controls the opening of the stomach into the small intestine?
     a.   pylorus
     b.   cardiac sphincter
     c.   duodenal bulb
     d.   pyloric sphincter

27. Which of the layers of the muscularis is present only in the stomach?
     a.   longitudinal muscle layer
     b.   circular muscle layer
     c.   oblique muscle layer
     d.   horizontal muscle layer

Student Name_____

True or false

28. ____T____ The folds in the lining of the stomach are called *rugae*.

29. ____T____ The cardiac sphincter controls the opening of the esophagus into the stomach.

30. ____T____ Parietal cells secrete hydrochloric acid and are thought to produce intrinsic factor.

Labeling—using the terms provided, label the following illustration of the stomach.

fundus	pylorus	pyloric sphincter
duodenal bulb	cardiac sphincter	oblique muscle layer
serosa	submucosa	body
esophagus	longitudinal muscle layer	circular muscle layer
lesser curvature	greater curvature	gastroesophageal opening
duodenum	mucosa	rugae

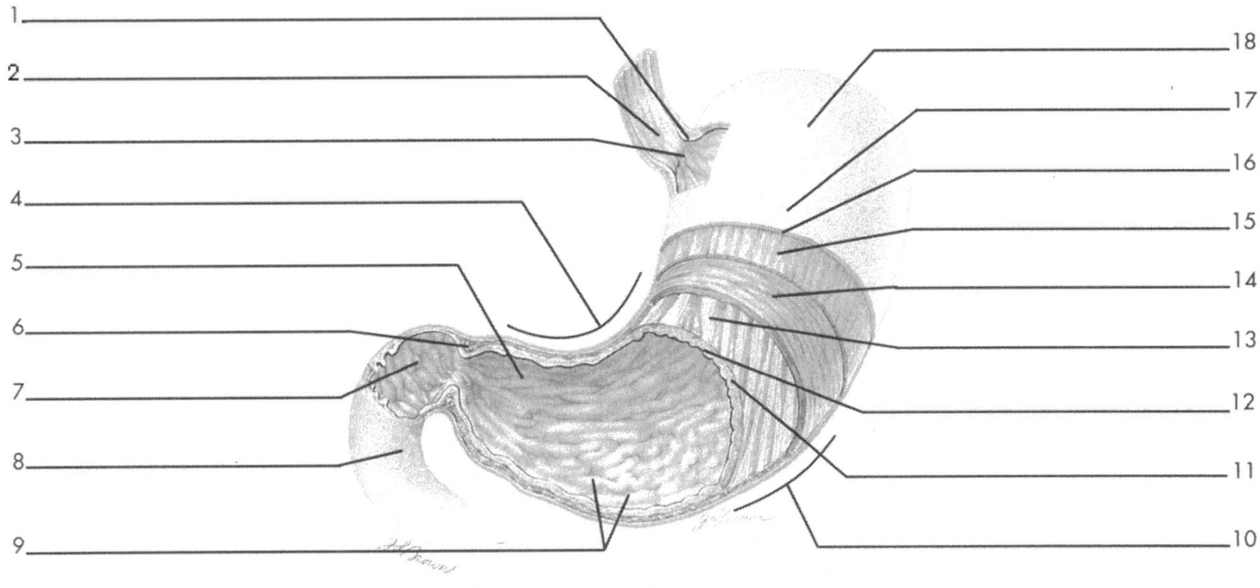

******If you had difficulty with this section, review pages **747-751**

IV SMALL INTESTINE, LARGE INTESTINE, APPENDIX, AND PERITONEUM

Multiple Choice—select the best answer.

31. The correct order of small intestine divisions, starting proximal to the stomach, are:
    a. ileum, duodenum, jejunum.
    b. duodenum, ileum, jejunum.
    c. duodenum, jejunum, ileum.
    d. ileum, jejunum, duodenum.

32. Beginning with the largest structures, which of the following is a correct description of the small intestine's adaptation for absorption?
    a. villi, microvilli, plicae
    b. plicae, villi, microvilli
    c. microvilli, villi, plicae
    d. microvilli, plicae, villi

33. Another term for hemorrhoids is:
    a. piles.   c. fissures.
    b. fistula.   d. proctitis.

34. The lesser omentum attaches the:
    a. transverse colon to the posterior abdominal wall.
    b. liver to the lesser curvature of the stomach.
    c. ileum and jejunum to the posterior abdominal wall.
    d. greater omentum to the posterior abdominal wall.

True or false

35. ___F___ The hepatic flexure of the large intestine is also called the *left colic flexure.*

36. ___F___ The nonpathogenic bacteria of the colon are thought to be produced in the sigmoid colon.

37. ___T___ The pouchlike structures of the large intestine are called *haustra.*

38. ___T___ Hemorrhoids are enlargements of veins in the anal canal.

Labeling—label the wall of the small intestine on the following illustration.

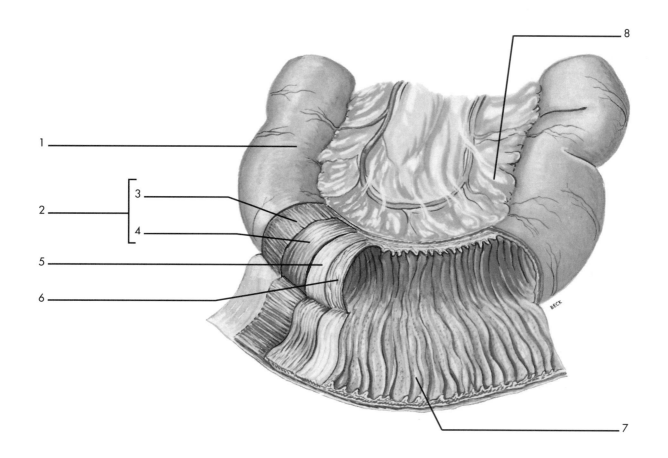

Student Name_____

Labeling—label the divisions of the large intestine on the following illustration.

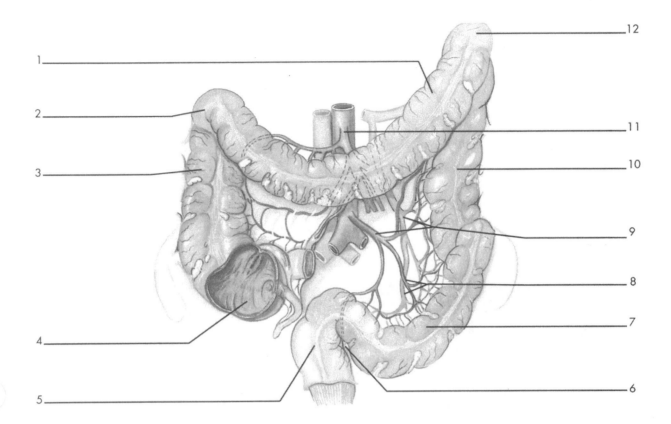

******If you had difficulty with this section, review pages **751-757**

V LIVER, GALLBLADDER, AND PANCREAS

Multiple Choice—select the best answer.

39. The anatomical units of the liver are called:
    a. lobes.
    b. lobules.
    c. sinusoids.
    d. none of the above.

40. Blood flows to hepatic lobules via branches of the:
    a. hepatic artery.
    b. hepatic portal vein.
    c. hepatic vein.
    d. both a and b.

41. A merger of the hepatic duct and cystic duct form the:
    a. common hepatic duct.
    b. common bile duct.
    c. right hepatic duct.
    d. left hepatic duct.

42. Bile salts aid in the absorption of:
    a. fat.   c. proteins.
    b. carbohydrates. d. waste products.

True or false

43.   _____T_____   The liver consists of two lobes separated by the falciform ligament.

44.   _____F_____   Bile is manufactured by the Kupffer cells of the liver.

45.   _____T_____   The pancreas is both an endocrine and exocrine gland.

46.   _____T_____   Surgical removal of the gallbladder is called *cholecystectomy.*

Labeling—label the gross structure of the liver on the following illustration.

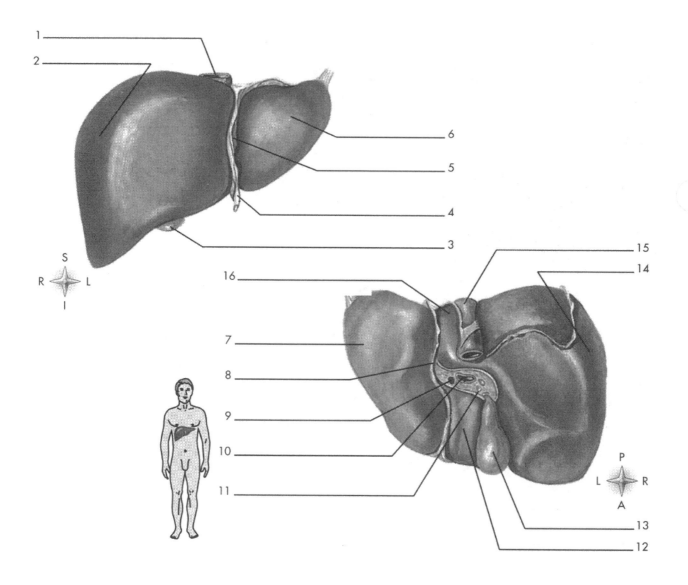

Student Name_____

Labeling—label the ducts on the following illustration of the common bile duct and its tributaries.

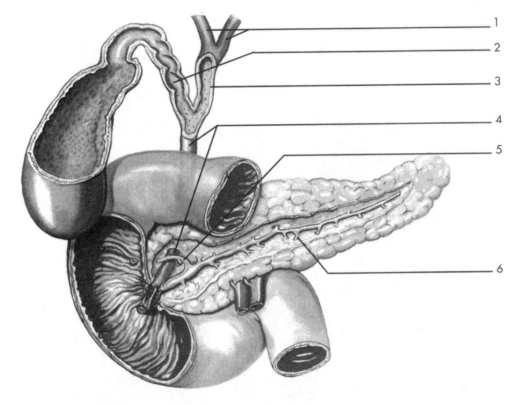

1

2

3

4

5

6

******If you had difficulty with this section, review pages **757-763**

VI   MECHANISMS OF DISEASE

Matching—identify the term on the left with the appropriate description on the right.

47. ____d____ hemorrhoids
48. ____g____ appendicitis
49. ____f____ pyloric stenosis
50. ____e____ ulcers
51. ____i____ *Helicobacter pylori*
52. ____a____ orthodontics
53. ____h____ anal fissures
54. ____b____ mumps
55. ____c____ proctitis
56. ____k____ gingivitis
57. ____j____ heartburn

a. corrects malocclusion
b. swelling of parotid glands
c. inflammation of rectal mucosa
d. dilated veins
e. triple therapy
f. obstructive narrowing
g. low incidence in elderly
h. minor laceration
i. causes peptic ulcers
j. gastric reflux
k. infection of gums

******If you had difficulty with this section, review pages **763-767**

Crossword Puzzle

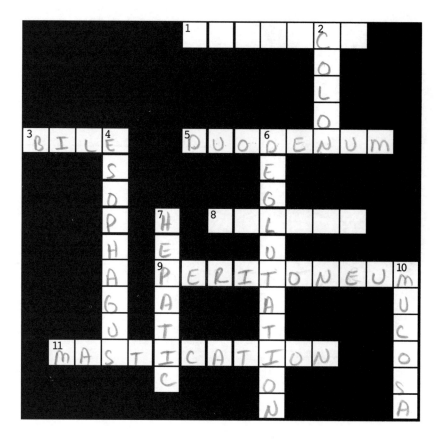

Across

1. Alimentary canal (abbrev., two words)
3. Stored in gallbladder
5. Division of small intestine
8. Small projection in small intestine
9. Large sheet of serous membrane
11. Chewing

Down

2. Large intestine
4. First segment of digestive tube
6. Swallowing
7. Refers to liver
10. Innermost layer of GI tract

APPLYING WHAT YOU KNOW

58. Brian is experiencing difficulty digesting fatty foods and is displaying a yellow discoloration of his skin. What may be causing his condition? What is the clinical term used to describe the yellow appearance of his skin and what is the physiology? How could doctors treat his condition and what are the names of the procedures?

59. Baby Billy has been regurgitating his bottle feeding at every meal. The milk is curdled, but does not appear to be digested. He has become dehydrated, so his mother, Amanda, is taking him to the pediatrician. What is a possible diagnosis from your textbook reading?

Student Name _____

DID YOU KNOW?

- The human stomach lining replaces itself every 3 days.
- If one were to unravel the entire human alimentary canal (esophagus, stomach, small and large intestines), it would reach the height of a three-story building.

ONE LAST QUICK CHECK ✔

Multiple Choice—select the best answer.

60. The first baby tooth, on an average, appears at age:
    - a. 2 months.
    - b. 1 year.
    - c. 1 month.
    - d. 6 months.

61. The portion of the tooth that is covered with enamel is the:
    - a. pulp cavity.
    - b. neck.
    - c. root.
    - d. crown.

62. Which of the following teeth is missing from the deciduous arch?
    - a. central incisor
    - b. canine
    - c. second premolar
    - d. first molar

63. The permanent central incisor erupts between the ages of _____.
    - a. 9 and 13
    - b. 5 and 6
    - c. 7 and 10
    - d. 7 and 8

64. A general term for infection of the gums is:
    - a. dental caries.
    - b. leukoplakia.
    - c. Vincent's angina.
    - d. gingivitis.

65. The ducts of the _____ glands open into the floor of the mouth.
    - a. sublingual
    - b. submandibular
    - c. parotid
    - d. carotid

66. The volume of saliva secreted per day is about:
    - a. 1/2 pint.
    - b. 1 pint.
    - c. 1 liter.
    - d. 1 gallon.

67. Another name for the third molar is:
    - a. central incisor.
    - b. wisdom tooth.
    - c. canine.
    - d. lateral incisor.

68. After food has been chewed, it is formed into a small rounded mass called a:
    - a. moat.
    - b. chyme.
    - c. bolus.
    - d. protease.

69. Which one is *NOT* part of the small intestine?
    - a. jejunum
    - b. ileum
    - c. cecum
    - d. duodenum

70. The union of the cystic duct and hepatic duct forms the:
    - a. common bile duct.
    - b. major duodenal papilla.
    - c. minor duodenal papilla.
    - d. pancreatic duct.

71. Each villus in the intestine contains a lymphatic vessel or _____ that serves to absorb lipid or fat materials from the chyme.
    - a. plica
    - b. lacteal
    - c. villa
    - d. microvilli

72. *Cholelithiasis* is the term used to describe:
    - a. biliary colic.
    - b. jaundice.
    - c. portal hypertension.
    - d. gallstones.

73. The largest gland in the body is the:
    - a. pituitary.
    - b. thyroid.
    - c. liver.
    - d. thymus.

True or false

74. ___F___   The splenic flexure is the bend between the ascending colon and the transverse colon.

75. ___F___   The splenic colon is the S-shaped segment that terminates in the rectum.

76. ___T___   The function of the appendix is uncertain.

77. ___T___   The oral cavity is also known as the *buccal cavity.*

78. ___T___   The esophagus is voluntary in the upper third, mixed in the middle, and involuntary in the lower third.

79. ___T___   The stomach secretes the intrinsic factor.

80. ___T___   The mesentery is a fan-shaped projection of the parietal peritoneum.

81. ___T___   The liver is an exocrine gland.

CHAPTER 26

PHYSIOLOGY OF THE DIGESTIVE SYSTEM

Digestion is the process of breaking down complex nutrients into simpler units suitable for absorption. It involves two major processes: mechanical and chemical. Mechanical digestion occurs during mastication and the churning and propelling mechanisms that occur along the alimentary canal. Chemical digestion occurs with the help of the many digestive enzymes and various substances that are added to the nutrients as they progress the length of the digestive tube. These substances include saliva and gastric, pancreatic, and intestinal enzymes. Delicate nervous and hormonal reflex mechanisms control the flow of these juices so that the proper amount is released at the appropriate time.

Absorption is the passage of substances (digested foods, water, salts, and vitamins) through the intestinal mucosa and into the blood or lymph. After the body has determined the nutrients necessary for absorption, it sends the residue of digestion to the final segment of the GI tract to be eliminated as feces.

Your review of this system will help you understand the mechanical and chemical processes necessary to convert food into energy sources and compounds necessary for survival.

I DIGESTION

Multiple Choice—select the best answer.

1. Which of the following describes the pharyngeal stage of deglutition?
   a. mouth to oropharynx
   b. oropharynx to esophagus
   c. esophagus to stomach
   d. none of the above

2. Which step of deglutition is under voluntary control?
   a. oral
   b. pharyngeal
   c. esophageal
   d. all of the above

3. The final product of carbohydrate digestion is a:
   a. disaccharide.
   b. monosaccharide.
   c. polysaccharide.
   d. fatty acid.

4. Enzymes that catalyze the hydrolysis of proteins are:
   a. proteases.
   b. amylases.
   c. lactases.
   d. lipases.

5. A micelle is:
   a. a disaccharide attached to the brush border of the small intestine.
   b. a tiny sphere of lipid and water.
   c. a thick, milky material comprised of food and digestive enzymes.
   d. synonymous with *bolus.*

6. Which of the following is *NOT* true concerning the gastric emptying of water?
   a. Large volumes of water leave the stomach more rapidly than small volumes.
   b. Warm fluids empty more quickly than cool fluids.
   c. High-solute concentration fluids empty slower than dilute concentrations.
   d. All of the above are true.

7. The process of fat emulsification consists of:
   a. chemically breaking down fat molecules.
   b. absorption of fats.
   c. breaking down fats into small droplets.
   d. the secretion of digestive juices for fat digestion.

True or false

8. _____ Peristalsis can be described as a mixing movement.

9. _____ The volumes of the stomach and the duodenum are approximately equal.

10. _____ Enzymes are organic catalysts.

11. _____ Digestive enzymes catalyze chemical reactions with great efficiency within a wide range of pH.

12. _____ Cellulose resists digestion and is eliminated in feces.

13. _____ Water is readily absorbed in the stomach.

14. _____ Amino acids are the end product of protein digestion.

******If you had difficulty with this section, review pages **771-781**

II SECRETION AND CONTROL OF DIGESTIVE GLAND SECRETION

Multiple Choice—select the best answer.

15. The principle enzyme of saliva is:
    a. protease.
    b. amylase.
    c. lipase.
    d. salivase.

16. Which of the following is true?
    a. Saliva contains large amounts of lipase.
    b. Pepsinogen is converted into pepsin by hydrochloric acid.
    c. Chief cells secrete pepsin.
    d. Zymogenic cells produce intrinsic factor.

17. Which of the following is present in bile?
    a. lecithin
    b. gastrin
    c. bile salts
    d. both a and c

18. The hormone that stimulates the gallbladder to release bile is:
    a. enterogastrone.
    b. insulin.
    c. gastrin.
    d. cholecystokinin-pancreozymin.

True or false

19. _____ Pancreatic juice is secreted by exocrine acinar cells of the pancreas.

20. _____ Olfactory and visual stimuli are factors concerning the control of digestive gland secretion.

21. _____ The cephalic phase is initiated by the presence of food in the stomach.

22. _____ Chyme is liquefied food found in the stomach.

******If you had difficulty with this section, review pages **778-784**

Student Name_____

III ABSORPTION AND ELIMINATION

Multiple Choice—select the best answer.

23. Fats are absorbed primarily into which of the following structures?
    a.   blood in intestinal capillaries
    b.   lymph in intestinal lacteals
    c.   none of the above

24. Movement of lower colon and rectum contents at a rate slower than normal can cause:
    a.   defecation.   c.   diarrhea.
    b.   constipation.   d.   both b and c.

25. Which blood vessel carries absorbed nutrients from the GI tract to the liver?
    a.   hepatic artery   c.   portal vein
    b.   hepatic vein   d.   inferior vena cava

True or false

26. _____   Both water and sodium are absorbed via simple diffusion.

27. _____   The majority of substances are absorbed in the small intestine.

28. _____   Cholera is an intestinal infection that kills more than 600,000 infants and children worldwide each year.

29. _____   Micelles, formed from bile salts, carry fatty acids from emulsified droplets to the plasma membrane of absorptive cells.

30. _____   Impaired fat absorption produces large, greasy, foul-smelling stools known as *steatorrhea*.

******If you had difficulty with this section, review pages **784-789**

IV MECHANISMS OF DISEASE

Matching—select the best term in the left column for the description in the right column.

31. _____   gastroenteritis
32. _____   anorexia
33. _____   emesis
34. _____   Zantac
35. _____   *Helicobacter pylori*
36. _____   diverticulosis
37. _____   colitis
38. _____   hepatitis
39. _____   pancreatic cancer
40. _____   cirrhosis

a.   reduces the formation of HCl in the stomach
b.   outpouchings of the intestinal wall
c.   inflammation of the liver
d.   chronic loss of appetite
e.   degenerative liver condition
f.   cause of ulcers
g.   vomiting
h.   stomach inflammation
i.   inflammation of large intestine
j.   a form of adenocarcinoma

******If you had difficulty with this section, review pages **789-791**

Crossword Puzzle

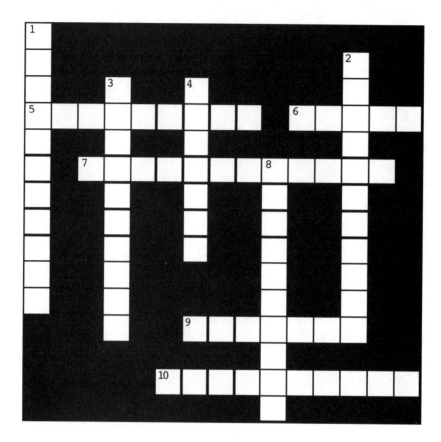

Across

5. Process of taking food into the GI tract
6. Food leaving the stomach
7. Mixing movement
9. GI hormones
10. Chemical process in digestion

Down

1. Wavelike ripple of organ
2. Fat droplet
3. Expelling feces
4. Fat droplet surrounded by bile salts
8. Movement of nutrients into internal environment

APPLYING WHAT YOU KNOW

41. Mrs. Haygood was diagnosed with an ulcer of the digestive system. What kind of symptoms might she display? Where along her alimentary canal is this lesion most likely to reside? What are the two accepted mechanisms of this disease? How should her doctor treat her condition?

42. Cliff and Pete like to play soccer vigorously in the heat of the day. What kind of recommendations should they observe concerning the replacement of fluids? Be sure to consider parameters such as fluid temperature, volume, and solute concentration.

Student Name_____

DID YOU KNOW?

- There are 35 million digestive glands in the stomach.
- Even if the stomach, the spleen, 75% of the liver, 80% of the intestines, one kidney, one lung, and virtually every organ from the pelvic and groin area are removed, the human body can still survive!

ONE LAST QUICK CHECK ✔

Multiple Choice—select the best answer.

43. During the process of digestion, stored bile is poured into the duodenum by which of the following?
    a. gallbladder
    b. liver
    c. pancreas
    d. spleen

44. The portion of the alimentary canal that mixes food with gastric juice and breaks it down into a mixture called *chyme* is the:
    a. gallbladder.
    b. small intestine.
    c. stomach.
    d. large intestine.

45. What is the middle portion of the small intestine called?
    a. jejunum
    b. ileum
    c. duodenum
    d. cecum

46. Duodenal ulcers appear in which of the following?
    a. stomach
    b. small intestine
    c. large intestine
    d. esophagus

47. Protein digestion begins in the:
    a. esophagus.
    b. small intestine.
    c. stomach.
    d. large intestine.

48. The enzyme pepsin is concerned primarily with the digestion of which of the following?
    a. sugars.
    b. starches.
    c. proteins.
    d. fats.

49. The enzyme amylase converts which of the following?
    a. starches to sugars
    b. sugars to starches
    c. proteins to amino acids
    d. fatty acids and glycerols to fats

50. Which of the following substances does *NOT* contain any enzymes?
    a. saliva
    b. bile
    c. gastric juice
    d. intestinal juice

51. Which of the following is a simple sugar?
    a. maltose
    b. sucrose
    c. lactose
    d. glucose

52. Fats are broken down into:
    a. amino acids.
    b. simple sugars.
    c. fatty acids.
    d. disaccharides.

53. Which one is *NOT* part of the small intestine?
    a. jejunum
    b. ileum
    c. colon
    d. duodenum

54. The union of the cystic duct and hepatic duct form the:
    a. common bile duct.
    b. major duodenal papilla.
    c. minor duodenal papilla.
    d. pancreatic duct.

55. The process of swallowing is known as:
    a. mastication.
    b. segmentation.
    c. peristalsis.
    d. deglutition.

56. Peristalsis begins in the:
    a. mouth.
    b. pharynx.
    c. esophagus.
    d. stomach.

True or false

57. _____ The mechanical process that occurs in the rectum is churning.

58. _____ Enzymes are functional proteins that catalyze chemical reactions.

59. _____ The hormones secretin and CCK stimulate ejection of bile.

60. _____ Vitamins A, D, E, and K are known as the *fat-soluble vitamins*.

61. _____ Constipation occurs with increased motility of the small intestine.

Student Name_____

CHAPTER 27

NUTRITION AND METABOLISM

Most of us love to eat, but do the foods we enjoy provide us with the basic food types necessary for good nutrition? The body, a finely tuned machine, requires a balance of carbohydrates, fats, proteins, vitamins, and minerals to function properly. These nutrients must be digested, absorbed, and circulated to cells constantly to accommodate the numerous activities that occur throughout the body. The use the body makes of foods once these processes are completed is called "metabolism."

Although the body relies on many organs to prepare nutrients for us, the liver plays a major role in the metabolism of food. It helps maintain a normal blood glucose level, removes toxins from the blood, processes blood immediately after it leaves the gastrointestinal tract, and initiates the first steps of protein and fat metabolism.

The study of metabolism is not complete without a discussion of the basal metabolic rate (BMR). The BMR is the rate at which food is catabolized under basal conditions. The total metabolic rate (TMR) is the amount of energy, expressed in calories, used by the body each day. This chapter also demonstrates the use of metabolic testing to measure thyroid functioning.

Finally, the hypothalamus appears to be a critical component in determining appetite and satiety. While many theories suggest various ways that the hypothalamus might perform these functions, it is imperative that we acknowledge its importance in nutrition and metabolism. Review of this chapter is necessary to provide you with an understanding of the "fuel," or nutrition, necessary to maintain your complex homeostatic machine—the body.

I   OVERVIEW OF NUTRITION AND METABOLISM

Multiple Choice—select the best answer.

1. The universal biological currency is:
   a. ATP.
   b. ADP.
   c. carbohydrates.
   d. NADH.

2. *Nutrition* refers to the:
   a. complex set of chemical processes that make life possible.
   b. breaking down of food into small molecular compounds.
   c. release of energy in two main forms.
   d. food we eat and the nutrients they contain.

True or false

3. _____ Catabolism is a process that breaks down molecules into smaller molecular compounds.

4. _____ Metabolism is identical in all cells.

******If you had difficulty with this section, review pages **795-797**

II   CARBOHYDRATES

Multiple Choice—select the best answer.

5.   Glucose, fructose, and galactose are important:
a.   monosaccharides.
b.   disaccharides.
c.   polysaccharides.
d.   starches.

6.   The carbohydrate most useful to the human cell is:
a.   cellulose.   c.   fructose.
b.   glucose.   d.   galactose.

7.   The process of glucose phosphorylation forms the molecule:
a.   ATP.
b.   ADP.
c.   glucose-6-phosphate.
d.   glycogen.

8.   The breakdown of one glucose molecule into two pyruvic acid molecules is called:
a.   glycolysis.   c.   glycogenolysis.
b.   glycogenesis.   d.   glycogen.

9.   The amount of heat necessary to raise the temperature of 1 g of water by 1° C is a:
a.   calorie.
b.   Celsius.
c.   kilocalorie.
d.   none of the above.

10.   To enter the citric acid cycle, glucose must be transformed into:
a.   pyruvic acid.   c.   ATP.
b.   acetyl-CoA.   d.   NADH.

11.   Which of the following defines *glycogenesis?*
a.   process of glycogen formation
b.   joining of glucose molecules
c.   catabolism of glycogen
d.   both a and b

12.   Which of the following hormones helps glucose enter cells, and therefore decreases blood glucose?
a.   glucagon   c.   epinephrine
b.   insulin   d.   growth hormone

True or false

13.   _____   Glycolysis is an anaerobic process.

14.   _____   *Kilocalorie* and *calorie* are synonymous terms.

15.   _____   Glycolysis occurs in the mitochondria, whereas the citric acid cycle occurs in the cytoplasm.

16.   _____   Erythrocytes rely upon aerobic respiration.

17.   _____   The process of gluconeogenesis synthesizes new glucose molecules.

18.   _____   Glycogenesis is a homeostatic mechanism that functions when blood glucose levels increase above normal.

19.   _____   Hyperglycemia occurs when the blood glucose dips below the normal set point level.

20.   _____   The conversion of proteins to glucose is an example of gluconeogenesis.

21.   _____   Glucagon stimulates glycogenolysis in the liver.

22.   _____   ACTH decreases blood glucose concentration.

Student Name_____

23. _____ Disaccharides do *NOT* need to be chemically digested before they can be absorbed.

24. _____ The *citric acid cycle*, the *TCA cycle*, and the *Krebs cycle* are all synonymous.

25. _____ *Oxidative phosphorylation* refers to the joining of a phosphate group to ADP to form ATP.

26. _____ The breakdown of ATP molecules provides 50% of all of the energy that does cellular work.

27. _____ Glycogenolysis is consistent in all cells.

******If you had difficulty with this section, review pages **797-808**

III LIPIDS

Multiple Choice—select the best answer.

28. _____ contains fatty acid chains in which all available bonds of its hydrocarbon chain are filled with hydrogen atoms.
    a. Saturated fat   c. Cholesterol
    b. Unsaturated fat d. both a and b

29. The most common lipids in the diet are:
    a. phospholipids.   c. triglycerides.
    b. cholesterol.   d. prostaglandins.

30. A high risk of atherosclerosis is associated with a high blood concentration of:
    a. LDL.   c. CVA.
    b. HDL.   d. both a and b.

31. All of the following hormones control lipid metabolism *EXCEPT:*
    a. ACTH.   c. epinephrine.
    b. glucocorticoids. d. insulin.

32. Which of the following lab results would indicate high risk for atherosclerosis?
    a. 100 mg LDL/100 ml of blood
    b. 180 mg HDL/100 ml of blood
    c. 60 mg HDL/100 ml of blood
    d. 200 mg LDL/100 ml of blood

True or false

33. _____ A diet high in saturated fats and cholesterol tends to increase blood concentration of high-density lipoproteins.

34. _____ Lipid catabolism yields 9 kcal/g.

35. _____ Essential fatty acids are not synthesized by the body and must be obtained through the diet.

36. _____ Lipids are transported in the blood as chylomicrons, lipoproteins, and free fatty acids.

37. _____ The liver is the chief site of ketogenesis.

******If you had difficulty with this section, review pages **808-811**

IV   PROTEINS

Multiple Choice—select the best answer.

38. Which of the following is a nonessential amino acid?
    a.   lysine   c.   tryptophan
    b.   alanine   d.   valine

39. The process by which proteins are synthesized by the ribosomes in all cells is called:
    a.   protein catabolism.
    b.   protein anabolism.
    c.   protein metabolism.
    d.   both a and b.

40. Which of the following hormones tends to promote protein anabolism?
    a.   testosterone
    b.   growth hormone
    c.   thyroid hormone
    d.   all of the above

True or false

41. _____   In protein metabolism, catabolism is primary and anabolism is secondary.

42. _____   Foods from animal sources high in proteins contain the essential amino acids.

43. _____   Glucocorticoids are protein catabolic hormones.

44. _____   Growth and pregnancy usually result in a negative nitrogen balance.

45. _____   The first step in protein catabolism takes place in the liver and is called *deamination*.

V   VITAMINS AND MINERALS

Multiple Choice—select the best answer.

46. Which of the following plays an important role in detecting light in the sensory cells of the eye?
    a.   vitamin D   c.   biotin
    b.   retinal   d.   pantothenic acid

47. Which of the following vitamins is fat-soluble?
    a.   vitamin A
    b.   vitamin B
    c.   vitamin C
    d.   none of the above

48. Which of the following illnesses can result from an iodine deficiency?
    a.   anemia
    b.   bone degeneration
    c.   goiter
    d.   acid-base imbalance

True or false

49. _____   Athletic performance can be enhanced by vitamin supplementation.

50. _____   Vitamin E is thought to neutralize free radicals.

Student Name_____

51. _____ Vitamin C deficiency could result in scurvy.

52. _____ Coenzymes are inorganic catalysts.

******If you had difficulty with this section, review pages **811-817**

VI   METABOLIC RATE AND MECHANISMS FOR REGULATING FOOD INTAKE

Multiple Choice—select the best answer.

53. Which of the following is *NOT* a condition required for the basal metabolic rate?
    a. The individual is lying down and not moving.
    b. The individual is sleeping.
    c. It has been 12 to 18 hours since the individual's last meal.
    d. The individual is in a comfortable, warm environment.

54. Which of the following does *NOT* influence BMR?
    a. age
    b. gender
    c. ethnicity
    d. size

55. One pound of adipose tissue equals:
    a. 1000 kcal.
    b. 350 kcal.
    c. 3500 kcal.
    d. 10,000 kcal.

56. The appetite center is most likely located in the:
    a. cerebrum.
    b. hypothalamus.
    c. small intestine.
    d. stomach.

True or false

57. _____ Males have a BMR approximately 15 to 20% higher than females.

58. _____ Increases in blood temperature and glucose concentration may be linked to satiety.

59. _____ Body weight is linked to both energy input and energy output.

60. _____ When body temperature decreases, metabolism increases.

61. _____ Metabolic rate is the amount of energy released in the body in a given time by anabolism.

******If you had difficulty with this section, review pages **817-822**

VII MECHANISMS OF DISEASE

Matching—choose the correct response.

62. _____ characterized by a refusal to eat

63. _____ results from a deficiency of calories in general and protein in particular

64. _____ inborn error of metabolism

65. _____ advanced form of PCM

66. _____ not a disorder but may be a symptom of abnormal behavior

67. _____ binge-purge syndrome

68. _____ abdominal bloating

a.   phenylketonuria
b.   anorexia nervosa
c.   bulimia
d.   obesity
e.   PCM
f.   marasmus
g.   ascites

******If you had difficulty with this section, review pages **822-825**

Crossword Puzzle

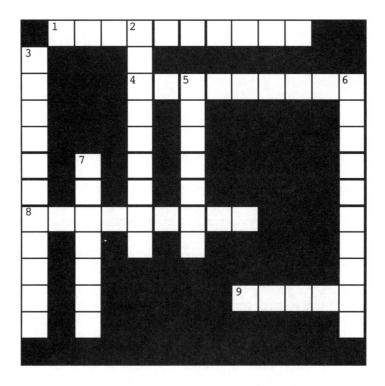

Across

1.   Decomposition process
4.   Synthesis process
8.   The food and nutrients we eat
9.   Discovered citric acid cycle

Down

2.   Does not require oxygen
3.   Forms body fat from food
5.   Requires oxygen
6.   Chemical processes that make life possible
7.   Organ molecule needed to assist enzyme functioning

Student Name_____

APPLYING WHAT YOU KNOW

69. Dr. Reeder was concerned about Myrna. Her daily food intake provided fewer calories than her TMR. If this trend continues, what will be the result? If it continues over a long period of time, what eating disorder might Myrna develop?

70. Paul was experiencing fatigue and a blood test revealed that he was slightly anemic. What mineral(s) will his doctor most likely prescribe? What dietary sources might you suggest that he emphasize in his daily diet?

DID YOU KNOW?

- The body's daily requirement of vitamins and minerals is less than a thimbleful.
- The average person consumes 2000 to 2500 calories a day but if you had the metabolism of a shrew you would need to consume approximately 200,000 calories a day! Smaller animals have higher metabolic rates because they have to work harder to keep their bodies warm.

ONE LAST QUICK CHECK ✓

Multiple Choice—select the best answer.

71. What is the process by which pyruvic acid is broken down into carbon dioxide and high-energy electrons called?
    a. glycogenesis   c. glycolysis
    b. citric acid cycle   d. pyruvic acid cycle

72. The anabolism of glucose produces which of the following?
    a. glycogen   c. renin
    b. amino acid   d. starch

73. Which of the following is a major hormone in the body that aids carbohydrate metabolism?
    a. oxytocin   c. insulin
    b. prolactin   d. ADH

74. The total metabolic rate is which of the following?
    a. the amount of fats we consume in a 24-hour period
    b. the same as the BMR
    c. the amount of energy expressed in calories used by the body per day
    d. cannot be calculated

75. When your consumption of calories equals your TMR, your weight will do which of the following?
    a. increase
    b. remain the same
    c. fluctuate
    d. decrease

76. What is the primary molecule the body usually breaks down as an energy source?
    a. amino acids   c. maltose
    b. pepsin   d. glucose

77. When glucose is *NOT* available, the body will next catabolize which of the following energy sources?
    a. fats   c. minerals
    b. proteins   d. vitamins

Circle the word or phrase that does not belong.

78. glycolysis   citric acid cycle   ATP   bile

79. adipose   amino acids   triglycerides   lipid

80. A   D   M   K

81. iron   protein   amino acids   essential

82. ACTH   insulin   growth hormone   epinephrine

83. sodium   calcium   zinc   folic acid

84. thiamine   niacin   ascorbic acid   riboflavin

Matching—identify the term that best matches the definition.

85. _____ preferred energy food   a.   carbohydrate
                                                  b.   fat
86. _____ amino acids   c.   protein
                                                  d.   vitamins
87. _____ fat soluble   e.   minerals

88. _____ required for nerve conduction

89. _____ glycolysis

90. _____ inorganic elements found
                  naturally in the earth

91. _____ pyruvic acid

CHAPTER 28

URINARY SYSTEM

Living produces wastes. Wherever people live or work or play, wastes accumulate. To keep these areas healthy, there must be a method of disposing of these wastes such as a sanitation department.

Wastes also accumulate in your body. The conversion of food and gases into substances and energy necessary for survival results in waste products. A large percentage of these wastes is removed by the urinary system.

Two vital organs, the kidneys, cleanse the blood of the many waste products that are continually produced as a result of the metabolism of food in the body cells. They eliminate these wastes in the form of urine.

Urine formation is the result of three processes: filtration, reabsorption, and secretion. These processes occur in successive portions of the microscopic units of the kidneys known as *nephrons*. The amount of urine produced by the nephrons is controlled primarily by the hormones ADH and aldosterone. After the urine is produced, it is drained from the renal pelvis by the ureters to flow into the bladder. The bladder then stores the urine until it is voided through the urethra.

If waste products are allowed to accumulate in the body, they soon become poisonous, a condition called *uremia*. A knowledge of the urinary system is necessary to understand how the body rids itself of waste and avoids toxicity.

I ANATOMY OF THE URINARY SYSTEM

Multiple Choice—select the best answer.

1. Which of the following is regulated by the kidneys?
   a. water content of the blood
   b. blood pH level
   c. blood ion concentration
   d. all of the above

2. The medial surface of each kidney has a notch called the:
   a. medulla.   c. hilum.
   b. cortex.   d. pelvis.

3. At the beginning of the "plumbing system" of the urinary system, urine leaving the renal papilla is collected in the cuplike structures called:
   a. renal columns.   c. calyces.
   b. renal pyramids. d. ureters.

4. The functional unit of the kidney is the:
   a. renal corpuscle.
   b. nephron.
   c. juxtaglomerular apparatus.
   d. Bowman's capsule.

5. Which of the following is a component of the renal corpuscle?
   a. glomerulus
   b. Bowman's capsule
   c. afferent arteriole
   d. both a and b

6. Which of the following structures secretes renin when blood pressure in the afferent arteriole drops?
   a. renal tubule
   b. proximal convoluted tubule
   c. juxtaglomerular apparatus
   d. both a and b

7. Substances pass from the glomerulus and into the Bowman's capsule by:
    a. diffusion.   c. filtration.
    b. active transport. d. osmosis.

8. The juxtaglomerular cells reside in the:
    a. afferent arteriole.
    b. efferent arteriole.
    c. proximal convoluted tubule.
    d. distal convoluted tubule.

True or false

9. _____   The left kidney is often slightly larger and positioned slightly lower than the right kidney.

10. _____   Blood is brought to the kidneys by the renal vein.

11. _____   *Micturition* and *urination* are synonymous terms.

12. _____   The glomerulus is one of the most important capillary networks for survival.

13. _____   Once urine enters the renal pelvis, it then travels to the renal calyces.

14. _____   As the basic functional unit of the kidney, the nephron's function is blood processing and urine formation.

15. _____   The kidneys are covered with visceral peritoneum.

Labeling—using the terms provided, label the following illustration of the kidney.

renal pelvis	hilum	capsule (fibrous)
renal papilla of pyramid	ureter	medulla
minor calyces	renal sinus	major calyces
renal column	interlobular arteries	medullary pyramid
cortex		

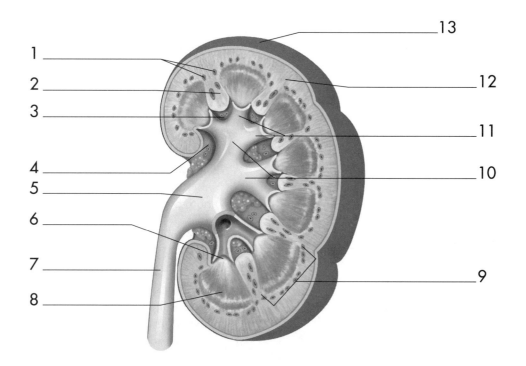

Student Name_____

Labeling—using the terms provided, label the following illustration of the nephron.

vasa recta
glomerulus
afferent arteriole
arcuate artery and vein
descending limb of Henle's loop

pyramid (medulla)
proximal tubule
efferent arteriole
interlobular vein and artery
ascending limb of Henle's loop

Henle's loop
collecting tubule
distal convoluted tubule
juxtamedullary nephron
cortical nephron

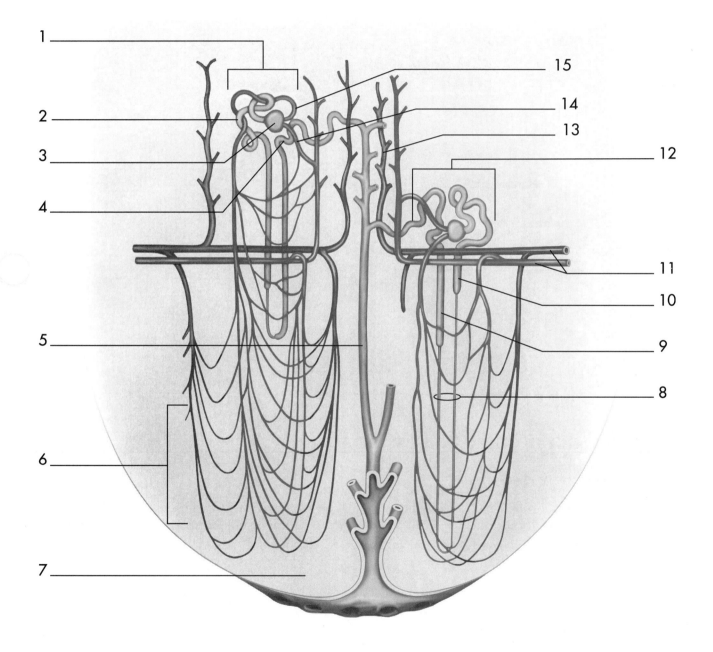

Labeling—label the following structure of the male urinary bladder.

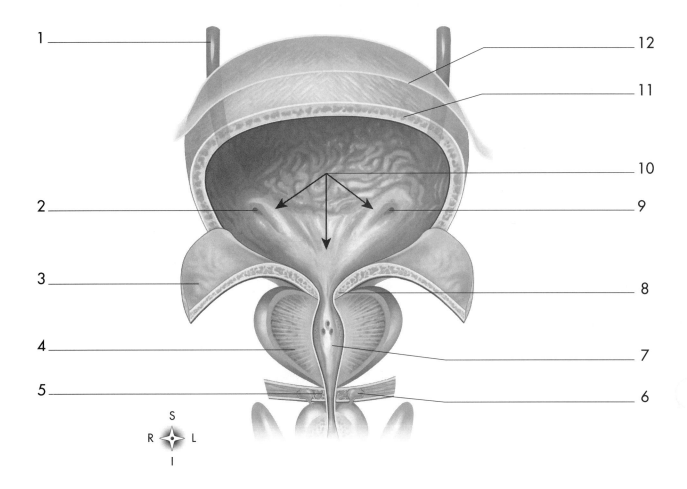

******If you had difficulty with this section, review pages **829-838**

II   PHYSIOLOGY OF THE URINARY SYSTEM

Multiple Choice—select the best answer.

16. Which of the following is *NOT* one of the processes of urine formation?
    a. filtration
    c. reabsorption
    b. diffusion
    d. secretion

17. The movement of water and solutes from the plasma in the glomerulus, across the glomerular-capsular membrane, and into the capsular space of the Bowman's capsule, is termed:
    a. filtration.
    c. reabsorption.
    b. diffusion.
    d. secretion.

18. The movement of molecules out of the peritubular blood and into the tubule for excretion is:
    a. filtration.
    c. reabsorption.
    b. diffusion.
    d. secretion.

19. Under normal conditions most water, electrolytes, and nutrients are reabsorbed in the:
    a. proximal convoluted tubule.
    b. distal convoluted tubule.
    c. loop of Henle.
    d. collecting duct.

20. Which of the following is considered a countercurrent structure?
    a. glomerulus
    b. proximal convoluted tubule
    c. loop of Henle
    d. distal convoluted tubule

21. Water loss from the blood is reduced by:
    a. ADH.   c. aldosterone.
    b. ANH.   d. both a and c.

22. *Dysuria* is a term describing:
    a. blood in the urine.
    b. pus in the urine.
    c. painful urination.
    d. absence of urine.

23. All of the following are normal contents of urine *EXCEPT*:
    a. nitrogenous wastes.
    b. hormones.
    c. pigments.
    d. plasma proteins.

24. Which of the following is *NOT* symptomatic of diabetes mellitus?
    a. copious urination
    b. glycosuria
    c. anuria
    d. diuresis

True or false

25. _____ Kidney failure means homeostatic failure, and if not relieved, inevitable death.

26. _____ Postexercise proteinuria is considered serious and often indicative of kidney disease.

27. _____ Fluid exiting the loop of Henle becomes less concentrated with Na^+ and Cl^- ions.

28. _____ A hydrostatic pressure gradient drives the filtration out of the plasma and into the nephron.

29. _____ The efferent arteriole has a larger diameter than the afferent arteriole.

30. _____ Stress causes an increase in glomerular hydrostatic pressure.

31. _____ In the renal tubule, Na^+ is reabsorbed via active transport.

32. _____ Glomerular filtration separates only harmful substances from the blood.

33. _____ Urine consists of approximately 75% water.

34. _____ Urine has a pH of 4.6 to 8.0 and is generally alkaline.

35. _____ Gout is a condition characterized by excessive levels of uric acid in the blood.

******If you had difficulty with this section, review pages **838-850**

III   MECHANISMS OF DISEASE

Matching—select the correct disorder from the choices provided.

36. _____ urine backs up into the kidneys causing swelling of the renal pelvis and calyces

37. _____ kidney stones

38. _____ final stage of chronic renal failure

39. _____ involuntary retention of urine with subsequent distention of the bladder

40. _____ inflammation of the bladder

41. _____ inflammation of the renal pelvis and connective tissues of the kidney

42. _____ an abrupt reduction in kidney function characterized by oliguria and a sharp rise in nitrogenous compounds in the blood

43. _____ progressive condition resulting from gradual loss of nephrons

44. _____ intense kidney pain caused by destruction of the ureters by large kidney stones

45. _____ most common form of kidney disease caused by a delayed immune response to strepto-coccal infection

46. _____ albumin in the urine

47. _____ inflammation of the urethra that commonly results from bacterial infection

a.   pyelonephritis
b.   renal colic
c.   renal calculi
d.   acute glomerulonephritis
e.   proteinuria
f.   uremia
g.   neurogenic bladder
h.   acute renal failure
i.   hydronephrosis
j.   chronic renal failure
k.   cystitis
l.   urethritis

******If you had difficulty with this section, review pages **850-853**

Student Name _____

Crossword Puzzle

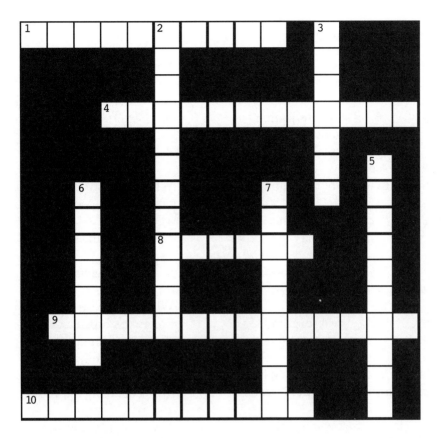

Across

1. Capillary network in renal corpuscles
4. Movement of molecules back into the blood
8. Tube from kidney to bladder
9. Mouth of nephron (two words)
10. Outer region of kidney (two words)

Down

2. Inner region of kidney (two words)
3. Opening from bladder to exterior
5. Osmotic concentration of a solution
6. Functional unit of kidney
7. Amount of substance removed from blood by kidneys per minute

APPLYING WHAT YOU KNOW

48. Mr. Dietz, an accident victim, was admitted to the hospital several hours ago. His chart indicates that he had been hemorrhaging at the scene of the accident. Nurse Petersen has been closely monitoring his urinary output and has noted that it has dropped to 10 ml/hr (the normal urine output for a healthy adult is approximately 30 to 60 ml/hr). What might explain this drop in urine output?

49. Christine developed chronic renal failure. Describe the progression of each of the three phases of chronic renal failure.

DID YOU KNOW?

- If the tubules in a kidney were stretched and untangled, there would be 70 miles of them.
- While examining urine, German chemist Hennig Brand discovered phosphorus.

ONE LAST QUICK CHECK ✔

Multiple Choice—select the best answer.

50. Which of the following processes is used by the artificial kidney to remove waste materials from the blood?
    a. pinocytosis
    b. dialysis
    c. catheterization
    d. active transport

51. Failure of the kidneys to remove wastes from the blood will result in which of the following?
    a. retention
    b. anuria
    c. incontinence
    d. uremia

52. Hydrogen ions are transferred from blood into the urine during which of the following processes?
    a. secretion
    b. filtration
    c. reabsorption
    d. all of the above

53. Which of the following conditions would be considered normal in an infant under 2 years of age?
    a. retention
    b. cystitis
    c. incontinence
    d. anuria

54. Which of the following steps involved in urine formation allows the blood to retain most body nutrients?
    a. secretion
    b. filtration
    c. reabsorption
    d. all of the above

55. Voluntary control of micturition is achieved by the action of which of the following?
    a. internal urethral sphincter
    b. external urethral sphincter
    c. trigone
    d. bladder muscles

56. What is the structure that carries urine from the kidney to the bladder called?
    a. urethra
    b. Bowman's capsule
    c. ureter
    d. renal pelvis

57. What are the capillary loops contained within Bowman's capsule called?
    a. convoluted tubules
    b. glomeruli
    c. limbs of Henle
    d. collecting ducts

58. The triangular divisions of the medulla of the kidney are known as:
    a. pyramids.
    b. papillae.
    c. calyces.
    d. nephrons.

59. The trigone is located in the:
    a. kidney.
    b. bladder.
    c. ureter.
    d. urethra.

269

Student Name_____

Matching—select the best answer from the right column to describe the terms on the left.

60. _____ hematuria

61. _____ anuria

62. _____ nephritis

63. _____ micturition

64. _____ oliguria

65. _____ polyuria

66. _____ incontinence

67. _____ proteinuria

68. _____ rugae

69. _____ urethra

70. _____ BUN

a. involuntary voiding
b. passes through prostate gland
c. absence of urine
d. urination
e. blood in the urine
f. inflammation of the kidney
g. large amount of protein in urine
h. large amount of urine
i. folds that line the bladder
j. scanty amount of urine
k. test for renal dysfunction

CHAPTER 29

FLUID AND ELECTROLYTE BALANCE

Referring to the very first chapter in your text, you will recall that survival depends on the body's ability to maintain or restore homeostasis. Specifically, *homeostasis* means that the body fluids remain constant within very narrow limits. These fluids are classified as either intracellular fluid (ICF) or extracellular fluid (ECF). As their names imply, intracellular fluid lies within the cells and extracellular fluid is located outside the cells. A balance between these two fluids is maintained by several body mechanisms. Among them are: 1) the adjustment of fluid output to fluid intake under normal circumstances; 2) the concentration of electrolytes; 3) the capillary blood pressure; and 4) the concentration of proteins in the blood. Comprehension of how these mechanisms maintain and restore fluid balance is necessary for an understanding of the complexities of homeostasis and its relationship to the survival of the individual.

I OVERVIEW OF FLUID AND ELECTROLYTE BALANCE

Multiple Choice—select the best answer.

1. The majority of total body water is found in the:
   a. plasma.
   b. interstitial fluid.
   c. intracellular fluid.
   d. extracellular fluid.

2. The most abundant intracellular cation is:
   a. Na^+.   c. K^+.
   b. Cl^-.   d. Mg^{++}.

3. The most abundant extracellular cation is:
   a. Na^+.   c. K^+.
   b. Cl^-.   d. Mg^{++}.

4. The most abundant anion in extracellular fluids is:
   a. Na^+.   c. K^+.
   b. Cl^-.   d. Mg^{++}.

5. Electrolyte reactivity is measured in:
   a. mg/100 L.
   b. milliequivalents.
   c. mEq/L.
   d. both b and c.

6. Which of the following mechanisms varies fluid output so that it equals input?
   a. antidiuretic device
   b. aldosterone mechanism
   c. renin-angiotensin mechanism
   d. both b and c

7. Which of the following is *NOT* one of the seven basic solutions used for parenteral therapy?
   a. ammonium chloride
   b. carbohydrate in water
   c. liquid protein
   d. Ringer's solution

True or false

8. _____ Obese people have a higher water content per kilogram of body weight than slender people.

9. _____ When compared chemically, plasma and interstitial fluid are nearly identical.

10. _____ Fluid intake usually equals fluid output.

11. _____ Electrolytes are substances that bind in water.

12. _____ Thirst is associated with any condition that decreases total volume of body water.

13. _____ Water exits the body only through the urinary and digestive systems.

14. _____ *Hypervolemia* refers to excess blood volume.

******If you had difficulty with this section, review pages **857-863**

II MECHANISMS THAT MAINTAIN HOMEOSTASIS OF TOTAL FLUID VOLUME

Multiple Choice—select the best answer.

15. The two factors that determine urine volume are:
    a. the amount of ADH and aldosterone secretion.
    b. the amount of ACTH and ADH secretion.
    c. fluid intake and ADH secretion.
    d. the glomerular filtration rate and the rate of water reabsorption by the renal tubules.

16. Which of the following is an example of obligatory fluid output?
    a. water vapor in expired air
    b. water diffusion through the skin
    c. both a and b
    d. none of the above

True or false

17. _____ If a person takes nothing by mouth for several days, fluid output decreases to zero to compensate and maintain homeostasis.

18. _____ Dehydration is often detected by loss of skin elasticity.

******If you had difficulty with this section, review pages **863-865**

Student Name_____

III REGULATION OF WATER AND ELECTROLYTE LEVELS IN PLASMA, INTERSTITIAL FLUID, AND INTRACELLULAR FLUID

Multiple Choice—select the best answer.

19. Blood hydrostatic pressure:
    a. tends to force fluid out of capillaries and into interstitial fluid.
    b. tends to force fluid out of interstitial fluid and into capillaries.
    c. allows for an equilibrium across the capillary membrane.
    d. none of the above.

20. Which of the following is *NOT* a symptom of severe dehydration?
    a. dim vision
    b. cessation of urine formation
    c. increased body temperature
    d. crackled skin

21. The formula representing Starling's law of the capillaries is:
    a. (BHP + BCOP) – (IFCOP + IFHP) = EFP.
    b. (BHP + IFHP) – (IFCOP + BCOP) = EFP.
    c. (BHP + IFCOP) – (IFHP + BCOP) = EFP.

22. Which large molecules are retained by the selectively permeable cell membrane?
    a. sodium ions   c. proteins
    b. potassium ions   d. water

True or false

23. _____ *Edema* can be defined as "the presence of abnormally large amounts of fluid in the intercellular spaces of the body."

24. _____ The most common cause of edema is glomerulonephritis.

25. _____ The most significant player regulating intracellular fluid composition is the plasma membrane.

26. _____ Osmotic pressure is influenced by large protein molecules in the intracellular fluid.

******If you had difficulty with this section, review pages **866-869**

IV REGULATION OF SODIUM AND POTASSIUM LEVELS IN BODY FLUIDS

True or false

27. _____ The release of ADH causes an increase in the reabsorption of sodium and water by the renal tubules.

28. _____ Over 8 liters of various internal secretions are produced daily.

29. _____ Potassium deficit is termed *hypokalemia*.

30. _____ Extracellular fluid depletion is said to be the "last line of defense" against dehydration.

31. _____ By volume, intestinal secretions are the largest sodium-containing internal secretions.

******If you had difficulty with this section, review pages **869-872**

V MECHANISMS OF DISEASE

Matching—identify the best answer on the right for the terms on the left.

32. _____ hypovolemia

33. _____ hyperkalemia

34. _____ hyponatremia

35. _____ diaphoresis

36. _____ hypervolemia

a. dehydration
b. excessive perspiration
c. excess fluid volume
d. increased serum potassium
e. decrease serum sodium

True or false

37. _____ Skin turgor is an important indicator of fluid volume stability.

38. _____ Cushing's syndrome can cause hypokalemia.

39. _____ Overuse of diuretics can result in hyponatremia.

40. _____ Hyperkalemia is *NOT* a serious threat to the body.

******If you had difficulty with this section, review pages **872-874**

Student Name_____

Crossword Puzzle

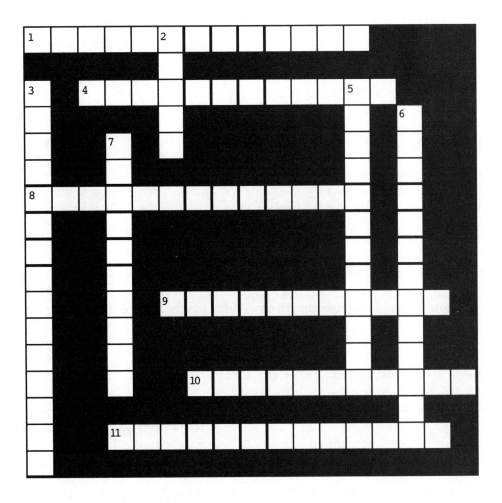

Across

1. Detect decreased pressure of blood when dehydration occurs
4. Fluid volume excess
8. Fluid located within cells
9. Excessive loss of fluid from the body
10. Low serum potassium
11. Water found outside the cells

Down

2. Swelling
3. MEq
5. Fluid that surrounds the cells
6. Chloride deficiency
7. Administration of fluids by injection

APPLYING WHAT YOU KNOW

41. Ms. Titus was asked to keep an accurate record of her fluid intake and output. She was concerned because the two did not balance, even though the physician assured her that she had no kidney pathology. What is a possible explanation for this?

42. Jack Sprat was 6' 5" and weighed 185 lbs. His wife was 5' 6" and weighed 185 lbs. Whose body contained more water?

DID YOU KNOW?

- The best fluid replacement drink is to add 1/2 tsp of table salt to one quart of water.
- If all of the water were drained from the body of an average 160-pound man, the body would weigh 64 pounds.

ONE LAST QUICK CHECK ✔

Circle the correct answer.

43. The largest volume of water by far lies (inside or outside) cells.

44. Interstitial fluid is (intracellular or extracellular).

45. Plasma is (intracellular or extracellular).

46. Obese people have a (lower or higher) water content per pound of body weight than thin people.

47. Infants have (more or less) water in comparison to body weight than adults of either sex.

48. In general, as age increases, the amount of water per pound of body weight (increases or decreases).

Multiple Choice—select the best answer.

49. Which one of the following is *NOT* a positively charged ion?
    a. chloride
    b. calcium
    c. sodium
    d. potassium

50. Which one of the following is *NOT* a negatively charged ion?
    a. chloride
    b. bicarbonate
    c. phosphate
    d. sodium

51. The smallest amount of water comes from:
    a. water in foods that are eaten.
    b. ingested food.
    c. water formed from catabolism.
    d. none of the above.

52. The greatest amount of water lost from the body is from the:
    a. lungs.
    b. skin by diffusion.
    c. skin by sweat.
    d. feces.
    e. kidneys.

53. Excessive water loss and fluid imbalance can result from which of the following?
    a. diarrhea
    b. vomiting
    c. severe burns
    d. all of the above

54. What factor is primarily responsible for moving water from interstitial fluid into blood?
    a. aldosterone secretions
    b. pressure in blood capillaries
    c. protein concentration of blood plasma
    d. antidiuretic hormone secretions

55. If blood sodium concentration decreases, what does blood volume do?
    a. increases
    b. decreases
    c. remains the same
    d. none of the above

56. Which of the following is true of body water?
    a. It is obtained from the liquids we drink.
    b. It is obtained from the foods we eat.
    c. It is formed by the catabolism of food.
    d. All of the above are true.

57. Edema may result from which of the following?
    a. retention of electrolytes
    b. decreased blood pressure
    c. increased concentration of blood plasma proteins
    d. all of the above

58. The most abundant and important positive plasma ion is which of the following?
    a. sodium.   c. calcium.
    b. chloride.   d. oxygen.

59. Which of the following is true when extracellular fluid volume decreases?
    a. aldosterone secretion increases
    b. kidney tubule reabsorption of sodium increases
    c. urine volume decreases
    d. all of the above are true

True or false

60. _____ Interstitial fluid contains hardly any protein anions.

61. _____ No net transfer of water occurs between blood and interstitial fluid as long as effective filtration (EFP) equals 0.

62. _____ Any change in the solute concentration of extracellular fluid will have a direct effect on water movement across the cell membrane in one direction or another.

CHAPTER 30

ACID-BASE BALANCE

It has been established in previous chapters that an equilibrium between intracellular and extra-cellular fluid volume must exist for homeostasis. Equally important to homeostasis is the chemical acid-base balance of the body fluids. The degree of acidity or alkalinity of a body fluid is expressed in pH value. The neutral point, where a fluid would be neither acid nor alkaline, is pH 7. Increasing acidity is expressed as less than 7, and increasing alkalinity as greater than 7. Examples of body fluids that are acidic are gastric juice (1.6) and urine (6.0). Blood, on the other hand, is considered alkaline with a pH of 7.4.

Buffers are substances that prevent a sharp change in the pH of a fluid when an acid or base is added to it. They are one of several mechanisms that are constantly monitoring the pH of fluids in the body. If for any reason these mechanisms do not function properly, a pH imbalance occurs. These two kinds of imbalances are known as *alkalosis* and *acidosis*.

Maintaining the acid-base balance of body fluids is a matter of vital importance. If this balance varies even slightly, necessary chemical and cellular reactions cannot occur. Your review of this chapter is necessary to understand the delicate fluid balance necessary for survival.

I   MECHANISMS THAT CONTROL pH OF BODY FLUIDS

Multiple Choice—select the best answer.

1. As pH goes down:
    a.   a solution becomes more basic.
    b.   a solution's hydrogen ion concentration decreases.
    c.   a solution becomes more acidic.
    d.   a solution thickens.

2. The most acidic body substance of the following is:
    a.   gastric juice.   c.   bile.
    b.   pancreatic juice. d.   urine.

3. Which of the following is an acid-forming food?
    a.   grapefruit   c.   orange juice
    b.   meat   d.   coffee

4. Which of the following are base-forming foods?
    a.   fruits   c.   eggs
    b.   vegetables   d.   both a and b

5. Which of the following describes the narrow pH range of blood?
    a.   7.21 to 7.49   c.   7.36 to 7.41
    b.   7.00 to 7.20   d.   7.50 to 7.77

6. An acid-forming element is:
    a.   sulfur.   c.   potassium.
    b.   calcium.   d.   sodium.

7. Acidic ketone bodies are associated with cellular metabolism of:
    a.   proteins.   c.   fats.
    b.   carbohydrates.   d.   minerals.

True or false

8. _____   Blood is slightly alkaline.

9. _____   Citrus fruits, such as oranges and grapefruit, have a significant effect on acid-base balance.

10. _____   Chemical buffer systems are fast-acting.

11. _____   The carbon dioxide present in venous blood causes it to become slightly more basic than arterial blood.

12. _____   A vegetarian diet would tend to produce an alkaline state in body fluids.

13. _____   The respiratory and urinary systems can serve as physiological buffer systems.

******If you had difficulty with this section, review pages **878-880**

II   BUFFER MECHANISMS FOR CONTROLLING pH OF BODY FLUIDS

Multiple Choice—select the best answer.

14. Potassium salts of hemoglobin inside the red blood cell primarily buffer:
    a.   carbonic acid.   c.   phosphoric acid.
    b.   lactic acid.   d.   sulfuric acid.

15. A serious complication of vomiting is:
    a.   carbonic acid.
    b.   bicarbonate deficit.
    c.   metabolic alkalosis.
    d.   metabolic acidosis.

True or false

16. _____   The process of exchanging a bicarbonate ion formed in the red blood cell with a chloride ion from the plasma is called *chloride shift.*

17. _____   Buffers control pH in a manner that requires no other mechanism of pH control to maintain homeostasis.

18. _____   The blood buffer system normally converts a strong acid to a weak acid.

19. _____   Bicarbonate loading by athletes has proven to be mildly successful in diminishing the muscle soreness and fatigue associated with strenuous exercise.

20. _____   Elevated CO_2 levels result in increased formation of carbonic acid in red blood cells.

******If you had difficulty with this section, review pages **880-884**

Student Name_____

III RESPIRATORY AND URINARY MECHANISMS OF pH CONTROL

Multiple Choice—select the best answer.

21. With each expiration, which substances leave the body?
    a. CO_2
    b. H_2O
    c. O_2
    d. both a and b

22. All of the following would increase the respiration rate *EXCEPT*:
    a. decreased blood pH.
    b. decreased carbon dioxide.
    c. increased arterial blood CO_2.
    d. all increase respirations.

23. The kidney tubules secrete hydrogen ions in exchange of:
    a. K^+.
    b. Na^+.
    c. Ca^{++}.
    d. Cl^-.

24. Acidosis causes:
    a. hyperventilation.
    b. hypoventilation.
    c. an increase in blood pH.
    d. increase in potassium ion excretion.

25. A decrease in blood pH accelerates tubule excretion of:
    a. hydrogen.
    b. ammonia.
    c. both a and b.
    d. none of the above.

True or false

26. _____ Prolonged hyperventilation may increase blood pH enough to cause alkalosis.

27. _____ Respiratory mechanisms are much more effective in expelling hydrogen ions than are urinary mechanisms.

28. _____ The more hydrogen ions secreted by the renal tubule, the fewer potassium ions secreted.

29. _____ Intravenous administration of normal saline is used for metabolic acidosis.

30. _____ An increase in blood pH above normal (alkalosis) causes hypoventilation.

******If you had difficulty with this section, review pages **884-888**

IV MECHANISMS OF DISEASE

Matching—write the letter of the correct term on the blank next to the appropriate definition.

31. _____ result of untreated diabetes

32. _____ sodium lactate

33. _____ bicarbonate deficit

34. _____ bicarbonate excess

35. _____ rapid breathing

36. _____ carbonic acid excess

37. _____ carbonic acid deficit

a. metabolic acidosis
b. metabolic alkalosis
c. respiratory acidosis
d. respiratory alkalosis
e. treatment for metabolic and respiratory acidosis
f. uncompensated metabolic acidosis
g. hyperventilation

******If you had difficulty with this section, review pages **888-891**

Crossword Puzzle

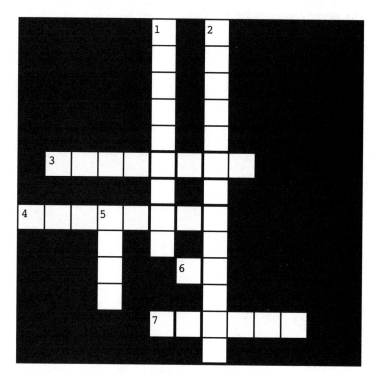

Across

3. May be caused by prolonged hypoventilation
4. pH greater than 7.0
6. Degree of acidity or alkalinity
7. Prevents swing in pH

Down

1. Complication of vomiting
2. Maintains electrical neutrality of red blood cells (two words)
5. pH less than 7.0

APPLYING WHAT YOU KNOW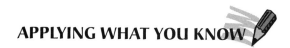

38. Desi was pregnant and was experiencing repeated vomiting episodes for several days. Her doctor became concerned, admitted her to the hospital, and began intravenous administrations of normal saline. How will this help Desi?

39. Ginny had a minor bladder infection. She had heard that this is often the result of the urine being less acidic than necessary and that she should drink cranberry juice to correct the acid problem. She had no cranberry juice, so she decided to substitute orange juice. What was wrong with this substitution?

DID YOU KNOW?

• English ships carried limes to protect the sailors from scurvy. American ships carried cranberries.

Student Name_____

ONE LAST QUICK CHECK ✔

Multiple Choice—select the best answer.

40. What happens as blood flows through lung capillaries?
    a. Carbonic acid in blood decreases.
    b. Hydrogen ions in blood decrease.
    c. Blood pH increases from venous to arterial blood.
    d. All of the above are true.

41. Which of the following organs is considered the most effective regulator of blood carbonic acid levels?
    a. kidneys   c. lungs
    b. intestines   d. stomach

42. Which of the following organs is considered the most effective regulator of blood pH?
    a. kidneys   c. lungs
    b. intestines   d. stomach

43. What is the pH of the blood?
    a. 7.0 to 8.0   c. 6.2 to 7.4
    b. 7.6 to 7.8   d. 7.3 to 7.4

44. If the ratio of sodium bicarbonate to carbonate ions is lowered (perhaps 10 to 1) and blood pH is also lowered, what is the condition called?
    a. uncompensated metabolic acidosis
    b. uncompensated metabolic alkalosis
    c. compensated metabolic acidosis
    d. compensated metabolic alkalosis

45. If a person hyperventilates for a given time period, which of the following will probably develop?
    a. metabolic acidosis
    b. metabolic alkalosis
    c. respiratory acidosis
    d. respiratory alkalosis

46. Which of the following is a characteristic of a buffer system in the body?
    a. It occurs in the case of prolonged vomiting.
    b. It results when the bicarbonate ion is present in excess.
    c. Therapy includes intravenous administration of normal saline.
    d. All of the above are true.

47. In the presence of a strong acid which of the following is true?
    a. Sodium bicarbonate will react to produce carbonic acid.
    b. Sodium bicarbonate will react to produce more sodium bicarbonate.
    c. Carbonic acid will react to produce sodium bicarbonate.
    d. Carbonic acid will react to form more carbonic acid.

Matching—select the best answer for each item on the left.

48. _____ pH lower than 7.0

49. _____ pH higher than 7.0

50. _____ buffers

51. _____ decrease in respirations

52. _____ increase in respirations

53. _____ metabolic acidosis

54. _____ metabolic alkalosis

55. _____ lactic acid

a. untreated diabetes mellitus
b. excessive vomiting
c. alkaline solution
d. "fixed" acid
e. barbiturate overdose
f. fever
g. acidic solution
h. prevent sharp pH changes

CHAPTER 31

MALE REPRODUCTIVE SYSTEM

The reproductive system consists of those organs that participate in propagating the species. It is a unique body system in that its organs differ between the two sexes, and yet the goal of creating a new being is the same. Of interest also is the fact that this system is the only one not necessary to the survival of the individual, and yet survival of the species depends on the proper functioning of the reproductive organs. The male reproductive system is divided into the external genitals, testes, duct system, and accessory glands. The testes, or gonads, are considered essential organs because they produce the sex cells—sperm—which join with the female sex cells—ova—to form a new human

being. They also secrete testosterone, the male sex hormone, which is responsible for the physical transformation of a boy to a man.

Sperm are formed in the testes by the seminiferous tubules. From there they enter a long narrow duct, the epididymis. They continue onward through the vas deferens into the ejaculatory duct, down the urethra, and out of the body. Throughout this journey, various glands secrete substances that add motility to the sperm and create a chemical environment conducive to reproduction.

A knowledge of the male reproductive system is necessary to understand the role of the male and the phenomena necessary to produce an offspring.

I MALE REPRODUCTIVE ORGANS

Multiple Choice—select the best answer.

1. The male gonads are known as the:
    a. testes.
    c. epididymis.
    b. prostate.
    d. perineum.

2. The region within a "triangle" created by the ischial tuberosities and the symphysis is the:
    a. anal triangle.
    b. urogenital triangle.
    c. perineal triangle.
    d. testicular triangle.

3. Which of the following is *NOT* a supporting structure?
    a. penis
    c. prostate
    b. scrotum
    d. spermatic cord

4. Each testicular lobule contains:
    a. seminiferous tubules.
    b. interstitial cells.
    c. Leydig cells.
    d. all of the above.

5. The blood-testis is formed by tight junctions between which cells?
    a. Leydig cells
    c. Sertoli cells
    b. interstitial cells
    d. all of the above

6. Sperm production occurs in the:
    a. seminiferous tubules.
    b. interstitial cells.
    c. Sertoli cells.
    d. prostate.

7. Which hormone is responsible for the stimulation of sperm production?
    a. FSH
    c. testosterone
    b. LH
    d. both b and c

8. Which of the following is *NOT* a specific region of a spermatozoon?
    a. head
    c. body
    b. middle piece
    d. tail

True or false

9. _____ The testes perform two primary functions: spermatogenesis and secretion of hormones.

10. _____ Testosterone is secreted by the anterior pituitary.

11. _____ Testicular cancer is the most common neoplasm in elderly men.

12. _____ *Capacitation* refers to the release of enzymes contained within the acrosome.

13. _____ *Sertoli cells* and *efferent ductules* are synonymous.

14. _____ The bulbourethral glands are a supporting structure of the male reproductive system.

15. _____ Testosterone is sometimes referred to as "the anabolic hormone."

Labeling—label the following sagittal section of the pelvis depicting placement of male reproductive organs.

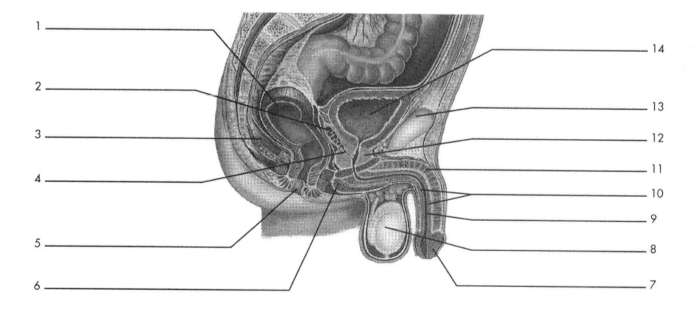

Student Name_____

Labeling—using the terms provided, label the following tubules of the testis and epididymis.

seminiferous tubules   septum   ductus deferens (vas)
tunica albuguinea   spermatic cord (nerves and   testis
epididymis   blood vessels
lobule

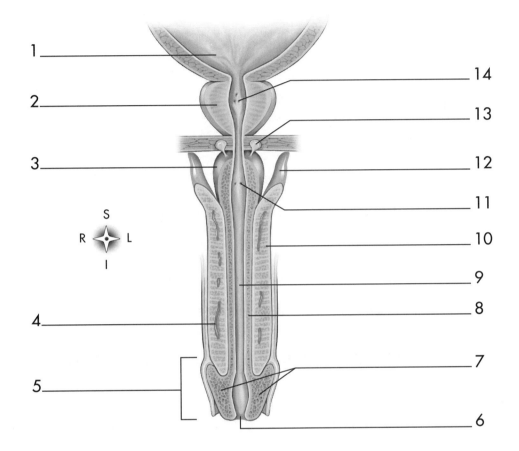

******If you had difficulty with this section, review pages **896-902**

II   REPRODUCTIVE DUCTS AND ACCESSORY REPRODUCTIVE GLANDS

Multiple Choice—select the best answer.

16. Which of the following is *NOT* a function of
     the epididymis?
     a.   a duct through which sperm travel on
          their journey to the exterior of the body
     b.   production of spermatozoa
     c.   maturation of spermatozoa
     d.   secretion of a portion of seminal fluid

17. The ejaculatory ducts are formed by the union
     of the:
     a.   seminal vesicles and ampulla.
     b.   vas deferens and urethra.
     c.   seminal vesicles and vas deferens.
     d.   seminal vesicles and urethra.

18. Which of the following accessory reproductive glands produce(s) a secretion rich in fructose?
    a. seminal vesicles
    b. prostate
    c. bulbourethral gland
    d. Cowper's gland

19. Which of the following accessory glands secrete(s) an alkaline substance?
    a. seminal vesicles
    b. bulbourethral gland
    c. all of the above
    d. none of the above

20. The most common cancer in American men is cancer of the:
    a. testes.
    b. prostate.
    c. penis.
    d. urinary bladder.

True or false

21. _____ The duct of the vas deferens is an extension of the tail of the epididymis.

22. _____ Sperm may be stored in the epididymis for up to a month with no loss of fertility.

23. _____ A vasectomy is a procedure intended to render a man sterile.

24. _____ Prostate specific antigen (PSA) is present in the blood of men with prostate cancer.

******If you had difficulty with this section, review pages **900-905**

III   SUPPORTING STRUCTURES, SEMINAL FLUID, AND MALE FERTILITY

Multiple Choice—select the best answer.

25. The greatest amount of seminal fluid is secreted by the:
    a. prostate.
    b. testes.
    c. seminal vesicles.
    d. epididymis.

26. Elevation of the testes is caused by contraction of the:
    a. dartos fascia and muscle.
    b. cremaster muscle.
    c. corpora cavernosa.
    d. corpus spongiosum.

27. Functional sterility results when sperm count falls below:
    a. 5 million/ml of semen.
    b. 25 million/ml of semen.
    c. 100 million/ml of semen.
    d. 500 million/ml of semen.

28. Which of the following factors related to sperm does *NOT* affect male fertility?
    a. size
    b. shape
    c. texture
    d. motility

True or false

29. _____ The urethra lies within the corpora cavernosa.

30. _____ The terminal end of the corpus spongiosum forms the glans penis.

31. _____ *Emission* and *ejaculation* are synonymous terms.

Student Name _____

Labeling—using the terms provided, label the following parts of the penis.

corpus cavernosum
bulb
glans penis
bulbourethral gland
deep artery

openings of ejaculatory ducts
prostate
urethra
crus penis
corpus spongiosum

foreskin (prepuce)
external urethral orifice
bladder
opening of Cowper glands

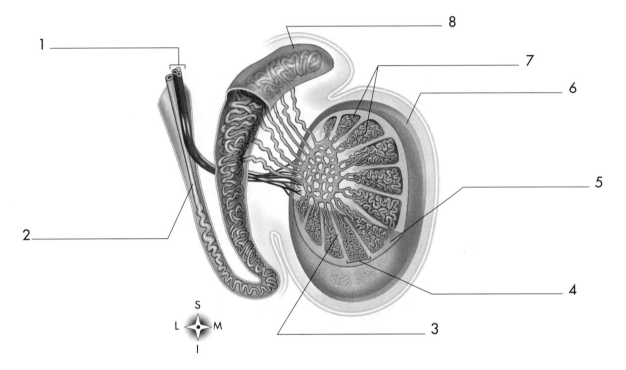

******If you had difficulty with this section, review pages **905-907**

IV   MECHANISMS OF DISEASE

Fill in the blanks.

32.   Decreased sperm production is called _____.

33.   Testes normally descend into the scrotum about _____ before birth.

34.   If a baby is born with undescended testes, a condition called _____ results.

35.   A common noncancerous condition of the prostate in older men is known as _____

_____ _____.

36.   _____ is a condition in which the foreskin fits so tightly over the glans that it

cannot retract.

37.   Failure to achieve an erection of the penis is called _____ or _____

_____.

38.   An accumulation of fluid in the scrotum is known as a _____.

39.   An _____ _____ results when the intestines push through the weak area of the abdominal wall that separates the abdominopelvic cavity from the scrotum.

******If you had difficulty with this section, review pages **907-909**

Crossword Puzzle

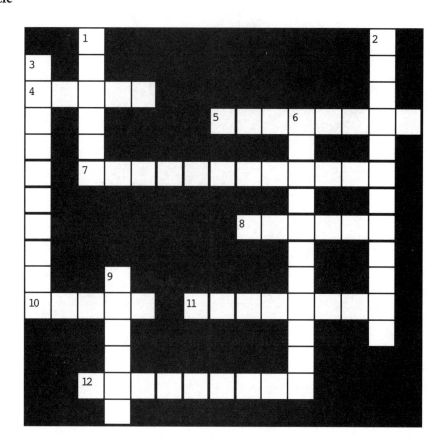

Across

4.   Male organ of copulation
5.   Accessory reproductive gland
7.   Provide protection for germ cells (two words)
8.   Sex cell
10.   Ejaculate from the penis
11.   Male sex hormone
12.   Reproductive organs

Down

1.   Sex glands where reproductive cells are formed
2.   Androgen
3.   Genital duct
6.   Mature male gametes
9.   Male gonads

APPLYING WHAT YOU KNOW

40.   Trent is an infant who was born with undescended testes. What is the clinical term for his condition? How easily is this diagnosed? What can Trent's doctor do to treat his condition? How serious is his condition if left untreated? What are his chances of normal testicular and sexual development?

Student Name _____

41. John noticed an unusual swelling of his scrotum. What possible conditions may he be experiencing? Also, he did notice that the swelling occurred after a day of heavy lifting while moving out of his apartment. Based on this detail, which condition is he more likely to be experiencing? Describe the anatomy of this condition. How will the doctor treat John?

DID YOU KNOW?

- The testes produce approximately 50 million sperm per day. Every 2 to 3 months they produce enough cells to populate the entire earth.
- Men reach the peak of their sexual powers in their late teens or early twenties, and then begin to slowly decline. Women however, do not reach their sexual peak until their late twenties or early thirties, and then remain at this level through their late fifties or early sixties.

ONE LAST QUICK CHECK ✔

Multiple Choice—select the best answer.

42. Sperm cells are suspended outside the body cavity to do which of the following?
    a. protect them from trauma
    b. keep them cooler
    c. keep them supplied with a greater number of blood vessels
    d. protect them from infection

43. What is the removal of the foreskin from the glans penis called?
    a. vasectomy   c. circumcision
    b. sterilization   d. ligation

44. The testes are surrounded by a tough membrane called the:
    a. ductus deferens.
    b. tunica albuginea.
    c. septum.
    d. seminiferous membrane.

45. The _____ lie near the septa that separate the lobules.
    a. ductus deferens   c. interstitial cells
    b. sperm   d. nerves

46. Sperm are found in the walls of the:
    a. seminiferous tubule.
    b. interstitial cells.
    c. septum.
    d. blood vessels.

47. The scrotum provides an environment that is approximately _____ for the testes.
    a. the same as the body temperature
    b. 5° warmer than the body temperature
    c. 3° warmer than the body temperature
    d. 3° cooler than the body temperature

48. The _____ produce(s) testosterone.
    a. seminiferous tubules
    b. prostate gland
    c. bulbourethral glands
    d. interstitial cells

49. The part of the sperm that contains genetic information that will be inherited is the:
    a. tail.   c. middle piece.
    b. acrosome.   d. head.

50. Which one of the following is *NOT* a function of testosterone?
    a. It causes a deepening of the voice.
    b. It promotes the development of the male accessory organs.
    c. It has a stimulatory effect on protein catabolism.
    d. It causes greater muscular development and strength.

51. Sperm production is called:
    a. spermatogonia.   c. spermatogenesis.
    b. spermatids.   d. spermatocyte.

52. The section of the sperm that contains enzymes that enable it to break down the covering of the ovum and permit entry should contact occur is the:
    a. acrosome.   c. tail.
    b. middle piece.   d. stem.

Matching—insert the letter in the space next to the appropriate description.

53. _____ continuation of ducts that start in the epididymis

54. _____ erectile tissue

55. _____ also known as *bulbourethral*

56. _____ narrow tube that lies along the top and behind the testes

57. _____ doughnut-shaped gland beneath the bladder

58. _____ union of the vas deferens with the ducts from the seminal vesicles

59. _____ mixture of sperm and secretions of accessory sex glands

60. _____ contributes 60% of the seminal fluid volume

61. _____ removed during circumcision

62. _____ enclose the vas deferens, blood vessels, lymphatics, and nerves

a. epididymis
b. vas deferens
c. ejaculatory duct
d. prepuce
e. seminal vesicles
f. prostate gland
g. Cowper's gland
h. corpus spongiosum
i. semen
j. spermatic cord

CHAPTER 32

FEMALE REPRODUCTIVE SYSTEM

The female reproductive system is truly extraordinary and diverse. It produces ova, receives the penis and sperm during intercourse, is the site of conception, houses and nourishes the embryo during the prenatal development, and nourishes the infant after birth.

Because of its diversity, the physiology of the female is generally considered to be more complex than that of the male. Much of the activity of this system revolves around the menstrual cycle and the monthly preparation that the female undergoes for a possible pregnancy.

The organs of this system are divided into essential organs and accessory organs of reproduction. The essential organs of the female are the ovaries. Just as with the male, the essential organs of the female are referred to as the *gonads*. The gonads of the female produce ova and are responsible for producing hormones necessary for the appearance of the secondary sex characteristics.

The menstrual cycle of the female typically covers a period of 28 days. Each cycle consists of three phases: menstrual period, postmenstrual phase, and premenstrual phase. Changes in the blood levels of the hormones that are responsible for the menstrual cycle also cause physical and emotional changes in the female. A knowledge of these phenomena and the female system are responsible to complete your understanding of the reproductive system.

I OVERVIEW OF THE FEMALE REPRODUCTIVE SYSTEM

Multiple Choice—select the best answer.

1.   Which of the following is **NOT** an accessory organ of reproduction in women?
    a.   ovaries   c.   vagina
    b.   uterus   d.   vulva

2.   The term that refers to the external female genitalia is:
    a.   vagina.
    b.   vulva.
    c.   perineum.
    d.   urogenital triangle.

True or false

3.   _____   Mammary glands are referred to as *additional sex glands*.

4.   _____   An episiotomy is associated with the perineum.

Labeling—match each term with its corresponding number in the following frontal section of the female pelvic organs.

fundus of uterus   cervix of uterus   body of uterus
cervical canal   myometrium   fimbriae
vagina   fallopian tube (uterine tube)   follicle
endometrium

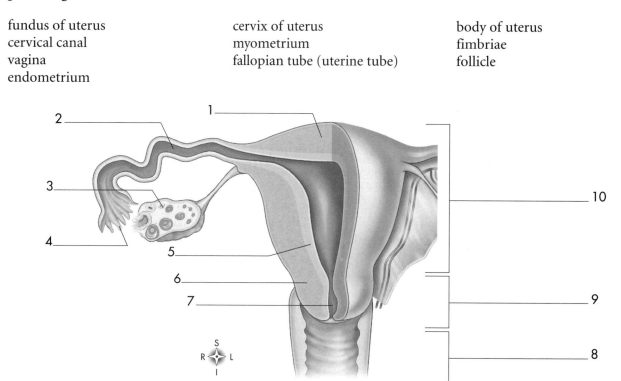

Labeling—label the following sagittal section of the pelvis showing the female reproductive organs.

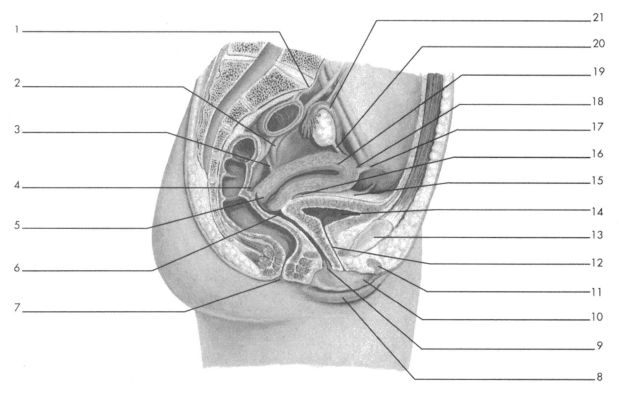

******If you had difficulty with this section, review pages **912-914**

Student Name _____

II INTERNAL FEMALE GENITALS

Multiple Choice—select the best answer.

5. The ovaries are homologous to the male:
    a. prostate.
    c. vas deferens.
    b. testes.
    d. seminal vesicle.

6. Cells of ovarian tissue secrete:
    a. estradiol.
    c. progesterone.
    b. estrone.
    d. all of the above.

7. The bulging upper component of the uterus is the:
    a. cervix.
    c. body.
    b. fundus.
    d. fornix.

8. The innermost lining of the uterus is the:
    a. endometrium.
    b. myometrium.
    c. perimetrium.
    d. parietal peritoneum.

9. The portion of the uterus that opens into the vagina is the:
    a. internal os.
    c. fornix.
    b. external os.
    d. cervix.

10. The fringelike projections of the uterine tubes are called the:
    a. isthmus.
    c. infundibulum.
    b. ampulla.
    d. fimbriae.

Matching—insert the letter of the correct structure in the blank next to the description.

11. _____ isthmus

12. _____ myometrium

13. _____ terminal end of birth canal

14. _____ site of menstruation

15. _____ intermediate portion called the *ampulla*

16. _____ consists of body, fundus, and cervix

17. _____ site of fertilization

18. _____ also known as *oviduct*

19. _____ receptacle for sperm

a. uterine tubes
b. uterus
c. vagina

True or false

20. _____ Ovarian follicles contain oocytes.

21. _____ *Retroflexion* refers to the normal position of the uterus in relation to the vagina and urinary bladder.

22. _____ The afterbirth is also referred to as the *fornix*.

23. _____ The "G spot" may be responsible for the female "ejaculate" reported to occur in some women during orgasm.

******If you had difficulty with this section, review pages **914-920**

III   EXTERNAL FEMALE GENITALS AND BREASTS

Multiple Choice—select the best answer.

24. The female organ that is homologous to the male corpora cavernosa and glans penis is the:
    a. labia minora.   c. clitoris.
    b. labia majora.   d. vulva.

25. The area between the labia minora is the:
    a. vulva.   c. mons pubis.
    b. vestibule.   d. "G spot."

26. Which of the following is *NOT* a structure of the vulva?
    a. vagina   c. urinary meatus
    b. labia majora   d. vestibule

27. Which of the following hormones are *NOT* involved with lactation?
    a. thyroxin   c. estrogen
    b. oxytocin   d. progesterone

True or false

28. _____ The mons pubis serves as a boundary between the external and internal female genitals.

29. _____ The larger the breasts, the greater amount of glandular tissue present.

30. _____ Milk secretion from the breasts begins about 3 or 4 hours after giving birth.

31. _____ Milk ejection is stimulated by oxytocin.

32. _____ Human milk provides active immunity to the offspring in the form of maternal antibodies present in the milk.

******If you had difficulty with this section, review pages **920-922**

IV   FEMALE REPRODUCTIVE CYCLES

Multiple Choice—select the best answer.

33. Menses occurs on days _____ of a new cycle.
    a. 1 to 5
    b. 1 to 14
    c. 6 to 14
    d. none of the above

34. Ovulation usually occurs on cycle day _____ of a 28-day cycle.
    a. 1   c. 14
    b. 7   d. 28

35. Failure to have a menstrual cycle is termed:
    a. infertility.   c. menses.
    b. menarche.   d. amenorrhea.

36. Which of the following hormones triggers ovulation?
    a. estrogen
    b. progesterone
    c. luteinizing hormone
    d. follicle-stimulating hormone

37. The average age at which menopause occurs is:
    a. 40 years.   c. 55 to 60 years.
    b. 45 to 50 years.   d. 60 to 65 years.

Student Name _____

True or false

38. _____ The time of ovulation can be easily predicted by simply knowing the length of a previous cycle.

39. _____ Cyclical changes in the ovaries result from cyclical changes in the amounts of gonadotropins secreted by the anterior pituitary.

40. _____ Contraceptive pills and implants function by preventing ovulation.

41. _____ The first menstrual flow is known as the *climacteric*.

42. _____ The LH surge occurs at the beginning of the menstrual cycle.

******If you had difficulty with this section, review pages **922-930**

V   MECHANISMS OF DISEASE

Matching—choose the correct response.

43. _____ often occurs from STDs or from a "yeast infection"

44. _____ benign tumor of smooth muscle and fibrous connective tissue; also known as a *fibroid tumor*

45. _____ absence of normal menstruation

46. _____ yeast infection characterized by leukorrhea

47. _____ caused by infestation by the itch mite

48. _____ venereal disease

49. _____ results from pathogenic organisms transmitted from another person; e.g., STD

50. _____ painful menstruation

51. _____ asymptomatic in most women and nearly all men

52. _____ results from a hormonal imbalance rather than from an infection or disease condition

53. _____ screening test for cervical cancer

54. _____ causes blisters on the skin of the genitals; the blisters may disappear temporarily, but reoccur, especially as a result of stress

a. amenorrhea
b. dysmenorrhea
c. exogenous infection
d. DUB
e. myoma
f. vaginitis
g. sexually transmitted disease (STD)
h. Candidiasis
i. scabies
j. Pap smear
k. genital herpes
l. Trichomoniasis

******If you had difficulty with this section, review pages **930-933**

Crossword Puzzle

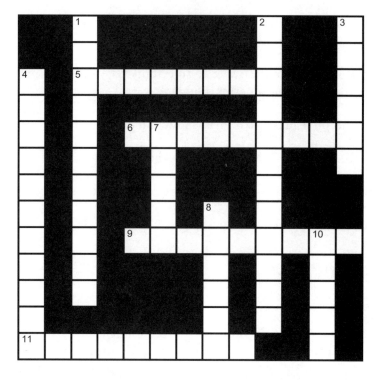

Across

5. Female sex hormone
6. Release of ovum
9. Secretion of milk
11. Climacteric

Down

1. Fallopian tube (two words)
2. Menarche
3. Lower portion of birth canal
4. Lining of uterus
7. External genitalia
8. Womb
10. Female gonad

APPLYING WHAT YOU KNOW

55. Prior to having children, Carmela used oral contraceptives to prevent an unwanted pregnancy with her husband. Describe the physiological mechanism of action of oral contraceptives. After having three children by the age of 35, the couple decided that Carmela would have a tubal ligation. Describe how this procedure prevents pregnancy.

56. Mary contracted gonorrhea. By the time she made an appointment to see her doctor, it had spread to her abdominal organs. How is this possible when gonorrhea is a disease of the reproductive system?

DID YOU KNOW?

- During menstruation, the sensitivity of a woman's middle finger is reduced.
- During pregnancy, the uterus expands to 500 times its normal size.
- There are an estimated 925,000 daily occurrences of STD transmission and 550,000 daily pregnancies worldwide.

Student Name _____

ONE LAST QUICK CHECK ✔

Matching—select the best answer for the descriptions.

57. _____ essential organ of reproduction

58. _____ external reproductive organ

59. _____ pregnancy in a location other than the uterus

60. _____ term of pregnancy

61. _____ inflammation of the uterine tube

62. _____ erotic zone

63. _____ middle pain

64. _____ menopause

65. _____ displaced endometrial tissue

66. _____ thin, yellow secretion

a. salpingitis
b. vulva
c. mittelschmerz
d. colostrum
e. ectopic
f. G spot
g. ovary
h. endometriosis
i. climacteric
j. gestation

Fill in the blanks.

67. The _____ _____ phase occurs between ovulation and

the onset of the menses.

68. _____ stimulates breast alveoli to secrete milk.

69. _____ stimulates breast alveoli to eject milk.

70. Sexual cell division is known as _____.

71. Immediately after ovulation, cells of the ruptured follicle enlarge and become transformed into the

_____ _____.

72. _____ measures blood levels of gonadotropins.

73. _____ is marked by the passage of one full year without menstruation.

74. _____ are the most common of all communicable diseases.

75. _____ uterine ligaments hold the uterus in its normal position by anchoring it in the pelvic cavity.

76. The _____ permits exchange of materials between the offspring's blood and the maternal blood.

Student Name_____

CHAPTER 33

GROWTH AND DEVELOPMENT

Millions of fragile microscopic sperm swim against numerous obstacles to reach the ova and create a new life. At birth, the newborn will fill his lungs with air and cry lustily, signaling to the world that he is ready to begin the cycle of life. This cycle will be marked by ongoing changes, periodic physical growth, and continuous development.

This chapter reviews the more significant events that occur in the normal growth and devel-opment of an individual from conception to death. Realizing that each person is unique, we nonethe-less can discover amid all the complexities of humanity some constants that are understandable and predictable.

A knowledge of human growth and develop-ment is essential in understanding the commonal-ties that influence individuals as they pass through the cycle of life.

I   A NEW HUMAN LIFE

Multiple Choice—select the best answer.

1. Which of the following processes reduces the number of chromosomes in each daughter cell to half the number present in the parent?
    a. mitosis
    c. prophase
    b. meiosis
    d. telophase

2. Forty-six chromosomes per body cell is known as the _____ number of chromo-somes.
    a. haploid
    c. tetrad
    b. diploid
    d. both a and c

3. Each primary spermatocyte undergoes meiotic division I to form:
    a. four haploid secondary spermatocytes.
    b. four diploid secondary spermatocytes.
    c. one diploid secondary spermatocytes.
    d. two haploid secondary spermatocytes.

4. A mature follicle ready to burst open from the ovary's surface is a:
    a. Graafian follicle.
    b. theca cell.
    c. zygote.
    d. first polar body.

5. Fertilization occurs in the:
    a. ovary
    c. uterus
    b. fallopian tubes
    d. vagina

6. The phenomenon of "crossing over" takes place during:
    a. meiosis I only.
    b. meiosis II only.
    c. both meiosis I and meiosis II.
    d. both meiosis and mitosis.

True or false

7. _____ Sex cells contain 23 chromosomes and are therefore referred to as *diploid*.

8. _____ The process of "crossing over" allows for almost infinite variety to the genetic makeup of an individual.

301

9. _____ Completion of meiosis II in the released oocyte requires the head of a sperm cell to enter the oocyte.

10. _____ *Zygote* is the term used to describe the ovulated ovum that is awaiting fertilization.

11. _____ *Insemination* and *fertilization* are synonymous terms.

12. _____ The ovum can live for up to 3 days.

13. _____ During oogenesis, the cytoplasm is not equally divided among daughter cells.

14. _____ Sperm cells can live in the female reproductive tract for up to 3 days.

******If you had difficulty with this section, review pages **937-944**

II   PRENATAL PERIOD

Multiple Choice—select the best answer.

15. About 3 days after fertilization, the zygote forms into a solid mass of cells called a:
    a. morula.
    b. blastocyst.
    c. inner cell mass.
    d. embryo.

16. The outer wall of the blastocyst is referred to as the:
    a. yolk sac.
    b. trophoblast.
    c. chorion.
    d. morula.

17. The "bag of waters" is also called the:
    a. amniotic sac.
    b. yolk sac.
    c. chorion.
    d. placenta.

18. Which of the following is *NOT* a primary germ layer?
    a. ectoderm
    b. exoderm
    c. endoderm
    d. mesoderm

19. By which month of fetal development are all organ systems formed and functioning?
    a. second
    b. third
    c. fourth
    d. fifth

True or false

20. _____ Placental tissue secretes large amounts of human chorionic gonadotropin (HCG) early in pregnancy.

21. _____ The yolk sac provides a critical role in the nutrition of the developing human offspring.

22. _____ The process by which the primary germ layers develop into many different kinds of tissues is called *organogenesis.*

23. _____ The blastocyst is a hollow ball of cells.

24. _____ Division of the cells of the zygote is called *cleavage.*

******If you had difficulty with this section, review pages **944-954**

Student Name_____

III BIRTH, OR PARTURITION, AND THE POSTNATAL PERIOD

Multiple Choice—select the best answer.

25. Stage two of labor is best described as the:
    a. onset of contractions until uterine dilation is complete.
    b. expulsion of the placenta through the vagina.
    c. time of maximum cervical dilation until the baby exits through the vagina.
    d. time after the baby exits through the vagina and the cervix regains normal aperture.

26. Fraternal twins:
    a. are also called *identical twins.*
    b. arise from the same zygote.
    c. arise from two different sperm and two different ova.
    d. arise from a single sperm.

27. The period of infancy lasts approximately from birth to:
    a. 4 weeks.   c. 12 months.
    b. 6 months.   d. 18 months.

28. A rare, inherited condition in which an individual appears to age rapidly is:
    a. senescence.   c. preeclampsia.
    b. progeria.   d. teratogenia.

29. Birth weight generally triples by:
    a. 6 months.   c. 18 months.
    b. 12 months.   d. 24 months.

True or false

30. _____ A cesarean section is a surgical procedure that delivers a newborn through an incision in the abdomen and uterine wall.

31. _____ When a single zygote divides early in its development and forms two separate individuals, it is referred to as *identical twinning.*

32. _____ Stage one of labor usually lasts from a few minutes to an hour.

33. _____ Neonates have both a lumbar and thoracic curve to their spines.

34. _____ Girls experience adolescent growth spurt before boys do.

******If you had difficulty with this section, review pages **954-959**

IV EFFECTS OF AGING

Multiple Choice—select the best answer.

35. A sound exercise program throughout life could reduce the effects of aging in which of the following body systems?
    a. cardiovascular   c. muscular
    b. skeletal   d. all of the above

36. Clouding of the lens of the eye is called:
    a. presbyopia.   c. glaucoma.
    b. myopia.   d. cataract.

True or false

37. _____   The number of functioning nephron units in the kidneys decreases by almost 50% between the ages of 30 and 75.

38. _____   Progesterone therapy may be used to relieve some symptoms of menopause.

******If you had difficulty with this section, review pages **959-962**

V   MECHANISMS OF DISEASE

Matching—select the best answer for the descriptions.

39. _____   pregnancy-induced hypertension

40. _____   placenta grows too close to the cervical opening

41. _____   miscarriage

42. _____   common type of ectopic pregnancy

43. _____   breast inflammation

44. _____   congenital abnormalities

45. _____   separation of placenta from uterine wall

46. _____   childbed fever

a.   placenta previa
b.   tubal pregnancy
c.   preeclampsia
d.   spontaneous abortion
e.   stillbirth
f.   birth defects
g.   puerperal fever
h.   mastitis
i.   teratogens
j.   abruptio placentae

******If you had difficulty with this section, review pages **962-964**

Student Name_____

Crossword Puzzle

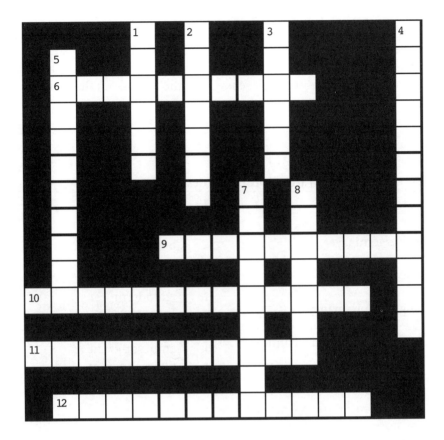

Across

6. Study of individual development before birth
9. Hollow ball that implants itself in the uterus
10. Conception
11. Birth
12. Process where germ layers develop into various tissues

Down

1. Solid mass formed by zygote
2. First 4 weeks of infancy
3. Fertilized ovum
4. Attachment of fertilized ovum in uterus
5. Older adulthood
7. Length of pregnancy
8. Develops from the trophoblast

APPLYING WHAT YOU KNOW

47. John is 70 years old. He has always enjoyed food and has a hearty appetite. Lately, however, he has complained that food "just doesn't taste as good anymore." What might be a possible explanation?

48. Mark and Patrick were identical twins. Christine gave birth to a baby boy and identified Mark as the father of the child on the birth certificate. Paternity testing later revealed that both twins were the father. How is this possible?

DID YOU KNOW?

- A 3-week-old embryo is no larger than a sesame seed. A 1-month old fetus's body is no heavier than an envelope and a sheet of paper. Its hand is no bigger than a teardrop.
- Between the ages of 30 and 70, a nose may lengthen and widen by as much as half an inch and the ears may be a quarter-inch longer because cartilage is one of the few tissues that continues to grow as we age.

ONE LAST QUICK CHECK ✔

Matching—choose the correct term for the appropriate description.

49. _____ "within a glass"

50. _____ inside germ layer

51. _____ before birth

52. _____ length of pregnancy

53. _____ fiberoptic viewing instrument

54. _____ process of birth

55. _____ surgical procedure in which a newborn is delivered through an incision in the abdomen and uterine wall

56. _____ study of how the primary germ layers develop into many different kinds of tissues

57. _____ fertilization until the end of the eighth week of gestation

58. _____ monitors progress of developing fetus.

a. laparoscope
b. gestation
c. antenatal
d. histogenesis
e. C-section
f. endoderm
g. in vitro
h. parturition
i. embryonic phase
j. ultrasonogram

Multiple Choice—select the best answer.

59. Degenerative changes in the urinary system that accompany old age include which of the following?
    a. decreased capacity of the bladder and the inability to empty or void completely
    b. decrease in the number of nephrons
    c. less blood flow through the kidneys
    d. all of the above

60. Any hardening of the arteries is referred to as which of the following?
    a. angioma   c. angina
    b. atherosclerosis d. arteriosclerosis

61. Which of the following is characteristic of the disorder called *presbyopia*?
    a. It is very characteristic of old age.
    b. If causes farsightedness in some individuals.
    c. It is characterized by a lens in the eye becoming hard and losing its elasticity.
    d. All of the above are true.

62. Which of the following events, if any, is NOT characteristic of adolescence?
    a. bone closure occurs
    b. secondary sexual characteristics develop
    c. very rapid growth occurs
    d. all of the above events are characteristic of adolescence

63. Which of the following structures is derived from ectoderm?
    a. lining of the lungs
    b. brain
    c. kidneys
    d. all of the above

Matching—select the best answer from the list of descriptions.

64. _____ atherosclerosis
65. _____ adolescence
66. _____ senescence
67. _____ progeria
68. _____ gerontology

a. older adulthood
b. study of aging
c. Hutchinson-Gilford disease
d. fat accumulation in arteries
e. secondary sexual characteristics

CHAPTER 34

GENETICS AND HEREDITY

Look about your classroom and you will notice various combinations of hair color, eye color, body size, skin tone, hair texture, sex, etc. Everyone has unique body features and this phenomenon alerts us to the marvel of genetics. Independent units, called *genes*, are responsible for the inheritance of biological traits. Genes determine the structure and function of the human body by producing specific regulatory enzymes. Some genes are dominant and some are recessive. Dominant genes produce traits that appear in the offspring and recessive genes have traits that do not appear in

the offspring when they are masked by a dominant gene.

Gene therapy is one of the latest advances of science. This revolutionary branch of medicine combines current technology with genetic research to unlock the secrets of the human body. Daily discoveries into the prevention, diagnosis, treatment, and cure of diseases and disorders are being revealed as a result of genetic therapy. A knowledge of genetics is necessary to understand the basic mechanism by which traits are transmitted from parents to offspring.

I   THE SCIENCE OF GENETICS; CHROMOSOMES AND GENES; GENE EXPRESSION

Multiple Choice—select the best answer.

1. When its genetic codes are being expressed, DNA is in a threadlike form called:
    a.   mRNA.
    b.   chromosomes.
    c.   chromatin.
    d.   tRNA.

2. DNA is arranged to form a larger structure called a:
    a.   gene.
    b.   genome.
    c.   chromosome.
    d.   gamete.

3. A person with a genotype expressed as *AA* is said to be:
    a.   heterozygous recessive.
    b.   heterozygous dominant.
    c.   homozygous recessive.
    d.   homozygous dominant.

4. Both males and females need at least:
    a.   one normal Y chromosome.
    b.   two normal X chromosomes.
    c.   one normal X chromosome.
    d.   two normal Y chromosomes.

5. The entire collection of genetic material in each typical cell of the human body is called the:
    a.   genome.
    b.   chromosome.
    c.   genotype.
    d.   phenotype.

6. Mutations are caused:
    a.   spontaneously.
    b.   by mutagens.
    c.   by environmental agents that damage DNA.
    d.   all of the above.

7. Red-green color blindness is an example of an X-linked recessive condition. If X is normal, X1 is recessive, and Y is normal, an individual with the genotype XX1 will be:
    a.   a normal male.
    b.   a color-blind male.
    c.   a normal female and a carrier.
    d.   a normal female and not a carrier.

8. The scientific study of genetics began in the:
    a.   16th century.
    b.   17th century.
    c.   18th century.
    d.   19th century.

True or false

9. _____ Each of the 23 pairs of chromosomes always appear to be nearly identical to each other.

10. _____ The manner in which genotype is expressed is termed *phenotype.*

11. _____ *Sickle-cell trait* and *sickle-cell anemia* are synonymous terms.

12. _____ Normal males have the sex chromosome combination XX, whereas normal females have the sex chromosome combination XY.

13. _____ X-linked recessive traits appear much more frequently in males than in females.

14. _____ Statistical evidence supports the notion that having sexual intercourse on the day of ovulation increases the probability of conceiving a male.

15. _____ Each cell of the body, except gametes, contain 46 pairs of chromosomes.

16. _____ A person whose genotype is heterozygous for albinism will express the abnormal phenotype of albinism.

******If you had difficulty with this section, review pages **968-976**

II   MEDICAL GENETICS; PREVENTION AND TREATMENT OF GENETIC DISEASES

Multiple Choice—select the best answer.

17. Trisomy and monosomy result from:
    a. an error in meiosis called *disjunction.*
    b. an error in meiosis called *nondisjunction.*
    c. single-gene abnormality.
    d. chromosome breakage.

18. Trisomy 21 is also called:
    a. Klinefelter's syndrome.
    b. Down syndrome.
    c. Turner's syndrome.
    d. cystic fibrosis.

19. A person with the sex chromosomes XXY is afflicted with:
    a. Klinefelter's syndrome.
    b. Down syndrome.
    c. Turner's syndrome.
    d. cystic fibrosis.

20. Which of the following is *NOT* a recessive X-linked genetic disease?
    a. hemophilia
    b. red-green color blindness
    c. sickle-cell anemia
    d. cleft palate

21. Which of the following abnormal genes are linked to some form of cancer?
    a. codominant genes
    b. tumor suppressor genes
    c. oncogenes
    d. recessive genes

22. A grid used to determine the mathematical probability of inheriting genetic traits is called:
    a. a pedigree.
    b. a Punnett square.
    c. amniocentesis.
    d. a chorionic villus sampling.

23. Which of the following genetic diseases can be treated to some degree, if diagnosed early?
    a. PKU
    b. Turner's syndrome
    c. Klinefelter's syndrome
    d. all of the above

Student Name_____

24. In gene replacement therapy:
    a. genetically altered cells are introduced into the body.
    b. genetic disease is treated by inducing an alteration in metabolism.
    c. synthetic hormones are used to relieve symptoms.
    d. genes that specify production of abnormal, disease-causing proteins are replaced by normal or "therapeutic" genes.

25. Disorders that involve trisomy or monosomy can be detected after a _____ is produced.
    a. genotype   c. karyotype
    b. phenotype   d. polytype

26. Cells that display distinct chromosomes during collection via amniocentesis and chorionic villus sampling are in:
    a. prophase.   c. anaphase.
    b. metaphase.   d. telophase

True or false

27. _____ *Congenital disorders* and *inherited disorders* are synonymous terms.

28. _____ Sickle-cell trait is milder than sickle-cell anemia.

29. _____ Parkinson's disease is linked to an error in the nuclear DNA.

30. _____ A pedigree is a chart that illustrates genetic relationships in a family over several generations.

31. _____ Electrophoresis is a method for determining an individual's DNA sequence, or DNA "fingerprint."

32. _____ Cystic fibrosis is a blood-clotting disorder.

33. _____ Cleft palate is a recessive X-linked disorder.

34. _____ Chorionic villus sampling is a procedure newer than amniocentesis.

35. _____ "Genes are not there to cause disease."

******If you had difficulty with this section, review pages **976-987**

Crossword Puzzle

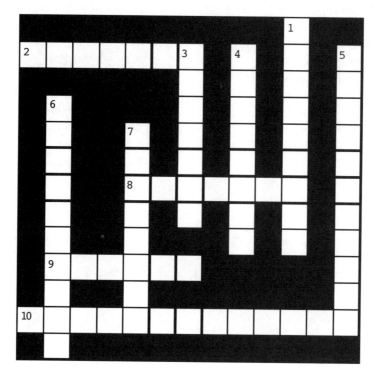

Across

2. Having half of the normal chromosomes
8. Triplet of autosomes
9. Entire collection of genetic material in each cell
10. Grid used to predict genetic traits (two words)

Down

1. Used to identify chromosomal disorders
3. Having a characteristic pair of chromosomes
4. Presence of one autosome
5. Equal effect of different dominant genes
6. Genotype with two identical forms of a gene
7. One of the 44 chromosomes (excluding sex chromosomes)

APPLYING WHAT YOU KNOW

36. Deb's mother has a dominant gene for dark skin color. Her father has a dominant gene for light skin color. What color will Deb's skin most likely be?

37. Mr. and Mrs. Mihm both carry recessive genes for cystic fibrosis. Using your knowledge of the Punnett square, estimate the probability of one of their offspring inheriting this condition.

DID YOU KNOW?

- Scientists estimate that they could fill a 1000-volume encyclopedia with the coded instructions in the DNA of a single human cell if the instructions could be translated into English.
- Identical twins do not have identical fingerprints. No two sets of prints are alike, including those of identical twins.

Student Name_____

ONE LAST QUICK CHECK ✔

Multiple Choice—select the best answer.

38. Independent assortment of chromosomes ensures:
    a. each offspring from a single set of parents is genetically unique.
    b. at meiosis each gamete receives the same number of chromosomes.
    c. that the sex chromosomes always match.
    d. an equal number of males and females are born.

39. Which of the following statements is *NOT* true of a pedigree?
    a. They are useful to genetic counselors in predicting the possibility of producing offspring with genetic disorders.
    b. They may allow a person to determine his or her likelihood of developing a genetic disorder later in life.
    c. They indicate the occurrence of those family members affected by a trait, as well as carriers of the trait.
    d. All of the above are true of a pedigree.

40. The genes that cause albinism are:
    a. codominant.   c. recessive.
    b. dominant.   d. AA.

41. During meiosis, matching pairs of chromosomes line up and exchange genes from their location to the same location on the other side; a process called:
    a. gene linkage.   c. cross-linkage.
    b. crossing-over.   d. genetic variation.

42. When a sperm cell unites with an ovum, a _____ is formed.
    a. zygote
    b. chromosome
    c. gamete
    d. none of the above

43. DNA molecules can also be called:
    a. a chromatin strand.
    b. a chromosome.
    c. a and b.
    d. none of the above.

44. Sex-linked traits:
    a. show up more often in females than in males.
    b. are nonsexual traits carried on sex chromosomes.
    c. are the result of genetic mutation.
    d. all of the above.

45. If a person has only X chromosomes, that person is:
    a. missing essential proteins.
    b. abnormal.
    c. female.
    d. male.

46. A karyotype:
    a. can detect trisomy.
    b. is useful for diagnosing a tubal pregnancy.
    c. is frequently used as a tool in gene augmentation therapy.
    d. can detect the presence of oncogenes.

47. Which of the following pairs is mismatched?
    a. osteogenesis imperfecta—dominant
    b. Turner's syndrome—trisomy
    c. PKU—recessive
    d. cystic fibrosis—recessive

Completion—using the terms below, complete the following statements.

48. Abnormal genes called _____ are believed to be related to cancer.

49. Fetal tissue may be collected by a procedure called _____.

50. An abnormal accumulation of phenylalanine results in _____.

51. The entire collection of genetic material in each cell is called the _____.

52. _____ is caused by recessive genes in chromosome pair seven.

53. A _____ is a person who has a recessive gene that is not expressed.

54. Absence of an essential lipid-producing enzyme may result in the recessive condition _____.

55. _____ is a recessive X-linked disorder characterized as a blood clotting disorder.

56. A gene capable of masking the effects of a recessive gene for the same trait is a _____ gene.

a. cystic fibrosis
b. males
c. phenylketonuria
d. carrier
e. genome
f. females
g. dominant
h. oncogenes
i. karyotype
j. Tay-Sachs disease
k. amniocentesis
l. hemophilia

ANSWER KEY

CHAPTER 1

Anatomy and Physiology and Characteristics of Life
1. b, p. 5
2. c, p. 6
3. a, p. 6
4. b, p. 7
5. c, p. 7

Levels of Organization
6. d, p. 8
7. a, p. 7
8. c, p. 7
9. c, p. 10
10. c, p. 10
11. d, p. 7
12. e, p. 9
13. a, p. 9
14. c, p. 9
15. b, p. 9
16. c, p. 10
17. a, p. 10
18. a, p. 10
19. b, p. 10
20. b, p. 10
21. f, p. 10
22. f, p. 10
23. e, p. 10
24. e, p. 10
25. f, p. 10
26. d, p. 10

Anatomical Position, Body Cavities, Body Regions, Anatomical Terms, and Body Planes
27. b, p. 11
28. a, p. 12
29. a, p. 11
30. d, p. 12
31. c, p. 12
32. c, p. 12
33. b, p. 12
34. b, p. 16
35. c, p. 16
36. d, p. 14
37. inferior, p. 14
38. anterior, p. 16
39. lateral, p. 16
40. proximal, p. 16
41. superficial, p. 16
42. equal, p. 16
43. anterior and posterior, p. 16
44. upper and lower, p. 16
45. frontal, p. 16
46. a, p. 11
47. b, p. 12
48. a, p. 11
49. a, p. 12
50. a, p. 11
51. a, p. 11

Homeostasis and Homeostatic Mechanisms of Control
52. a, p. 20
53. d, p. 23
54. a, p. 25
55. b, p. 25
56. f, p. 23
57. f, p. 24
58. t, p. 25
59. t, p. 25

Health Matters
60. b, p. 27
61. e, p. 27
62. a, p. 27
63. d, p. 27
64. c, p. 27
65. f, p. 27
66. h, p. 27
67. i, p. 27
68. g, p. 27
69. j, p. 27
70. pathophysiology
71. homeostasis
72. mutated
73. parasite
74. tumors
75. self-immunity

Applying What You Know
76. #1 on diagram
77. #2 on diagram
78. #3 on diagram

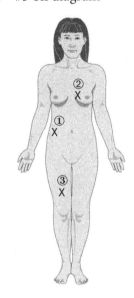

One Last Quick Check
79. a, p. 21
80. d, p. 13
81. d, p. 16
82. a, p. 6
83. b, p. 14
84. d, p. 12
85. d, p. 16
86. d, p. 14
87. a, p. 12
88. c, p. 16

Diagrams
Directions and Planes of the Body
1. transverse plane
2. lateral plane
3. coronal plane
4. medial
5. sagittal plane
6. inferior
7. distal
8. proximal
9. anterior (ventral)
10. superior

11. posterior (dorsal)

Body Cavities
1. cranial
2. spinal
3. pleural
4. thoracic
5. abdominal
6. pelvic
7. ventral
8. dorsal

CHAPTER 2

Basic Chemistry
1. c, p. 37
2. c, p. 37
3. c, p. 38
4. d, p. 39
5. c, p. 39
6. c, p. 41
7. b, p. 42
8. a, p. 43
9. t, p. 36
10. t, p. 38
11. f, p. 41
12. f, p. 42
13. t, p. 43
14. oxygen
15. calcium
16. potassium
17. sodium
18. magnesium
19. iron
20. selenium

Inorganic Molecules
21. b, p. 44
22. d, p. 44
23. c, p. 46
24. b, p. 46
25. c, p. 47
26. t, p. 46
27. t, p. 46
28. t, p. 46
29. t, p. 44
30. f, p. 45

Organic Molecules
31. c, p. 48
32. d, p. 48

33. c, p. 51
34. a, p. 52
35. c, p. 51
36. b, p. 57
37. c, p. 59
38. d, p. 59
39. a, p. 59
40. f, p. 57
41. t, p. 59
42. f, p. 52
43. t, p. 51
44. t, p. 55

Metabolism
45. a, p. 61
46. b, p. 62
47. c, p. 62
48. t, p. 62
49. t, p. 62
50. f, p. 62

Applying What You Know
51. (A) Basement (B) In-
creasing ventilation or
sealing the basement floors
52. Unsaturated fats can often
form a solid mass at higher
temperatures. Review
pages 56 and 57 for more
information.

One Last Quick Check
53. e, p. 39
54. b, p. 60
55. g, p. 39
56. a, p. 38
57. i, p. 50
58. f, p. 59
59. h, p. 44
60. c, p. 46
61. b, p. 49
62. c, p. 49
63. a, p. 49
64. c, p. 49
65. b, p. 48
66. c, p. 49
67. a, p. 55
68. b, p. 46
69. a, p. 46
70. b, p. 46
71. b, p. 46
72. a, p. 46

CHAPTER 3

Functional Anatomy of Cells
1. b, p. 73
2. d, p. 75
3. b, p. 80
4. d, p. 82
5. a, p. 80
6. a, p. 82
7. b, p. 83
8. f, p. 76
9. f, p. 83
10. f, p. 82
11. t, p. 82
12. f, p. 71
13. a, p. 83
14. d, p. 73
15. b, p. 75
16. f, p. 75
17. c, p. 77
18. h, p. 82
19. g, p. 75
20. e, p. 75

Cytoskeleton
21. cytoskeleton, p. 83
22. microfilaments, p.83
23. microtubules, p. 84
24. centrosome, p. 84
25. microvilli, cilia, flagella,
p. 85
26. gap junctions, p. 86
27. desmosomes, p. 86

Applying What You Know
28. (a) CD 36 (b) LDL (c)
stroke, diabetes, cancer,
muscular dystrophy
29. mitochondria

One Last Quick Check
30. b, p. 85
31. c, p. 86
32. b, p. 86
33. b, p. 77
34. b, p. 76
35. e, p. 73
36. d, p. 73
37. b, p. 73
38. a, p. 73
39. c, p. 73
40. composite, p. 69
41. hydrophilic, p. 75

42. signal transduction, p. 77
43. peroxisomes, p. 81
44. nucleus, p. 82

Diagrams

Microscope
1. ocular lens
2. mechanical stage
3. condenser lens
4. coarse focus
5. fine focus
6. light source
7. specimen on slide
8. objective lens

Cell Anatomy
1. centrosome
2. smooth endoplasmic reticulum
3. rough endoplasmic reticulum
4. nuclear envelope
5. nucleolus
6. microvilli
7. Golgi apparatus
8. cilia
9. mitochondria
10. ribosomes

CHAPTER 4

Movement of Substances Through Cell Membranes
1. d, p. 98
2. b, p. 95
3. c, p. 98
4. a, p. 96
5. b, p. 96
6. f, p. 96
7. t, p. 97
8. t, p. 98
9. t, p. 94
10. f, p. 95
11. b, p. 96
12. a, p. 95
13. c, p. 96
14. d, p. 91
15. e, p. 98

Cell Metabolism
16. b, p. 99

17. a, p. 105
18. c, p. 106
19. b, p. 108
20. c, p. 104
21. d, p. 106
22. t, p. 102
23. t, p. 99
24. f, p. 106
25. f, p. 99
26. t, p. 104
27. t, p. 103
28. f, p. 102

Growth and Reproduction of Cells
29. a, p. 110
30. a, p. 111
31. b, p. 112
32. c, p. 115
33. f, p. 112
34. t, p. 112
35. f, p. 111
36. t, p. 112
37. f, p. 115
38. e, p. 108
39. a, p. 107
40. c, p. 107
41. d, p. 107
42. f, p. 106
43. b, p. 108

Mechanisms of Disease
44. t, p. 116
45. t, p. 117
46. t, p. 116
47. f, p. 117
48. t, p. 117

Applying What You Know
49. diffusion
50. shrink

One Last Quick Check
51. b, p. 112
52. a, p. 106
53. a, p. 103
54. d, p. 97
55. d, p. 95
56. a, p. 95
57. c, p. 96
58. b, p. 96

59. c, p. 97
60. c, p. 92
61. a, p. 98
62. b, p. 96
63. a, p. 96
64. uracil (RNA contains the base uracil, not DNA)
65. thymine (the others refer to RNA)
66. interphase (the others refer to translation)
67. prophase (the others refer to anaphase)
68. gene (the others refer to stages of cell division)

Diagrams

Cellular Respiration
1. glucose
2. acetyl CoA
3. citric acid cycle
4. mitochondrion
5. ATP
6. oxygen O_2
7. water H_2O
8. aerobic
9. anaerobic
10. transition
11. pyruvic acid
12. lactic acid

DNA Molecule
1. hydrogen bonds
2. sugar
3. phosphate
4. cytosine
5. guanine
6. adenine
7. thymine

Mitosis
1. prophase
2. metaphase
3. anaphase
4. telophase

CHAPTER 5

Principal Types of Tissues
1. b, p. 123
2. c, p. 124

3.   d, p. 124
4.   b, p. 123
5.   b, p. 124
6.   a, p. 124
7.   t, p. 123
8.   f, p. 124
9.   f, p. 124
10. t, p. 124

Epithelial Tissue
11. d, p. 124
12. b, p. 134
13. b, p. 128
14. b, p. 127
15. c, p. 129
16. b, p. 131
17. a, p. 131
18. d, p. 131
19. a, p. 126
20. t, p. 124
21. f, p. 125
22. f, p. 131
23. b, p. 128
24. e, p. 129
25. d, p. 129
26. h, p. 130
27. a, p. 126
28. c, p. 128

Connective Tissue
29. a, p. 134
30. c, p. 132
31. b, p. 136
32. d, p. 134
33. c, p. 134
34. d, p. 137
35. a, p. 140
36. b, p. 140
37. a, p. 141
38. d, p. 142
39. t, p. 136
40. t, p. 140
41. f, p. 140
42. f, p. 140
43. t, p. 132
44. f, p. 138

Muscle Tissue
45. b, p. 143
46. c, p. 144
47. a, p. 144

48. b, p. 143
49. c, p. 143
50. c, p. 143

Nervous Tissue
51. d, p. 145
52. b, p. 145
53. c, p. 145
54. a, p. 145
55. e, p. 145

Tissue Repair
56. h, p. 142
57. d, p. 142
58. b, p. 146
59. a, p. 142
60. j, p. 142
61. f, p. 142
62. e, p. 142
63. g, p. 147
64. i, p. 142
65. c, p. 143

Body Membranes
66. a, p. 148
67. b, p. 147
68. f, p. 147
69. t, p. 148

Mechanisms of Disease
70. slowly
71. are not
72. papilloma
73. sarcoma
74. oncologist
75. cytotoxic

Applying What You Know
76. Too lean. Holly should be in the 20–22% range to be considered normal. Holly's obsession may put her at risk for other disease conditions because of the stress to her body of being "too lean."
77. Modalities—medical imaging, biopsy, and blood tests
     Tissues—epithelial, connective, and muscle

One Last Quick Check
78. squamous, p. 126
79. cuboidal, p. 126
80. columnar, p. 126
81. simple squamous, p. 126
82. simple cuboidal, p. 126
83. simple columnar, p. 126
84. stratified (transitional), p. 126
85. pseudostratified, p. 126
86. a, p. 134
87. d, p. 129
88. b, p. 132
89. c, p. 135
90. c, p. 136
91. b, p. 141
92. a, p. 147
93. c, p. 147

Diagrams
Tissue #1 is epithelial
1.   basement membrane
2.   cell nuclei
3.   cuboidal epithelial cells
4.   lumen of tubule
Tissue #2 is simple columnar epithelial
1.   goblet cells
2.   columnar epithelial cell
Tissue #3 is pseudostratified ciliated epithelium
1.   cilia
2.   columnar cell
3.   goblet cell
4.   basement membrane
5.   mucous glands
Tissue#4 is stratified squamous (keratinized) epithelium
1.   cornified layer
2.   basement membrane
3.   basal cells
4.   dermis
Tissue #5 is loose, ordinary (areolar) connective
1.   bundle of collagenous fibers
2.   elastic fibers
Tissue #6 is adipose
1.   storage area for fat
2.   plasma membrane
3.   nucleus of adipose
Tissue #7 is dense fibrous

(regular) connective
1. fibroblast
2. collagenous fibers

Tissue #8 is elastic cartilage
1. lacuna
2. chondrocyte
3. elastic fibers

Tissue # 9 is bone
1. osteon (haversian system)

Tissue # 10 is skeletal muscle
1. cross striations of muscle cell
2. nuclei of muscle cell
3. muscle fiber

Tissue # 11 is cardiac muscle
1. nucleus
2. intercalated disks

Tissue # 12 is nervous
1. nerve cell body
2. axon
3. dendrites

CHAPTER 6

Skin Function and Structure
1. b, p. 161
2. a, p. 161
3. d, p. 162
4. d, p. 162
5. a, p. 163
6. d, p. 166
7. c, p. 168
8. c, p. 168
9. b, p. 168
10. c, p. 169
11. f, p. 161
12. t, p. 167
13. t, p. 169
14. f, p. 164
15. t, p. 161

Functions of the Skin
16. d, p. 170
17. d, p. 170
18. c, p. 172
19. a, p. 172
20. b, p. 173
21. f, p. 172
22. f, p. 171
23. t, p. 172

Burns
24. a, p. 175
25. b, p. 175
26. f, p. 175
27. t, p. 175
28. c, p. 175
29. a, p. 175
30. d, p. 175
31. b, p. 175
32. e, p. 175

Appendages of the Skin
33. b, p. 176
34. a, p. 178
35. c, p. 180
36. b, p. 178
37. d, p. 178
38. t, p. 176
39. f, p. 177
40. t, p. 178
41. t, p. 178
42. t, p. 178

Mechanisms of Disease
43. f, p. 181
44. c, p. 182
45. a, p. 182
46. b, p. 182
47. g, p. 182
48. h, p. 182
49. d, p. 182
50. e, p. 182
51. fever or febrile
52. heat exhaustion
53. heat stroke
54. frostbite

Applying What You Know
55. 46%
56. fingerprints
57. It is theorized that adults who had more than two blistering sunburns before the age of 20 have a greater risk of developing melanoma than someone who experienced no burns. Bernie's exposure may have been during his youth or adolescence.

One Last Quick Check
58. a, p. 166
59. d, p. 179
60. b, p. 166
61. d, p. 175
62. b, p. 180
63. b, p. 163
64. c, p. 178
65. b, p. 170
66. a, p. 165
67. a, p. 171
68. c, p. 168
69. b, p. 168
70. e, p. 180
71. f, p. 176
72. g, p. 178
73. a, p. 162
74. d, p. 178
75. h, p. 179
76. i, p. 182
77. j, p. 182

Diagrams
Skin
1. opening of sweat ducts
2. hair shaft
3. stratum corneum
4. stratum granulosum
5. stratum basale
6. dermal papilla
7. Meissner corpuscle
8. sebaceous (oil) gland
9. hair follicle
10. hypodermis
11. dermis
12. epidermis

Rule of Nines
1. 4.5%
2. 4.5%
3. 18%
4. 4.5%
5. 1%
6. 9%
7. 9%
8. 9%
9. 9%
10. 4.5%
11. 4.5%
12. 18%
13. 4.5%

CHAPTER 7

Types of Bones

1. f, p. 190
2. k, p. 190
3. h, p. 190
4. e, p. 189
5. d, p. 190
6. i, p. 190
7. j, p. 190
8. c, p. 189
9. a, p. 190
10. b, p. 190
11. g, p. 190

Bone Tissue Structure, Function, and Homeostasis

12. d, p. 191
13. b, p. 192
14. c, p. 192
15. b, p. 195
16. b, p. 195
17. c, p. 196
18. t, p. 192
19. f, p. 195
20. t, p. 195
21. t, p. 196
22. f, p. 196
23. f, p. 190

Bone Development, Growth, Resorption, and Repair

24. b, p. 197
25. d, p. 197
26. a, p. 199
27. b, p. 201
28. b, p. 201
29. t, p. 197
30. f, p. 197
31. f, p. 200
32. t, p. 201
33. t, p. 200

Cartilage

34. b, p. 202
35. c, p. 203
36. b, p. 202
37. f, p. 202
38. t, p. 203
39. t, p. 203

Mechanisms of Disease

40. Osteochondroma
41. Osteosarcoma
42. Osteoporosis
43. Paget's disease
44. Osteomyelitis

Applying What You Know

45. (a) Osteoporosis
    (b) DXA—dual energy x-ray absorptiometry scan or bone density (RA) imagery of the wrist
    (c) hormonal therapy (HRT), bone-building nonhormonal drugs such as Fosamax or Miacalcin, vitamin (D) and mineral (calcium) therapy, and weight-bearing exercises.
46. The bones are responsible for the majority of our blood cell formation. Her disease condition might be inhibiting the production of blood cells.
47. Epiphyseal cartilage is present only while a child is still growing. It becomes bone in adulthood. It is particularly vulnerable to fractures in childhood and preadolescence.
48. Ms. Strickland's surgeon most likely used a synthetic skeletal repair material called "vitos" which facilitates fracture repairs. Unlike metal stabilizers, vitos "patches" degrade naturally in the body following surgery and do not require surgical removal.

One Last Quick Check

49. four, p. 189
50. medullary cavity, p. 190
51. articular cartilage, p. 190
52. endosteum, p. 190
53. hematopoiesis, p. 196
54. red bone marrow, p. 195
55. periosteum, p. 190
56. long, short, flat, and irregular, p. 189
57. calcium, p. 196
58. hyaline, p. 202
59. d, p. 192
60. b, p. 192
61. e, p. 192
62. a, p. 190
63. c, p. 202
64. i, p. 195
65. f, p. 192
66. j, p. 192
67. g, p. 202
68. h, p. 192

Diagrams

Long Bone

1. epiphysis
2. diaphysis
3. epiphysis
4. periosteum
5. yellow marrow
6. endosteum
7. medullary cavity
8. compact bone
9. red marrow cavities
10. epiphyseal plate
11. spongy bone
12. articular cartilage

Cross Section of Cancellous and Compact Bone

1. osteons (haversian systems)
2. periosteum
3. compact bone
4. medullary marrow cavity
5. Volkmann's canals
6. haversian canals
7. trabeculae
8. endosteum

CHAPTER 8

Divisions of the Skeleton

1. a, p. 213
2. a, p. 210
3. b, p. 210

4. a, p. 213
5. b, p. 213
6. b, p. 213
7. a, p. 213
8. b, p. 213
9. a, p. 213
10. b, p. 213

The Skull
11. c, p. 227
12. b, p. 227
13. a, p. 229
14. c, p. 214
15. a, p. 229
16. b, p. 220
17. f, p. 229
18. f, p. 228
19. t, p. 227
20. f, p. 230
21. t, p. 215

Sternum and Ribs
22. e, p. 235
23. c, p. 235
24. a, p. 235
25. d, p. 235
26. f, p. 232
27. b, p. 235
28. g, p. 235

The Appendicular Skeleton/ Upper Extremity
29. b, p. 236
30. d, p. 237
31. d, p. 237
32. t, p. 235
33. f, p. 236
34. t, p. 239
35. f, p. 236

The Appendicular Skeleton/ Lower Extremity
36. b, p. 241
37. a, p. 243
38. a, p. 241
39. c, p. 246
40. f, p. 241
41. f, p. 244
42. f, p. 244
43. f, p. 244

Skeletal Differences in Men and Women
44. b, p. 247
45. a, p. 247
46. a, p. 247
47. b, p. 247
48. a, p. 247
49. b, p. 247

Cycle of Life: Mechanisms of Disease
50. b, p. 249
51. c, p. 248
52. f, p. 249
53. t, p. 249

Applying What You Know
54. Bill could have possibly injured his humerus and his ulna.
55. (a) High heels cause a forward thrust to the body which forces an undue amount of weight on the heads of the metatarsals. (b) Metatarsals, tarsals, and phalanges

One Last Quick Check
56. coxal (all others refer to the spine)
57. axial (all others refer to the appendicular skeleton)
58. maxilla (all others refer to the cranial bones)
59. ribs (all others refer to the shoulder girdle)
60. vomer (all others refer to the bones of the middle ear)
61. ulna (all others refer to the coxal bone)
62. ethmoid (all others refer to the hand and wrist)
63. nasal (all others refer to cranial bones)
64. anvil (all others refer to the cervical vertebra)
65. c, p. 232
66. g, p. 243
67. j, l, m, k, p. 243

68. n, p. 237
69. i, p. 215
70. a, p. 244
71. p, p. 214
72. b, d, p. 215
73. f, p. 237
74. h, q, p. 243
75. o, t, p. 214
76. r, p. 227
77. s, e, p. 227

Diagrams
Anterior View of Skull
1. glabella
2. ethmoid bone
3. sphenoid bone
4. nasal bone
5. vomer
6. mental foramen
7. mandible
8. maxilla
9. perpendicular plate of ethmoid
10. optic foramen
11. parietal bone
12. frontal bone

Floor of Cranial Cavity
1. crista galli
2. optic foramen
3. internal auditory meatus
4. jugular foramen
5. foramen magnum
6. occipital bone
7. petrous portion of temporal bone
8. sella turcica
9. greater wing of sphenoid bone
10. lesser wing of sphenoid bone

Skull Viewed from Below
1. palatine process of maxilla
2. zygomatic arch
3. foramen ovale
4. styloid process
5. occipital condyle
6. foramen magnum
7. horizontal plate of palatine
8. zygomatic process of maxilla

9.   hard palate
10. incisive foramen

Left Half of Skull
1.   squamous suture
2.   parietal bone
3.   lambdoidal suture
4.   temporal bone (squamous portion)
5.   occipital bone
6.   external auditory meatus
7.   condyloid process
8.   mastoid process of temporal bone
9.   styloid process
10. pterygoid process
11. coronoid process
12. mandible
13. mental foramen
14. maxilla
15. zygomatic (malar) bone
16. nasal bone
17. lacrimal bone
18. ethmoid bone
19. sphenoid bone
20. frontal bone
21. coronal suture

Bones that Form the Orbit
1.   optic foramen
2.   superior orbital fissure
3.   ethmoid bone
4.   lacrimal bone
5.   maxilla
6.   inferior orbital fissure
7.   infraorbital foramen
8.   zygomatic bone
9.   sphenoid bone
10. frontal bone

Skull at Birth
1.   parietal bone
2.   occipital fontanel
3.   occipital bone
4.   mastoid fontanel
5.   sphenoid fontanel
6.   sagittal suture
7.   occipital fontanel
8.   occipital bone
9.   parietal bone
10. coronal suture

11. frontal fontanel
12. frontal bone
13. coronal suture
14. frontal fontanel

The Vertebral Column
1.   thoracic curvature
2.   intervertebral foramina
3.   pelvic curvature
4.   atlas
5.   axis
6.   cervical curvature
7.   lumbar curvature
8.   coccyx
9.   sacrum
10. lumbar vertebrae
11. thoracic vertebrae
12. cervical vertebrae

Vertebrae
Atlas
1.   transverse process
2.   transverse foramen
3.   anterior arch
4.   facet for dens
5.   vertebral foramen
6.   superior articular facet
7.   posterior arch

Cervical Vertebra
1.   spinous process
2.   lamina
3.   pedicle
4.   transverse foramen
5.   transverse process
6.   superior articular facet
7.   vertebral foramen

Lumbar Vertebra
1.   spinous process
2.   lamina
3.   transverse process
4.   pedicle
5.   superior articular facet
6.   vertebral foramen

Axis
1.   spinous process
2.   transverse process
3.   transverse foramen
4.   dens

5.   superior articular facet
6.   vertebral foramen
7.   posterior arch

Thoracic Vertebra
1.   spinous process
2.   lamina
3.   transverse process
4.   pedicle
5.   superior articular facet
6.   articular facet for tubercle of rib
7.   vertebral foramen

Sacrum and Coccyx
1.   superior articular facet
2.   articular surface
3.   median sacral crest
4.   sacral foramina
5.   sacral hiatus
6.   coccyx
7.   sacrum
8.   ala
9.   sacral canal

Thoracic Cage
1.   clavicle
2.   true ribs
3.   costal cartilage
4.   costosternal articulation
5.   false ribs
6.   floating ribs
7.   xiphoid process
8.   body
9.   manubrium
10. sternum
11. first thoracic vertebra
12. seventh cervical vertebra

Rib
1.   rib
2.   head
3.   neck
4.   transverse process
5.   sternal extremity
6.   body
7.   angle
8.   nonarticular part of tubercle
9.   neck
10. head

11. vertebral extremity
12. articular part of tubercle

Scapula
Anterior View
1. superior angle
2. superior border
3. coracoid process
4. acromion process
5. supraglenoid tubercle
6. glenoid cavity
7. infraglenoid tubercle
8. axillary border
9. inferior angle
10. vertebral border
11. costal surface

Posterior View
1. acromion process
2. coracoid process
3. spine
4. superior border
5. medial angle
6. vertebral border
7. inferior angle
8. dorsal surface
9. axillary border
10. glenoid cavity

Lateral View
1. coracoid process
2. glenoid cavity
3. infraglenoid tubercle
4. axillary border
5. inferior angle

Bones of the Arm
Anterior View
1. humerus
2. greater tubercle
3. lesser tubercle
4. lateral epicondyle
5. capitulum
6. coronoid fossa
7. medial epicondyle
8. styloid process of radius
9. radial tuberosity
10. radius
11. olecranon process
12. styloid process of ulna

Posterior View
1. head
2. anatomical neck
3. trochlea
4. olecranon fossa
5. coronoid process
6. head of radius
7. olecranon process

Bones of the Hand and Wrist
1. carpal bones
2. ulna
3. phalanges
4. metacarpal
5. radius

Coxal Bone
1. ilium
2. greater sciatic notch
3. ischium
4. obturator foramen
5. ischial tuberosity
6. pubis
7. acetabulum
8. iliac crest

Bones of the Thigh and Leg
1. greater trochanter
2. lateral epicondyle
3. medial epicondyle
4. femur
5. lesser trochanter
6. intertrochanteric line
7. neck
8. head
9. medial condyle
10. head of fibula
11. fibula
12. lateral malleolus
13. medial malleolus
14. tibia
15. crest
16. tibial tuberosity
17. medial condyle
18. intercondylar eminence

Foot
1. phalanges
2. metatarsals
3. tarsals
4. navicular

5. talus
6. calcaneus
7. cuboid

CHAPTER 9

Classification of Joints
1. b, p. 256
2. a, p. 256
3. a, p. 256
4. c, p. 257
5. c, p. 257
6. d, p. 258
7. c, p. 259
8. d, p. 259
9. t, p. 257
10. f, p. 258
11. t, p. 259
12. t, p. 255
13. f, p. 257
14. f, p. 258
15. f, p. 258
16. t, p. 259
17. a, p. 267
18. a, p. 267
19. b, p. 267
20. c, p. 256
21. c, p. 256
22. a, p. 267
23. b, p. 259
24. c, p. 256
25. b, p. 257
26. b, p. 267
27. a, p. 256
28. b, p. 257
29. d, p. 261
30. c, p. 261
31. b, p. 259
32. e, p. 258
33. d, p. 267
34. b, p. 260
35. a, p. 260
36. a, p. 260
37. f, p. 259

Representative Synovial Joints
38. c, p. 260
39. b, p. 261
40. b, p. 261
41. a, p. 261

42. d, p. 266
43. c, p. 265
44. b, p. 261
45. c, p. 266

Types and Range of Movement at Synovial Joints
46. e, p. 268
47. c, p. 269
48. f, p. 671
49. g, p. 269
50. b, p. 270
51. d, p. 270
52. a, p. 270
53. h, p. 270
54. i, p. 270
55. j, p. 271

Mechanisms of Disease
56. arthroscopy
57. osteoarthritis or degenerative joint disease
58. arthritis
59. gouty arthritis
60. sprain

Applying What You Know
61. (a) Nodular swelling, joint pain, tenderness, aching, stiffness, and limited motion. Systemic symptoms may also include fever, anemia, weight loss, profound fatigue, and possible pericarditis. (b) Small joints of the hand, wrist, and feet progressing often to the larger joints.
62. (a) Gouty arthritis (b) Swelling, tenderness, and pain, typically in the joints of the fingers, wrists, elbows, ankles, and knees. (c) Allopurinol (Zyloprim) is the drug of choice to treat this disease.

One Last Quick Check
63. diarthroses
64. synarthrotic
65. diarthrotic

66. ligaments
67. articular cartilage
68. least movable
69. largest
70. 2
71. mobility
72. pivot
73. t, p. 257
74. f, p. 257
75. f, p. 260
76. t, p. 269
77. t, p. 271
78. t, p. 271
79. f, p. 272
80. f, p. 272
81. f, p. 274
82. t, p. 264

Diagrams
Synovial Joint
1. bursa
2. articular cartilage
3. periosteum
4. joint capsule
5. nerve
6. synovial membrane
7. bone
8. joint cavity

Shoulder Joint
1. coracoid process of scapula
2. glenoid cavity
3. superior transverse ligament of scapula
4. articular cartilage of glenoid cavity
5. scapula
6. glenoidal labrum
7. humerus
8. head of humerus
9. articular cartilage of humerus
10. bursa
11. tendon of long head of biceps brachii m.
12. synovial cavity

Hip Joint
1. acetabular labrum
2. head
3. articular capsule
4. greater trochanter

5. femur
6. lesser trochanter
7. articular capsule
8. transverse acetabular ligament
9. ligamentum teres
10. articular cavity
11. acetabulum
12. ilium

Knee Joint
Anterior View
1. lateral condyle of femur
2. lateral meniscus
3. fibular collateral ligament
4. transverse ligament of knee
5. fibula
6. tibia
7. tibial tuberosity
8. tibial collateral ligament
9. medial meniscus
10. anterior cruciate ligament
11. medial condyle of femur
12. posterior cruciate ligament
13. femur

Knee Joint
Posterior View
1. femur
2. ligament of Wrisberg
3. medial condyle
4. medial meniscus
5. tibial collateral ligament
6. posterior cruciate ligament
7. tibia
8. fibula
9. fibular collateral ligament
10. lateral meniscus
11. lateral condyle
12. anterior cruciate ligament

Vertebrae
1. lamina
2. anterior longitudinal ligament
3. body of vertebra
4. intervertebral disk
5. posterior longitudinal ligament
6. ligamentum flavum
7. intervertebral foramen

8. supraspinous ligament
9. interspinous ligament
10. spinous process

CHAPTER 10

Skeletal Muscle Structure
1. c, p. 281
2. d, p. 282
3. a, p. 281
4. a, p. 283
5. d, p. 283
6. a, p. 284
7. f, p. 282
8. t, p. 283
9. t, p. 283
10. f, p. 283
11. t, p. 284

How Muscles Are Named
12. c, p. 285
13. a, p. 285
14. f, p. 285
15. e, p. 285
16. g, p. 285
17. b, p. 285
18. d, p. 285

Important Skeletal Muscles: Muscles of the Face and Neck
19. b, p. 287
20. e, p. 287
21. a, p. 287
22. c, p. 287
23. f, p. 288
24. d, p. 287

Important Skeletal Muscles: Trunk Muscles
25. t, p. 290
26. t, p. 290
27. f, p. 292
28. t, p. 289
29. t, p. 292

Important Skeletal Muscles: Upper Limb Muscles
30. a, p. 295
31. c, p. 293
32. a, p. 297
33. d, p. 297

34. f, p. 295
35. t, p. 301
36. t, p. 294
37. t, p. 295
38. f, p. 297

Important Skeletal Muscles: Lower Limb Muscles
39. d, p. 304
40. a, p. 304
41. c, p. 305
42. d, p. 304
43. a, p. 304
44. t, p. 302
45. f, p. 304
46. f, p. 304

Applying What You Know
47. (a) Carpal tunnel syndrome
(b) The wrist, hand, and fingers are affected due to tenosynovitis. Pain may radiate to the forearm and shoulder.
(c) Injections of anti-inflammatory agents or surgical removal of tissue pressing on median nerve.
48. deltoid area
49. See tables 10-2 to 10-15

One Last Quick Check
50. c, a, b, p. 305
51. a, p. 305
52. a, b, p. 297
53. a, p. 297
54. c, p. 305
55. b, f, p. 302
56. a, p. 295
57. a, d, p. 302
58. b, p. 297
59. b, p. 288
60. a, p. 293
61. b, p. 302
62. d, a, p. 282
63. d, p. 282
64. b, p. 283
65. a, p. 281
66. e, p. 283
67. c, p. 283

Diagrams
Facial Muscles
Lateral View
1. temporalis
2. masseter
3. sternocleidomastoid
4. orbicularis oris
5. buccinator
6. zygomaticus major
7. orbicularis oculi (palpebral portion)
8. orbicularis oculi
9. corrugator supercilii
10. occipitofrontalis (frontal portion)

Anterior View
1. occipitofrontalis (frontal portion)
2. orbicularis oculi
3. orbicularis oculi (palpebral portion)
4. orbicularis oris
5. buccinator
6. masseter
7. corrugator supercilii
8. temporalis

Muscles of the Thorax
1. external intercostals
2. diaphragm
3. central tendon of diaphragm
4. internal intercostals

Muscles of the Trunk and Abdominal Wall
1. rectus abdominis
2. rectus abdominis (covered by sheath)
3. external abdominal oblique
4. inguinal ligament
5. internal abdominal oblique
6. transverse abdominus
7. linea alba

Muscles Acting on the Shoulder Girdle
1. trapezius
2. seventh cervical vertebra

3. rhomboideus major
4. rhomboideus minor
5. levator scapulae
6. pectoralis minor (cut)
7. subscapularis
8. latissimus dorsi
9. serratus anterior
10. latissimus dorsi (cut)
11. pectoralis minor
12. teres major
13. teres minor
14. subscapularis

Rotator Cuff Muscles
1. clavicle
2. acromion process
3. infraspinatus
4. greater tubercle
5. teres minor
6. intertubercular (bicipital) groove
7. humerus
8. subscapularis
9. lesser tubercle
10. supraspinatus
11. coracoid process

Muscles that Move the Upper Arm
1. deltoideus (cut)
2. coracobrachialis
3. pectoralis major
4. serratus anterior
5. deltoideus
6. thoracolumbar fascia
7. latissimus dorsi
8. teres major
9. infraspinatus
10. rhomboideus major
11. teres minor
12. rhomboideus minor
13. supraspinatus
14. levator scapulae

Muscles of the Upper Arm
1. triceps brachii
2. brachioradialis
3. brachialis
4. biceps brachii (long head)
5. pectoralis major
6. deltoid
7. clavicle

8. biceps brachii
9. radius
10. pronator teres
11. ulna
12. brachialis
13. triceps brachii
14. teres major
15. coracobrachialis

Muscles that Act on the Forearm
1. coracoid process
2. supraglenoid tuberosity
3. tubercle of radius
4. biceps brachii (short head)
5. biceps brachii (long head)
6. olecranon process of ulna
7. triceps brachii (medial head)
8. triceps brachii: lateral (short head)
9. triceps brachii (long head)
10. posterior surface of humerus; lateral intermuscular septum
11. infraglenoid tubercle
12. coracoid process
13. coracobrachialis
14. medial surface of humerus
15. medial epicondyle of humerus
16. pronator teres
17. lateral surface of radius
18. coronoid process of ulna
19. brachialis
20. humerus (distal half)

Muscles of the Forearm
1. pronator teres
2. palmaris longus
3. flexor pollicis brevis
4. opponens pollicis
5. flexor digiti minimi
6. abductor digiti minimi
7. flexor carpi ulnaris
8. flexor carpi radialis
9. palmar interosseus
10. pronator quadratus
11. flexor digitorum profundus
12. supinator
13. brachioradialis
14. flexor digitorum superficialis
15. extensor carpi ulnaris

16. extensor pollicis brevis
17. extensor pollicis longus
18. abductor pollicis longus
19. extensor carpi radialis brevis
20. extensor carpi radialis longus
21. supinator (deep)

Muscles of the Upper Leg
1. tensor fasciae latae
2. iliotibial tract
3. vastus lateralis
4. vastus medialis
5. rectus femoris
6. sartorius
7. gracilis
8. iliopsoas
9. adductor brevis
10. adductor longus
11. adductor magnus
12. fibula
13. tibia
14. pectineus

Muscles of the Lower Leg
1. soleus
2. extensor digitorum longus
3. peroneus brevis
4. tibialis anterior
5. tibia
6. gastrocnemius
7. calcaneal tendon (Achilles tendon)
8. calcaneus

CHAPTER 11

Function of Skeletal Muscle Tissue
1. b, p. 312
2. a, p. 313
3. a, p. 314
4. d, p. 313
5. c, p. 315
6. a, p. 313
7. c, p. 314
8. a, p. 316
9. c, p. 316
10. b, p. 316
11. t, p. 315
12. f, p. 313
13. f, p. 314

14. t, p. 315
15. t, p. 313
16. t, p. 316
17. f, p. 313
18. f, p. 319
19. t, p. 319
20. t, p. 318

Function of Skeletal Muscle Organs
21. d, p. 322
22. d, p. 323
23. a, p. 322
24. d, p. 326
25. a, p. 324
26. c, p. 325
27. c, p. 325
28. f, p. 324
29. t, p. 325
30. t, p. 323
31. f, p. 324

Function of Cardiac and Smooth Muscle Tissue
32. c, p. 329
33. b, p. 329
34. b, p. 329
35. c, p. 329
36. a, p. 329
37. c, p. 329
38. a, p. 329
39. b, p. 329
40. a, p. 329
41. c, p. 329

Mechanisms of Disease
42. myalgia, p. 332
43. myoglobin, p. 332
44. poliomyelitis, p. 332
45. muscular dystrophy, p. 332
46. myasthenia gravis, p. 333

Applying What You Know
47. Linda may have more slow and intermediate fibers than fast fibers. The former are conducive to long races rather than short ones.
48. Muscles in a dead body may be stiff because individual muscle fibers ran out of the ATP required to "turn off" a muscle contraction.

One Last Quick Check
49. a, p. 326
50. b, p. 325
51. b, p. 325
52. d, p. 316
53. a, p. 322
54. d, p. 322
55. f, p. 316
56. t, p. 322
57. t, p. 324
58. t, p. 322
59. t, p. 333
60. t, p. 330
61. t, p. 328
62. t, p. 325
63. f, p. 319

Diagrams
Structure of Skeletal Muscle
1. muscle
2. fascia
3. tendon
4. bone
5. sarcoplasmic reticulum
6. T tubule
7. sarcomere
8. thick filament
9. Z disk
10. thin filament
11. Z line
12. myofibril
13. muscle fiber
14. fascicle
15. endomysium
16. perimysium
17. epimysium

Neuromuscular Junction and Skeletal Muscle Cell
1. motor neuron fiber
2. Schwann cell
3. sarcoplasm
4. acetylcholine receptor sites
5. synaptic cleft
6. motor endplate
7. synaptic vesicles
8. myelin sheath
9. sarcomere
10. sarcolemma
11. mitochondria
12. T tubule
13. sarcoplasmic reticulum
14. triad
15. myofibril

Motor Unit
1. myelin sheath
2. Schwann cell
3. neuromuscular junction
4. nucleus
5. muscle fibers
6. myofibrils
7. motor neuron

Cardiac Muscle Fiber
1. intercalated disks
2. sarcomere
3. sarcolemma
4. myofibril
5. mitochondrion
6. sarcoplasmic reticulum
7. T tubule
8. diad
9. nucleus

CHAPTER 12

Organization of the Nervous System
1. c, p. 344
2. f, p. 344
3. a, p. 344
4. h, p. 344
5. g, p. 344
6. b, p. 344
7. d, p. 344
8. e, p. 344

Cells of the Nervous System
9. b, p. 346
10. a, p. 346
11. d, p. 347
12. a, p. 346
13. c, p. 346
14. d, p. 347
15. a, p. 346
16. c, p. 347
17. c, p. 347
18. b, p. 348

19. a, p. 349
20. c, p. 350
21. d, p. 351

Nerves and Tracts
22. c, p. 350
23. b, p. 352
24. b, p. 352
25. d, p. 352
26. c, p. 352

Repair of Nerve Fibers
27. f, p. 353
28. t, p. 352
29. f, p. 353

Nerve Impulses
30. a, p. 353
31. b, p. 353
32. b, p. 354
33. a, p. 354
34. t, p. 353
35. f, p. 355
36. f, p. 354

Action Potential
37. b, p. 357
38. b, p. 356
39. c, p. 357
40. b, p. 357
41. t, p. 355
42. f, p. 357
43. t, p. 356
44. t, p. 358

Synaptic Transmission
45. c, p. 359
46. b, p. 361
47. a, p. 362
48. f, p. 359
49. t, p. 361
50. t, p. 359

Neurotransmitters
51. d, p. 363
52. b, p. 363
53. c, p. 365
54. c, p. 366
55. d, p. 365
56. f, p. 365
57. t, p. 366

Mechanisms of Disease
58. multiple sclerosis
59. glioma
60. glioblastoma multiforme
61. multiple neurofibromato-sis
62. glia

Applying What You Know
63. (a) Multiple sclerosis (b) CNS (c) Myelin loss and demyelination of the white matter in the CNS (d) No known cure (e) Cause is thought to be related to autoimmunity and viral infections.
64. CNS damage is most often permanent. Since the damage is suspected to involve the spinal cord—which is part of the CNS—the prognosis for repair is not good.

One Last Quick Check
65. presynaptic, p. 359
66. neurotransmitter, p. 363
67. communicate, p. 362
68. specifically, p. 362
69. pain, p. 366
70. sensory, p. 350
71. ganglion, p. 352
72. telodendria, p. 348
73. a, p. 347
74. b, p. 344
75. b, p. 345
76. a, p. 350
77. a, p. 344
78. b, p. 346
79. b, p. 346
80. a, p. 350
81. b, p. 347
82. a, p. 349

Diagrams
Typical Neuron
1. dendrite
2. Golgi apparatus
3. mitochondrion
4. cell body
5. nucleus
6. Nissl bodies
7. axon hillock
8. axon
9. Schwann cell
10. myelin sheath
11. axon collateral
12. node of Ranvier
13. telodendria
14. synaptic knobs

Myelinated Axon
1. node of Ranvier
2. neurilemma
3. neurofibrils
4. plasma membrane of axon
5. myelin sheath
6. nucleus of Schwann cell

Classification of Neurons
1. multipolar neuron
2. bipolar neuron
3. unipolar neuron

Reflex Arc
1. gray matter
2. interneuron
3. sensory neuron axon
4. cell body
5. spinal nerve
6. motor neuron axon
7. white matter
8. dendrite
9. synapse

Chemical Synapse
1. voltage-gated Ca^{++} channels
2. synaptic cleft
3. stimulus-gated Na^+ channels
4. presynaptic cell
5. postsynaptic cell
6. action potential
7. voltage-gated K^+ channels
8. synaptic knob

CHAPTER 13

Coverings of the Brain and Spinal Cord
1. a, p. 375

2. c, p. 375
3. b, p. 375
4. c, p. 375

Cerebrospinal Fluid
5. c, p. 377
6. a, p. 377
7. d, p. 378
8. d, p. 378
9. t, p. 377
10. t, p. 380

The Spinal Cord
11. b, p. 382
12. d, p. 382
13. a, p. 382
14. c, p. 382
15. b, p. 383
16. d, p. 383
17. c, p. 383
18. a, p. 383
19. e, p. 383

The Brain
20. b, p. 385
21. d, p. 386
22. a, p. 387
23. b, p. 390
24. d, p. 390
25. c, p. 391
26. b, p. 395
27. a, p. 397
28. b, p. 395
29. a, p. 397
30. t, p. 387
31. f, p. 395
32. f, p. 386
33. t, p. 391
34. t, p. 391

Somatic Sensory and Motor Pathways
35. c, p. 400
36. c, p. 400
37. a, p. 403
38. t, p. 400
39. f, p. 381

Mechanisms of Disease
40. d, p. 404
41. b, p. 404
42. a, p. 404

43. c, p. 404

Applying What You Know
44. hydrocephalus
45. (a) dementia
    (b) Alzheimer's disease

One Last Quick Check
46. h, p. 404
47. d, p. 404
48. e, p. 404
49. c, p. 398
50. j, p. 398
51. a, p. 398
52. b, p. 398
53. f, p. 397
54. i, p. 405
55. g, p. 404
56. e, p. 385
57. d, p. 386
58. a, p. 388
59. d, p. 389
60. e, p. 395
61. b, p. 393
62. c, p. 393
63. d, p. 387
64. c, p. 390
65. d, p. 395
66. d, p. 387

Diagrams
Coverings of the Brain
1. superior sagittal sinus (of dura)
2. subdural space
3. skull
4. falx cerebri
5. muscle
6. skin
7. subarachnoid space
8. arachnoid
9. periosteum
10. epidural space

Fluid Spaces of the Brain
1. cerebral hemisphere
2. anterior horn of lateral ventricle
3. interventricular foramen
4. third ventricle
5. inferior horn of lateral ventricle

6. fourth ventricle
7. pons
8. central canal of spinal cord
9. cerebellum
10. cerebral aqueduct
11. posterior horn of lateral ventricle

Flow of Cerebrospinal Fluid and the Layers of the Brain
1. arachnoid villus
2. choroid plexus of lateral ventricle
3. superior sagittal sinus
4. interventricular foramen
5. choroid plexus of third ventricle
6. cerebral aqueduct
7. choroid plexus of fourth ventricle
8. median foramen
9. central canal of spinal cord
10. dura mater
11. cisterna magna
12. lateral foramen
13. cerebral cortex
14. subarachnoid space
15. arachnoid layer
16. falx cerebri
17. pia mater

Spinal Cord
1. anterior median fissure
2. posterior column
3. gray matter
4. central canal
5. dorsal nerve root
6. spinal nerve
7. lateral column
8. anterior column
9. white matter
10. end of spinal column
11. filum terminale
12. cauda equina
13. lumbar enlargement
14. cervical enlargement

Spinal Cord Tracts
1. fasciculus cuneatus
2. posterior spinocerebellar
3. lateral spinothalamic
4. anterior spinocerebellar

5. spinotectal
6. anterior spinothalmic
7. tectospinal
8. vestibulospinal
9. recticulospinal
10. anterior corticospinal
11. rubrospinal
12. lateral corticospinal
13. fasciculus gracilis

Left Hemisphere of Cerebrum
1. central sulcus
2. superior frontal gyrus
3. frontal lobe
4. lateral fissure
5. temporal lobe
6. occipital lobe
7. parietooccipital fissure
8. parietal lobe
9. postcentral gyrus

Cerebral Cortex
1. precentral gyrus
2. premotor area
3. prefrontal area
4. Broca's area
5. transverse gyrus
6. auditory association area
7. primary auditory area
8. Wernicke's area
9. visual cortex
10. visual association area
11. somatic sensory association area
12. primary taste area
13. postcentral gyrus

CHAPTER 14

Spinal Nerves
1. a, p. 414
2. c, p. 414
3. a, p. 415
4. b, p. 417
5. a, p. 417
6. t, p. 414
7. t, p. 413
8. f, p. 419
9. f, p. 418
10. t, p. 417

Cranial Nerves
11. g, p. 424
12. a, p. 422
13. j, p. 425
14. h, p. 424
15. b, p. 422
16. e, p. 423
17. i, p. 424
18. c, p. 422
19. d, p. 423
20. f, p. 423
21. l, p. 425
22. k, p. 425

Somatic Motor Nervous System
23. b, p. 429
24. a, p. 431
25. a, p. 429

Autonomic Nervous System
26. c, p. 432
27. d, p. 433
28. b, p. 435
29. a, p. 438
30. b, p. 440
31. f, p. 432
32. f, p. 415
33. t, p. 431
34. f, p. 440
35. t, p. 433

Applying What You Know
36. (1) Sympathetic
    (2a) Muscular—skeletal muscles faster
    (b) Circulatory—stronger heartbeat, dilated blood vessels
    (c) Respiratory—dilated bronchi
    (d) Digestive—increased blood sugar levels
    (3) Dysfunction of the sympathetic effectors and perhaps even the ANS itself.
37. (a) Herpes zoster or shingles
    (b) Varicella zoster virus of chickenpox
    (c) It attacks a dermatome (T-4) and symptoms occur in that region.

(d) His immunological protective mechanism may have become diminished due to the stress.

One Last Quick Check
38. d, p. 431
39. e, p. 431
40. f, p. 431
41. b, p. 431
42. a, p. 431
43. c, p. 429
44. c, p. 433
45. b, p. 433
46. b, p. 433
47. d, p. 433
48. b, p. 438
49. a, p. 438
50. a, p. 438
51. b, p. 438
52. a, p. 438
53. b, p. 438
54. a, p. 438
55. a, p. 438
56. b, p. 438
57. b, p. 438
58. a, p. 421
59. b, p. 418
60. a, p. 425
61. b, p. 419
62. b, p. 413
63. a, p. 426
64. b, p. 414
65. b, p. 415

Diagrams
Spinal Nerves
1. cervical vertebrae
2. brachial plexus
3. thoracic vertebrae
4. lumbar vertebrae
5. sacrum
6. coccyx
7. cervical plexus
8. cervical nerves
9. thoracic nerves
10. dura mater
11. cauda equina
12. lumbar nerves
13. sacral nerves
14. coccygeal nerve

Cranial Nerves
1. trochlear nerve
2. optic nerve
3. oculomotor nerve
4. abducens nerve
5. facial nerve
6. vestibulocochlear nerve
7. vagus nerve
8. accessory nerve
9. hypoglossal nerve
10. glossopharyngeal nerve
11. trigeminal nerve
12. olfactory nerve

Patellar Reflex
1. gray matter
2. spinal cord
3. motor neuron
4. quadriceps muscle
5. patellar tendon
6. patella
7. stretch receptor
8. sensory neuron
9. dorsal root ganglion
10. interneuron

Autonomic Conduction Path
1. somatic motor neuron axon
2. collateral ganglion
3. postganglionic neuron axon
4. sympathetic ganglion
5. preganglionic sympathetic neuron axon

CHAPTER 15

Sensory Receptors
1. b, p. 448
2. d, p. 450
3. a, p. 450
4. b, p. 449
5. a, p. 452
6. f, p. 449
7. t, p. 450
8. f, p. 449
9. t, p. 453
10. t, p. 449

The Sense of Smell and the Sense of Taste
11. b, p. 453
12. a, p. 456
13. c, p. 456
14. b, p. 453
15. t, p. 453
16. f, p. 453
17. t, p. 453
18. f, p. 456

Sense of Hearing and Balance: The Ear
19. a, p. 457
20. c, p. 457
21. d, p. 457
22. d, p. 460
23. b, p. 460
24. b, p. 460
25. a, p. 456
26. t, p. 457
27. f, p. 457
28. t, p. 457
29. t, p. 459
30. f, p. 461

Vision: The Eye
31. c, p. 464
32. a, p. 464
33. a, p. 464
34. d, p. 465
35. d, p. 466
36. a, p. 464
37. c, p. 468
38. a, p. 469
39. c, p. 470
40. a, p. 467
41. f, p. 467
42. f, p. 467
43. t, p. 468
44. t, p. 468
45. f, p. 471
46. t, p. 470
47. t, p. 464
48. t, p. 469
49. f, p. 470
50. t, p. 475

Mechanisms of Disease
51. c, p. 473
52. a, p. 473
53. d, p. 473
54. e, p. 474
55. b, p. 473
56. f, p. 474
57. c, p. 474
58. e, p. 474
59. f, p. 475
60. a, p. 475
61. j, p. 474
62. b, p. 476
63. h, p. 474
64. g, p. 476
65. i, p. 476
66. d, p. 476

Applying What You Know
67. The eustachian tube connects the throat to the middle ear and provides a perfect pathway for the spread of infection.
68. (a) Legally blind (b) 20-200 (c) myopia (d) concave contact lenses or glasses

One Last Quick Check
69. a, p. 456
70. b, p. 457
71. a, p. 456
72. c, p. 472
73. b, p. 464
74. b, p. 452
75. d, p. 465
76. b, p. 464
77. d, p. 456
78. a, p. 456
79. t, p. 456
80. f, p. 476
81. t, p. 469
82. f, p. 460
83. t, p. 474
84. t, p. 464
85. t, p. 464
86. t, p. 450
87. t, p. 451
88. t, p. 460

Diagrams
Midsagittal Section of the Nasal Area
1. olfactory bulb
2. fibers of olfactory nerve

3. cribriform plate of ethmoid bone
4. olfactory tract
5. olfactory recess
6. nasopharynx
7. palate
8. nasal cavity
9. frontal bone

The Ear
1. auricle
2. temporal bone
3. external auditory meatus
4. tympanic membrane
5. semicircular canals
6. oval window
7. facial nerve
8. vestibular nerve
9. cochlear nerve
10. cochlea
11. vestibule
12. round window
13. auditory tube
14. stapes
15. incus
16. malleus

The Eye
1. lens
2. pupil
3. lacrimal caruncle
4. optic disk
5. optic nerve
6. central artery and vein
7. fovea
8. macula lutea
9. posterior chamber
10. sclera
11. choroid
12. retina
13. ciliary body
14. lower lid
15. iris
16. anterior chamber
17. cornea

Extrinsic Muscles of the Right Eye
1. superior oblique
2. medial rectus
3. superior rectus
4. optic nerve
5. levator palpebrae

superioris (cut)
6. lateral rectus
7. inferior oblique
8. trochlea

Lacrimal Apparatus
1. caruncle
2. lacrimal canals
3. lacrimal sac
4. nasolacrimal duct
5. puncta
6. lacrimal ducts
7. lacrimal gland

CHAPTER 16

The Endocrine System and Hormones
1. a, p. 484
2. c, p. 485
3. d, p. 486
4. c, p. 484
5. a, p. 486
6. d, p. 487
7. c, p. 486
8. a, p. 490
9. c, p. 491
10. b, p. 489
11. t, p. 485
12. t, p. 486
13. f, p. 489
14. f, p. 494
15. t, p. 484

Prostaglandins
16. b, p. 494
17. c, p. 495

Pituitary Gland
18. b, p. 496
19. a, p. 498
20. d, p. 500
21. c, p. 496
22. b, p. 500
23. a, p. 496
24. d, p. 496
25. c, p. 498
26. e, p. 498
27. h, p. 496
28. g, p. 501
29. f, p. 487

30. i, p. 498
31. b, p. 501

Pineal, Thyroid, and Parathyroid Glands
32. b, p. 502
33. b, p. 503
34. b, p. 502
35. b, p. 505
36. c, p. 505
37. t, p. 503
38. f, p. 505
39. t, p. 504
40. t, p. 502
41. f, p. 502

Adrenal Glands
42. b, p. 506
43. d, p. 506
44. a, p. 507
45. t, p. 506
46. f, p. 508
47. t, p. 508

Pancreatic Islets
48. c, p. 512
49. a, p. 512
50. t, p. 512
51. f, p. 512
52. b, p. 512
53. c, p. 512
54. a, p. 512
55. d, p. 512

Other Endocrine Glands and Tissues
56. a, p. 513
57. b, p. 513
58. c, p. 514
59. f, p. 514
60. t, p. 514
61. t, p. 514

Mechanisms of Disease
62. e, p. 519
63. h, p. 519
64. a, p. 519
65. c, p. 519
66. f, p. 519
67. g, p. 520
68. b, p. 520
69. d, p. 520

Applying What You Know

70. (a) hCG is high during early pregnancy (b) placenta (c) It forms on the lining of the uterus as an interface between the circulatory systems of the mother and the developing child. It is a temporary endocrine gland.

71. (a) Diabetes mellitus (b) inadequate amount or abnormal type of insulin (c) insulin

72. oxytocin

One Last Quick Check

73. a, p. 507
74. c, p. 501
75. d, p. 504
76. b, p. 497
77. d, p. 501
78. d, p. 500
79. b, p. 514
80. d, p. 508
81. d, p. 510
82. b, p. 494
83. j, p. 504
84. g, p. 501
85. h, p. 516
86. i, p. 496
87. b, p. 501
88. f, p. 512
89. a, p. 508
90. d, p. 501
91. e, p. 497
92. c, p. 507

Diagrams

Major Endocrine Glands

1. pineal
2. parathyroids
3. testes (male)
4. ovaries (female)
5. pancreas (islets)
6. adrenals
7. thymus
8. thyroid
9. pituitary
10. hypothalamus

Location and Structure of Pituitary Gland

1. optic chiasma
2. infundibulum
3. pituitary diaphragm
4. pituitary gland
5. nasal cavity
6. brainstem
7. hypothalamus
8. pineal gland
9. thalamus
10. pars anterior
11. pars intermedia
12. adenohypophysis
13. sphenoid bone
14. neurohypophysis
15. infundibulum
16. mammillary body
17. third ventricle
18. optic chiasma

Structure of Thyroid and Parathyroid Glands

1. epiglottis
2. hyoid bone
3. larynx
4. superior parathyroid gland
5. thyroid gland
6. inferior parathyroid glands
7. trachea

CHAPTER 17

Composition of Blood and Red Blood Cells

1. a, p. 530
2. a, p. 532
3. c, p. 532
4. b, p. 533
5. d, p. 535
6. t, p. 532
7. f, p. 540
8. t, p. 536
9. f, p. 537
10. f, p. 537

White Blood Cells and Platelets

11. d, p. 538
12. i, p. 538
13. b, p. 539

14. c, p. 538
15. f, p. 540
16. h, p. 540
17. j, p. 541
18. g, p. 541
19. a, p. 538
20. e, p. 538

Blood Types

21. b, p. 542
22. a, p. 544
23. a, p. 542
24. t, p. 544
25. f, p. 544
26. f, p. 544

Blood Plasma

27. t, p. 545
28. t, p. 545
29. f, p. 545

Blood Clotting (Coagulation)

30. b, p. 546
31. d, p. 548
32. c, p. 548

Mechanisms of Disease

33. Polycythemia
34. Aplastic anemia
35. pernicious anemia
36. sickle cell anemia
37. Leukopenia
38. thrombus
39. embolus
40. Hemophilia

Applying What You Know

41. Theoretically, infused red blood cells and elevation of hemoglobin levels after transfusion should increase oxygen consumption and muscle performance during exercise. In practice, however, the advantage appears to be minimal.

42. No. If Mrs. Payne were a negative Rh factor and her husband were a positive Rh factor, it would set up

the strong possibility of erythroblastosis fetalis.

43. Both procedures assist the clotting process.

One Last Quick Check
44. b, p. 550
45. b, p. 550
46. a, p. 539
47. a, p. 545
48. d, p. 545
49. a, p. 538
50. a, p. 551
51. d, p. 544
52. c, p. 533
53. b, p. 546
54. d, p. 540
55. f, p. 550
56. h, p. 542
57. a, p. 539
58. g, p. 550
59. c, p. 541
60. b, p. 542
61. e, p. 544
62. i, p. 542
63. j, p. 539

Diagram
1. basophil
2. neutrophil
3. eosinophil
4. lymphocyte
5. monocyte

CHAPTER 18

Heart
1. b, p. 557
2. c, p. 559
3. a, p. 561
4. a, p. 561
5. d, p. 562
6. d, p. 564
7. c, p. 564
8. d, p. 561
9. d, p. 561
10. b, p. 565
11. Trace the Blood Flow, p. 563
    tricuspid (3)
    pulmonary arteries (6)
    bicuspid (9)
    vena cava (1)
    right ventricle (4)
    aorta (12)
    pulmonary semilunar valve (5)
    left ventricle (10)
    right atrium (2)
    left atrium (8)
    aortic semilunar valve (11)
12. echocardiography, p. 564
13. cardiac enzyme studies, p. 564
14. cardiac nuclear scanning, p. 565
15. cardiopulmonary resuscitation (CPR), p. 557

Blood Vessels
16. d, p. 566
17. c, p. 566
18. e, p. 566
19. g, p. 566
20. f, p. 566
21. b, p. 566
22. a, p. 568
23. t, p. 567
24. f, p. 566
25. t, p. 567
26. f, p. 568

Major Blood Vessels
27. d, p. 571
28. c, p. 569
29. b, p. 569
30. d, p. 580
31. b, p. 581
32. b, p. 582
33. a, p. 583
34. d, p. 579
35. systemic circulation, p. 569
36. circle of Willis, p. 573
37. veins, p. 577
38. hepatic portal system, p. 579
39. ascites, p. 580
40. (a) umbilical arteries (b) umbilical veins, p. 581
41. veins, p. 577

Mechanisms of Disease
42. i, p. 585
43. b, p. 586
44. d, p. 586
45. e, p. 586
46. a, p. 565
47. c, p. 586
48. f, p. 587
49. g, p. 588
50. j, p. 588
51. h, p. 587
52. l, p. 565
53. k, p. 584

Applying What You know
54. Congestive heart failure. Left-sided heart failure often leads to right-sided heart failure. The combination of both problems may require a transplant, implant, or may lead to death.
55. coronary bypass surgery
56. Cardiac enzymes usually increase over the next few hours following a heart attack. These elevations suggest that Mr. Wertz may have had a myocardial infarction with resulting heart muscle damage.

One Last Quick Check
57. c, p. 569
58. d, p. 584
59. c, p. 557
60. d, p. 561
61. b, p. 587
62. b, p. 585
63. g, p. 571
64. a, p. 586
65. i, p. 581
66. c, p. 581
67. f, p. 586
68. b, p. 588
69. h, p. 569
70. d, p. 586
71. e, p. 569
72. j, p. 585

Diagrams
Heart
1. aorta
2. superior vena cava
3. right atrium

4. left AV (mitral or bicuspid) valve
5. right AV (tricuspid) valve
6. chordae tendineae
7. right ventricle
8. interventricular septum
9. papillary muscle
10. left ventricle
11. right ventricle
12. pulmonary veins
13. right atrium
14. openings of coronary arteries
15. pulmonary trunk
16. aortic semilunar valve
17. left atrium

Blood Vessels
1. tunica adventitia
2. tunica media
3. tunica intima
4. tunica adventitia
5. tunica media
6. tunica intima

Veins
1. facial
2. right brachiocephalic
3. right subclavian
4. superior vena cava
5. inferior vena cava
6. hepatic
7. hepatic portal
8. median cubital
9. superior mesenteric
10. common iliac
11. external iliac
12. femoral
13. great saphenous
14. small saphenous
15. dorsal venous arch
16. digital
17. posterior tibial
18. anterior tibial
19. fibular
20. popliteal
21. femoral
22. digital
23. internal iliac
24. common iliac
25. inferior mesenteric

26. splenic
27. median basilic
28. basilic
29. axillary
30. cephalic
31. internal jugular
32. external jugular
33. superior sagittal sinus

Arteries
1. right common carotid
2. brachiocephalic
3. axillary
4. brachial
5. superior mesenteric
6. abdominal aorta
7. common iliac
8. internal iliac
9. external iliac
10. deep medial circumflex femoral
11. deep femoral
12. femoral
13. popliteal
14. anterior tibial
15. peroneal
16. posterior tibial
17. arcuate
18. dorsal metatarsal
19. dorsal pedis
20. digital
21. palmar arch
22. ulnar
23. radial
24. arch of aorta
25. left subclavian
26. external carotid
27. internal carotid

Fetal Circulation
1. superior vena cava
2. foramen ovale
3. inferior vena cava
4. ductus venosus
5. umbilical vein
6. fetal umbilicus
7. umbilical cord
8. internal iliac arteries
9. common iliac artery
10. pulmonary trunk
11. ductus arteriosus

CHAPTER 19

Hemodynamics and the Heart as a Pump
1. b, p. 594
2. b, p. 594
3. a, p. 598
4. b, p. 598
5. a, p. 604
6. t, p. 602
7. f, p. 600
8. f, p. 600
9. t, p. 600
10. t, p. 602

Circulation and Blood Pressure
11. d, p. 605
12. c, p. 606
13. b, p. 606
14. d, p. 607
15. d, p. 609
16. a, p. 611
17. b, p. 617
18. c, p. 620
19. b, p. 608
20. d, p. 609
21. f, p. 605
22. t, p. 606
23. t, p. 606
24. t, p. 612
25. f, p. 612
26. f, p. 614
27. t, p. 617
28. t, p. 619
29. f, p. 620
30. t, p. 610

Mechanisms of Disease
31. septic shock
32. Cardiogenic shock
33. anaphylaxis; anaphylactic shock
34. Neurogenic shock
35. low blood volume
36. toxic shock syndrome

Applying What You Know
37. (a) Hypovolemic shock (b) The body might respond by increasing the heart rate, decreasing the urine

output and decreasing available fluids to the tissues.
38. (a) heart block (b) artificial pacemaker

One Last Quick Check
39. c, p. 622
40. a, p. 623
41. c, p. 623
42. c, p. 612
43. a, p. 623
44. e, p. 594
45. k, p. 594
46. a, p. 598
47. b, p. 600
48. c, p. 600
49. g, p. 602
50. i, p. 602
51. d, p. 607
52. h, p. 610
53. f, p. 611
54. j, p. 617
55. l, p. 620

Diagram
ECG Strip Recording
1. atrial depolarization
2. ventricular depolarization
3. ventricular repolarization

CHAPTER 20

Lymphatic Vessels, Lymph, and Circulation of Lymph
1. c, p. 629
2. b, p. 631
3. a, p. 631
4. d, p. 631
5. c, p. 631
6. b, p. 632
7. a, p. 632
8. t, p. 629
9. f, p. 629
10. t, p. 629
11. f, p. 630
12. t, p. 631
13. t, p. 632
14. t, p. 632

Lymph Nodes
15. b, p. 633
16. d, p. 634
17. a, p. 634
18. c, p. 634
19. f, p. 634
20. t, p. 633

Lymphatic Drainage of the Breast
21. a, p. 636
22. c, p. 635

Tonsils, Thymus, and Spleen
23. a, p. 636
24. c, p. 637
25. c, p. 636
26. f, p. 636
27. f, p. 637
28. t, p. 638

Mechanisms of Disease
29. Lymphoma
30. acute otitis media
31. blood poisoning
32. nasal
33. Hodgkin's and non-Hodgkin's

Applying What You Know
34. (a) Yes (b) Yes (c) The spleen destroys old blood cells and platelets. Preventing this will allow Nancy to preserve her own supply and avoid anemia.
35. Baby Wilson had no means of producing T cells, thus making him susceptible to several diseases. Isolation was a means of controlling his exposure to these diseases.

One Last Quick Check
36. b, p. 636
37. c, p. 638
38. c, p. 638
39. a, p. 636
40. c, p. 638
41. a, p. 637
42. a, p. 636

43. t, p. 631
44. t, p. 632
45. t, p. 632
46. f, p. 633
47. t, p. 635
48. f, p. 635
49. f, p. 637
50. f, p. 637

Diagrams
Principal Organs of the Lymphatic System
1. thymus gland
2. right lymphatic duct
3. thoracic duct
4. intestinal duct
5. appendix
6. bone marrow
7. inguinal lymph nodes
8. Peyer's patches in intestinal wall
9. spleen
10. mammary plexus
11. axillary lymph node
12. cervical lymph node
13. tonsils

Lymph Node
1. afferent lymph vessel
2. capsule
3. trabeculae
4. efferent lymph vessel
5. hilus
6. medullary cords
7. medullary sinus
8. cortical nodules
9. sinuses
10. germinal center

Lymphatic Drainage of Breast
1. supraclavicular nodes
2. midaxillary nodes
3. lateral axillary nodes
4. subscapular nodes
5. anterior axillary (pectoral) nodes
6. internal mammary nodes
7. interpectoral (Rotter) nodes

CHAPTER 21

Nonspecific Immunity
1. d, p. 645
2. c, p. 646
3. a, p. 649
4. a, p. 647
5. b, p. 648
6. f, p. 645
7. t, p. 645
8. f, p. 649
9. f, p. 649
10. t, p. 649

Specific Immunity
11. b, p. 649
12. b, p. 649
13. d, p. 650
14. a, p. 651
15. b, p. 655
16. b, p. 653
17. c, p. 651
18. b, p. 656
19. b, p. 653
20. b, p. 656
21. t, p. 653
22. f, p. 653
23. t, p. 655
24. t, p. 655
25. t, p. 660
26. t, p. 659
27. t, p. 659
28. t, p. 657
29. f, p. 660
30. f, p. 660

Mechanisms of Disease
31. f, p. 663
32. t, p. 663
33. t, p. 661
34. f, p. 662
35. f, p. 662

Applying What You Know
36. (a) Passive acquired immunity (b) active artificial immunity (c) Active immunity usually lasts longer than passive.
37. (a) AIDS
    (b) azidothymidine (AZT) and dideoxyinosine (DDI)

One Last Quick Check
38. a, p. 657
39. d, p. 663
40. b, p. 649
41. d, p. 651
42. b, p. 654
43. d, p. 656
44. c, p. 660
45. c, p. 645
46. a, p. 660
47. b, p. 660
48. d, p. 660

CHAPTER 22

Selye's Concept of Stress
1. b, p. 672
2. b, p. 671
3. b, p. 672
4. b, p. 670
5. d, p. 670
6. f, p. 673
7. f, p. 676
8. t, p. 673
9. f, p. 670
10. t, p. 673

Some Current Concepts About Stress
11. c, p. 674
12. d, p. 675
13. b, p. 676
14. t, p. 674
15. f, p. 676
16. f, p. 677
17. t, p. 675
18. f, p. 677

Applying What You Know
19. (a) Stress (b) See Figure 22-6, page 675 (c) Immune diseases, decreased quality of life, ulcers, hypertension, chemical dependency, impaired relationships, and loss of contact with reality.
20. (a) Sympathetic (b) No, digestion decreases under the influence of the sympathetic nervous system.

One Last Quick Check
21. General adaptation syndrome, p. 671
22. exhaustion, p. 673
23. corticotropin releasing hormone, p. 674
24. fight or flight reaction, p. 674
25. Psychophysiology, p. 677
26. f, p. 676
27. t, p. 669
28. t, p. 676
29. f, p. 678
30. t, p. 670

CHAPTER 23

Upper Respiratory Tract
1. a, p. 685
2. c, p. 684
3. d, p. 687
4. c, p. 687
5. a, p. 691
6. f, p. 686
7. f, p. 689
8. t, p. 689
9. f, p. 691
10. t, p. 691

Lower Respiratory Tract
11. a, p. 692
12. b, p. 696
13. c, p. 700
14. d, p. 700
15. f, p. 692
16. f, p. 692
17. t, p. 692
18. f, p. 698
19. f, p. 698
20. t, p. 697

Mechanisms of Disease
21. d, p. 703
22. g, p. 703
23. b, p. 701
24. a, p. 702
25. c, p. 701
26. f, p. 701
27. e, p. 701
28. h, p. 689

Applying What You Know

29. (a) epiglottis
     (b) *Haemophilus influenzae*
     type B
     (c) yes
30. (a) croup
     (b) no
31. During the day Mr.
     Gorski's cilia are paralyzed
     because of his heavy
     smoking. They use the
     time when Mr. Gorski is
     asleep to sweep accumula-
     tions of mucus and
     bacteria toward the
     pharynx. When Mr. Gorski
     awakes, these collections
     are waiting to be elimi-
     nated.

One Last Quick Check

32. a, p. 688
33. b, p. 690
34. a, p. 687
35. a, p. 686
36. a, p. 686
37. b, p. 690
38. b, p. 701
39. c, p. 690
40. a, p. 701
41. b, p. 701
42. a, p. 686
43. air distributor, p. 684
44. gas exchanger, p. 684
45. filters, p. 684
46. warms, p. 684
47. humidifies, p. 684
48. nose, p. 685
49. pharynx, p. 685
50. larynx, p. 685
51. trachea, p. 685
52. bronchi, p. 685
53. lungs, p. 685
54. alveoli, p. 698
55. Exchange, p. 700
56. respiratory membrane,
     p. 696
57. surface, p. 700

Diagrams

Respiratory System

1. upper respiratory tract
2. lower respiratory tract
3. alveolar duct
4. alveolar sac
5. bronchioles
6. primary bronchi
7. trachea
8. larynx
9. laryngopharynx
10. oropharynx
11. nasopharynx
12. nasal cavity

Nasal Cavity

1. cribriform plate of eth-
    moid bone
2. frontal sinus
3. superior turbinate
4. middle turbinate
5. inferior turbinate
6. vestibule
7. anterior naris
8. pharyngeal tonsil
9. posterior naris
10. sella turcica
11. sphenoid sinus

Divisions of Pharynx

1. opening of eustachian tube
2. soft palate
3. hyoid bone
4. lingual tonsil
5. vocal cords
6. trachea
7. esophagus
8. laryngopharynx
9. epiglottis
10. oropharynx
11. palatine tonsil
12. uvula
13. nasopharynx
14. pharyngeal tonsil

Paranasal Sinuses

1. sphenoid sinus
2. maxillary sinus
3. lacrimal sac
4. ethmoid air cells
5. superior turbinate
6. middle turbinate
7. inferior turbinate
8. oral cavity
9. maxillary sinus
10. sphenoid sinus
11. frontal sinus
12. ethmoid air cells
13. frontal sinus

Lobes and Fissures of the Lungs

1. superior lobe
2. middle lobe
3. inferior lobe
4. oblique fissure
5. horizontal fissure
6. oblique fissure
7. inferior lobe
8. superior lobe

CHAPTER 24

Pulmonary Ventilation

1. b, p. 709
2. c, p. 711
3. b, p. 711
4. c, p. 714
5. d, p. 716
6. d, p. 717
7. d, p. 716
8. d, p. 715
9. a, p. 708
10. d, p. 709
11. t, p. 709
12. f, p. 714
13. t, p. 716
14. t, p. 717
15. t, p. 714

Pulmonary Gas Exchange

16. a, p. 716
17. d, p. 719
18. c, p. 718
19. a, p. 718
20. t, p. 720
21. t, p. 717
22. f, p. 720
23. t, p. 718

**Blood Transportation of Gases
and Systemic Gas Exchange**

24. d, p. 721
25. b, p. 725
26. d, p. 725
27. c, p. 722
28. t, p. 721

29. f, p. 723
30. f, p. 725
31. t, p. 727

Regulation of Breathing

32. d, p. 727
33. b, p. 729
34. f, p. 727
35. t, p. 729

Mechanisms of Disease

36. COPD; chronic obstructive pulmonary disease
37. Bronchitis
38. Emphysema
39. Asthma

Applying What You Know

40. (a) obstructive pulmonary disorders (b) COPD which may include bronchitis, emphysema, and asthma (c) They obstruct inspiration and expiration. The primary difficulty is in emptying their lungs adequately which creates a buildup of CO_2 in the lungs.
41. The "diving reflex" was responsible for this phenomenon. It is a protective response of the body to cold water immersion that slows the metabolism and tissue requirements to enable survival.

One Last Quick Check

42. d, p. 708
43. c, p. 723
44. c, p. 721
45. b, p. 711
46. d, p. 715
47. d, p. 714
48. d, p. 714
49. e, p. 714
50. c, p. 714
51. a, p. 714
52. f, p. 716
53. d, p. 717
54. b, p. 721

55. i, p. 727
56. j, p. 729
57. g, p. 731
58. h, p. 731

Diagrams
Pulmonary Volumes
1. total lung capacity (TLC)
2. inspiratory reserve volume (IRV)
3. tidal volume (TV)
4. expiratory reserve volume (ERV)
5. residual volume (RV)
6. vital capacity (VC)

Respiratory Centers of Brainstem
1. limbic system
2. pneumotaxic center
3. respiratory centers
4. apneustic center
5. pons
6. inspiratory center
7. expiratory area
8. medulla
9. respiratory muscles
10. cortex

CHAPTER 25

Overview of the Digestive System

1. c, p. 741
2. b, p. 742
3. t, p. 740
4. f, p. 742
5. a, p. 741
6. a, p. 741
7. a, p. 741
8. b, p. 741
9. b, p. 741
10. b, p. 741
11. b, p. 741
12. b, p. 741
13. a, p. 741
14. a, p. 741

Mouth and Pharynx

15. d, p. 743
16. b, p. 743

17. c, p. 746
18. d, p. 747
19. b, p. 747
20. t, p. 746
21. f, p. 743
22. f, p. 747
23. t, p. 743
24. f, p. 743

Esophagus and Stomach

25. b, p. 747
26. d, p. 749
27. c, p. 750
28. t, p. 750
29. t, p. 749
30. t, p. 750

Small Intestine, Large Intestine, Appendix, and Peritoneum

31. c, p. 751
32. b, p. 751
33. a, p. 755
34. b, p. 757
35. f, p. 754
36. f, p. 756
37. t, p. 756
38. t, p. 755

Liver, Gallbladder, and Pancreas

39. b, p. 757
40. d, p. 757
41. b, p. 759
42. a, p. 760
43. t, p. 757
44. f, p. 759
45. t, p. 762
46. t, p. 760

Mechanisms of Disease

47. d, p. 766
48. g, p. 766
49. f, p. 766
50. e, p. 765
51. i, p. 765
52. a, p. 764
53. h, p. 766
54. b, p. 763
55. c, p. 766
56. k, p. 764
57. j, p. 764

Applying What You Know

58.   (a) cholelithiasis (b) jaundice (c) obstruction of the bile flow into the duodenum (d) cholecys- tectomy or ultrasound lithotripsy

59.   pylorospasm

One Last Quick Check

60.   d, p. 747
61.   d, p. 746
62.   c, p. 747
63.   d, p. 747
64.   d, p. 764
65.   a, p. 744
66.   c, p. 743
67.   b, p. 747
68.   c, p. 747
69.   c, p. 751
70.   a, p. 759
71.   b, p. 751
72.   d, p. 760
73.   c, p. 757
74.   f, p. 754
75.   f, p. 755
76.   t, p. 756
77.   t, p. 742
78.   t, p. 748
79.   t, p. 750
80.   t, p. 756
81.   t, p. 760

Diagrams

Digestive Organs

1.   parotid gland
2.   submandibular gland
3.   pharynx
4.   esophagus
5.   liver
6.   transverse colon
7.   ascending colon
8.   ileum
9.   cecum
10.   vermiform appendix
11.   rectum
12.   sigmoid colon
13.   descending colon
14.   stomach
15.   sublingual gland
16.   tongue

Tooth

1.   crown
2.   neck
3.   root
4.   bone
5.   cementum
6.   peridontal membrane
7.   peridontal ligament
8.   root canal
9.   gingiva (gum)
10.   pulp cavity with nerves and vessels
11.   dentin
12.   enamel
13.   cusp

Stomach

1.   lower esophageal sphincter
2.   esophagus
3.   gastroesophageal opening
4.   lesser curvature
5.   pylorus
6.   pyloric sphincter
7.   duodenal bulb
8.   duodenum
9.   rugae
10.   greater curvature
11.   submucosa
12.   mucosa
13.   oblique muscle layer
14.   circular muscle layer
15.   longitudinal muscle layer
16.   serosa
17.   body
18.   fundus

Wall of Small Intestine

1.   serosa
2.   muscularis
3.   longitudinal muscle
4.   circular muscle
5.   submucosa
6.   mucosa
7.   plica (fold)
8.   mesentery

Divisions of Large Intestine

1.   transverse colon
2.   hepatic flexure
3.   ascending colon
4.   cecum

5.   rectum
6.   superior rectal artery and vein
7.   sigmoid colon
8.   sigmoid artery and vein
9.   inferior mesenteric artery and vein
10.   descending colon
11.   superior mesenteric artery
12.   splenic flexure

Liver

1.   inferior vena cava
2.   right lobe
3.   gallbladder
4.   round ligament
5.   falciform ligament
6.   left lobe
7.   left lobe
8.   falciform ligament
9.   hepatic artery
10.   hepatic portal vein
11.   common hepatic duct
12.   quadrate lobe
13.   gallbladder
14.   right lobe proper
15.   inferior vena cava
16.   caudate lobe

Common Bile Duct and Its Tributaries

1.   right and left hepatic ducts
2.   cystic duct
3.   common hepatic duct
4.   common bile duct
5.   accessory duct of pancreas
6.   pancreatic duct

CHAPTER 26

Digestion

1.   b, p. 772
2.   a, p. 772
3.   b, p. 777
4.   a, p. 774
5.   b, p. 777
6.   b, p. 781
7.   c, p. 777
8.   f, p. 773
9.   f, p. 774
10.   t, p. 774

11. f, p. 775
12. t, p. 778
13. f, p. 781
14. t, p. 777

Secretion and Control of Digestive Gland Secretion
15. b, p. 779
16. b, p. 779
17. d, p. 781
18. d, p. 782
19. t, p. 780
20. t, p. 781
21. f, p. 783
22. t, p. 779

Absorption and Elimination
23. b, p. 784
24. b, p. 787
25. c, p. 786
26. f, p. 784
27. t, p. 786
28. f, p. 786
29. f, p. 786
30. t, p. 785

Mechanisms of Disease
31. h, p. 789
32. d, p. 789
33. g, p. 789
34. a, p. 789
35. f, p. 789
36. b, p. 790
37. i, p. 790
38. c, p. 790
39. j, p. 790
40. e, p. 790

Applying What You Know
41. (a) pain in the abdomen with possible hemorrhage
(b) duodenum or possibly the stomach
(c) *Helicobacter pylori* bacterium and hyperacidity
(d) drugs that reduce hydrochloric acid formation and antibiotics to kill the bacteria

42. Replacement of fluids should focus on large amounts of cool, diluted, or isotonic fluids.

One Last Quick Check
43. a, p. 777
44. c, p. 774
45. a, p. 774
46. b, p. 789
47. c, p. 788
48. c, p. 788
49. a, p. 779
50. b, p. 779
51. d, p. 776
52. c, p. 785
53. c, p. 775
54. a, p. 781
55. d, p. 772
56. c, p. 775
57. f, p. 775
58. t, p. 776
59. t, p. 784
60. t, p. 786
61. f, p. 789

CHAPTER 27

Overview of Nutrition and Metabolism
1. a, p. 796
2. d, p. 795
3. t, p. 796
4. f, p. 797

Carbohydrates
5. a, p. 797
6. b, p. 797
7. c, p. 798
8. a, p. 798
9. a, p. 798
10. b, p. 798
11. d, p. 803
12. b, p. 806
13. t, p. 798
14. t, p. 798
15. f, p. 799
16. f, p. 802
17. t, p. 806
18. t, p. 803

19. f, p. 807
20. t, p. 806
21. t, p. 808
22. f, p. 806
23. f, p. 797
24. t, p. 799
25. t, p. 799
26. f, p. 799
27. f, p. 805

Lipids
28. a, p. 808
29. c, p. 808
30. a, p. 809
31. c, p. 811
32. d, p. 809
33. f, p. 809
34. t, p. 810
35. t, p. 810
36. t, p. 808
37. t, p. 810

Proteins
38. b, p. 811
39. b, p. 812
40. d, p. 813
41. f, p. 812
42. t, p. 812
43. t, p. 812
44. f, p. 813
45. t, p. 812

Vitamins and Minerals
46. b, p. 815
47. a, p. 815
48. c, p. 817
49. f, p. 815
50. t, p. 815
51. t, p. 816
52. f, p. 813

Metabolic Rate and Mechanisms for Regulating Food Intake
53. b, p. 817
54. c, p. 819
55. c, p. 820
56. b, p. 820
57. f, p. 819
58. t, p. 820
59. t, p. 820

60. f, p. 819
61. f, p. 817

Mechanisms of Disease
62. b, p. 822
63. e, p. 823
64. a, p. 822
65. f, p. 823
66. d, p. 823
67. c, p. 823
68. g, p. 823

Applying What You Know
69. weight loss and anorexia nervosa
70. Iron would be the first mineral of choice. It is found in meat, eggs, vegetables, and legumes. Copper sources which might also help the anemia would be seafood, organ meats, and legumes.

One Last Quick Check
71. b, p. 799
72. a, p. 803
73. c, p. 806
74. c, p. 819
75. b, p. 820
76. d, p. 797
77. a, p. 797
78. bile (all others refer to carbohydrate metabolism)
79. amino acids (all others refer to fat metabolism)
80. M (all others refer to vitamins)
81. iron (all others refer to protein metabolism)
82. insulin (all others tend to increase blood glucose)
83. folic acid (all others are minerals)
84. ascorbic acid (all others refer to the B-complex vitamins)
85. a, p. 797
86. c, p. 811
87. d, p. 815
88. e, p. 815

89. a, p. 798
90. e, p. 815
91. a, p. 798

CHAPTER 28

Anatomy of the Urinary System
1. d, p. 829
2. c, p. 830
3. c, p. 830
4. b, p. 836
5. d, p. 836
6. c, p. 837
7. c, p. 836
8. a, p. 838
9. f, p. 830
10. f, p. 830
11. t, p. 836
12. t, p. 836
13. f, p. 830
14. t, p. 836
15. f, p. 830

Physiology of the Urinary System
16. b, p. 838
17. a, p. 840
18. d, p. 845
19. a, p. 841
20. c, p. 842
21. d, p. 846
22. c, p. 851
23. d, p. 848
24. c, p. 846
25. t, p. 838
26. f, p. 839
27. t, p. 843
28. t, p. 838
29. f, p. 840
30. f, p. 840
31. t, p. 846
32. f, p. 839
33. f, p. 848
34. f, p. 848
35. t, p. 848

Mechanisms of Disease
36. i, p. 850
37. c, p. 851
38. g, p. 851
39. f, p. 852

40. k, p. 851
41. a, p. 851
42. h, p. 852
43. j, p. 852
44. b, p. 851
45. d, p. 852
46. e, p. 851
47. l, p. 851

Applying What You Know
48. Hemorrhage causes a drop in blood pressure, which decreases the urine output and can eventually lead to kidney failure.
49. Stage I—Often asymptomatic because healthy nephrons compensate for the ones destroyed by disease
Stage 2—Renal insufficiency; BUN increases, polyuria and dehydration may occur
Stage 3—Uremia; high BUN, loss of kidney function, oliguria, edema, hypertension, and eventual death if an artificial kidney or transplant not available.

One Last Quick Check
50. b, p. 849
51. d, p. 852
52. a, p. 845
53. c, p. 845
54. c, p. 841
55. b, p. 836
56. c, p. 834
57. b, p. 836
58. a, p. 830
59. b, p. 835
60. e, p. 851
61. c, p. 851
62. f, p. 851
63. d, p. 836
64. j, p. 851
65. h, p. 851
66. a, p. 850
67. g, p. 851
68. i, p. 835

69. b, p. 835
70. k, p. 840

Diagrams
Kidney
1. interlobular arteries
2. renal column
3. renal sinus
4. hilum
5. renal pelvis
6. renal papilla of pyramid
7. ureter
8. medulla
9. medullary pyramid
10. major calyces
11. minor calyces
12. cortex
13. capsule (fibrous)

Nephron
1. cortical nephron
2. proximal tubule
3. glomerulus
4. distal convoluted tubule
5. collecting tubule
6. vasa recta
7. pyramid (medulla)
8. Henle's loop
9. ascending limb of Henle's loop
10. descending limb of Henle's loop
11. arcuate artery and vein
12. juxtamedullary nephron
13. interlobular artery and vein
14. afferent arteriole
15. efferent arteriole

Male Urinary Bladder
1. ureter
2. opening of ureter
3. rugae
4. prostate
5. external urinary sphincter
6. bulbourethral gland
7. prostatic urethra
8. internal urinary sphincter
9. opening of ureter
10. trigone
11. smooth muscle
12. cut edge of peritoneum

CHAPTER 29

Overview of Fluid and Electrolyte Balance
1. c, p. 858
2. c, p. 860
3. a, p. 860
4. b, p. 860
5. d, p. 861
6. d, p. 862
7. c, p. 859
8. f, p. 858
9. t, p. 860
10. t, p. 862
11. f, p. 859
12. t, p. 863
13. f, p. 862
14. t, p. 861

Mechanisms that Maintain Homeostasis of Total Fluid Volume
15. d, p. 864
16. c, p. 863
17. f, p. 863
18. t, p. 865

Regulation of Water and Electrolyte Levels in Plasma, Interstitial Fluid, and Intracellular Fluid
19. a, p. 866
20. c, p. 870
21. c, p. 867
22. c, p. 869
23. t, p. 867
24. f, p. 867
25. t, p. 867
26. t, p. 869

Regulation of Sodium and Potassium Levels in Body Fluids
27. f, p. 869
28. t, p. 872
29. t, p. 872
30. f, p. 870
31. t, p. 872

Mechanisms of Disease
32. a, p. 872
33. d, p. 873

34. e, p. 873
35. b, p. 873
36. c, p. 873
37. t, p. 873
38. f, p. 873
39. t, p. 873
40. f, p. 873

Applying What You Know
41. Ms. Titus could not accurately measure water intake created by foods or catabolism, nor could she measure output created by lungs, skin, or the intestines.
42. Jack's body contained more water. Obese people have a lower water content than slender people.

One Last Quick Check
43. inside
44. extracellular
45. extracellular
46. lower
47. more
48. decreases
49. a, p. 860
50. d, p. 860
51. c, p. 862
52. e, p. 862
53. d, p. 873
54. c, p. 860
55. b, p. 860
56. d, p. 861
57. a, p. 867
58. a, p. 860
59. d, p. 862
60. t, p. 860
61. t, p. 867
62. t, p. 869

CHAPTER 30

Mechanisms that Control pH of Body Fluids
1. c, p. 878
2. a, p. 879
3. b, p. 879

4. d, p. 878
5. c, p. 878
6. a, p. 879
7. c, p. 879
8. t, p. 878
9. f, p. 879
10. t, p. 880
11. f, p. 878
12. t, p. 879
13. t, p. 880

Buffer Mechanisms for Controlling pH of Body Fluids

14. a, p. 882
15. c, p. 881
16. t, p. 882
17. f, p. 884
18. t, p. 880
19. f, p. 882
20. t, p. 882

Respiratory and Urinary Mechanisms of pH Control

21. d, p. 884
22. b, p. 884
23. b, p. 886
24. a, p. 884
25. c, p. 886
26. t, p. 884
27. f, p. 884
28. t, p. 886
29. f, p. 881
30. t, p. 884

Mechanisms of Disease

31. f, p. 889
32. e, p. 888
33. a, p. 889
34. b, p. 889
35. g, p. 889
36. c, p. 890
37. d, p. 890

Applying What You Know

38. Normal saline contains chloride ions, which replace bicarbonate ions and thus relieve the bicarbonate excess that occurs during severe vomiting.

39. Most citrus fruits, although acid tasting, are fully oxidized with the help of buffers during metabolism and have little effect on acid-base balance. Cranberry juice is one of the few exceptions.

One Last Quick Check

40. a, p. 884
41. c, p. 884
42. a, p. 884
43. d, p. 880
44. a, p. 884
45. d, p. 884
46. d, p. 881
47. a, p. 881
48. g, p. 878
49. c, p. 878
50. h, p. 880
51. e, p. 890
52. f, p. 890
53. a, p. 889
54. b, p. 889
55. d, p. 883

CHAPTER 31

Male Reproductive Organs

1. a, p. 896
2. b, p. 897
3. c, p. 897
4. d, p. 897
5. c, p. 898
6. a, p. 899
7. a, p. 900
8. c, p. 902
9. t, p. 899
10. f, p. 899
11. f, p. 900
12. t, p. 900
13. f, p. 897
14. f, p. 897
15. t, p. 900

Reproductive Ducts and Accessory Reproductive Glands

16. b, p. 900
17. c, p. 903

18. a, p. 904
19. c, p. 904
20. b, p. 904
21. t, p. 902
22. t, p. 903
23. t, p. 903
24. t, p. 904

Supporting Structures, Seminal Fluid, and Male Fertility

25. c, p. 906
26. b, p. 905
27. b, p. 906
28. c, p. 906
29. f, p. 905
30. t, p. 905
31. f, p. 906

Mechanisms of Disease

32. oligospermia
33. 2 months
34. cryptorchidism
35. benign prostatic hypertrophy
36. Phimosis
37. impotence; erectile dysfunction
38. hydrocele
39. inguinal hernia

Applying What You Know

40. (a) cryptorchidism (b) easily detected by palpation of the scrotum (c) surgery or testosterone injections (d) early detection results in normal testicular and sexual development.

41. (a) hydrocele or inguinal hernia (b) inguinal hernia (c) Swelling of the scrotum occurs when the intestine pushes through the weak area of the abdominal wall that separates the abdominopelvic cavity from the scrotum. (d) external supports or surgical repair

One Last Quick Check
42. b, p. 905
43. c, p. 905
44. b, p. 897
45. c, p. 897
46. a, p. 899
47. d, p. 905
48. d, p. 899
49. d, p. 900
50. c, p. 900
51. c, p. 899
52. a, p. 900
53. b, p. 902
54. h, p. 905
55. g, p. 904
56. a, p. 900
57. f, p. 904
58. c, p. 903
59. i, p. 906
60. e, p. 906
61. d, p. 905
62. j, p. 905

Diagrams
Male Pelvis—Sagittal Section
1. rectum
2. seminal vesicle
3. levator ani muscle
4. ejaculatory duct
5. anus
6. bulbocavernosus muscle
7. glans
8. testis
9. urethra
10. corpus spongiosum
11. corpus cavernosum
12. prostate gland
13. symphysis pubis
14. urinary bladder

Tubules of Testis and Epididymis
1. nerves and blood vessels of spermatic cord
2. ductus (vas) deferens
3. septum
4. lobule
5. tunica albuquinea
6. testis
7. seminiferous tubules
8. epididymis

Penis
1. bladder
2. prostate
3. bulb
4. deep artery
5. foreskin (prepuce)
6. external urethral orifice
7. glans penis
8. corpus spongiosum
9. urethra
10. corpus cavernosum
11. opening of Cowper's glands
12. crus penis
13. bulbourethral gland
14. openings of ejaculatory ducts

CHAPTER 32

Overview of the Female Reproductive System
1. a, p. 913
2. b, p. 913
3. t, p. 913
4. t, p. 914

Internal Female Genitals
5. b, p. 914
6. d, p. 915
7. b, p. 916
8. a, p. 916
9. b, p. 916
10. d, p. 918
11. a, p. 918
12. b, p. 916
13. c, p. 920
14. b, p. 917
15. a, p. 918
16. b, p. 916
17. a, p. 918
18. a, p. 918
19. c, p. 920
20. t, p. 914
21. f, p. 917
22. f, p. 920
23. t, p. 919

External Female Genitals and Breasts
24. c, p. 920
25. b, p. 920
26. a, p. 920
27. a, p. 921
28. f, p. 920
29. f, p. 920
30. f, p. 922
31. t, p. 922
32. f, p. 922

Female Reproductive Cycle
33. a, p. 923
34. c, p. 924
35. d, p. 930
36. c, p. 925
37. b, p. 927
38. f, p. 924
39. t, p. 925
40. t, p. 931
41. f, p. 927
42. f, p. 926

Mechanisms of Disease
43. f, p. 930
44. e, p. 931
45. a, p. 930
46. h, p. 930
47. i, p. 932
48. g, p. 931
49. c, p. 930
50. b, p. 930
51. l, p. 932
52. d, p. 930
53. j, p. 931
54. k, p. 932

Applying What You Know
55. (a) Contraceptive pills contain synthetic progesterone-like compounds such as progestin, sometimes combined with synthetic estrogens. By sustaining a high blood concentration of these substances, contraceptive pills prevent the monthly development of a follicle. With no ovum to be expelled, ovulation does not occur, and therefore pregnancy cannot occur. (b) Tubal ligation involves

tying a piece of suture material around each uterine tube in two places, then cutting the tube between these two points. Sperm and eggs are thus prevented from meeting. This procedure is a surgical sterilization.

56. The uterine tubes are not attached to the ovaries and infections can exit at this area and enter the abdominal cavity.

One Last Quick Check
57. g, p. 913
58. b, p. 913
59. e, p. 914
60. j, p. 917
61. a, p. 918
62. f, p. 919
63. c, p. 923
64. i, p. 927
65. h, p. 931
66. d, p. 922
67. premenstrual or postovulatory
68. Prolactin
69. Oxytocin
70. meiosis
71. corpus luteum
72. Radioimmunoassay
73. Menopause
74. STDs
75. Eight
76. placenta

Diagrams
Female Pelvic Organs
1. fundus of uterus
2. uterine tube (fallopian)
3. follicle
4. fimbriae
5. endometrium
6. myometrium
7. cervical canal
8. vagina
9. cervix of uterus
10. body of uterus

Sagittal Section of Female Pelvis
1. sacral promontory
2. ureter
3. sacrouterine ligament
4. posterio cul-de-sac
5. cervix
6. fornix of vagina
7. anus
8. labium majus
9. vagina
10. labium minus
11. clitoris
12. urethra
13. symphysis pubis
14. urinary bladder
15. parietal peritoneum
16. anterior cul-de-sac
17. round ligament
18. fundus of uterus
19. body of uterus
20. ovarian ligament
21. uterine tube

CHAPTER 33

A New Human Life
1. b, p. 939
2. b, p. 939
3. d, p. 940
4. a, p. 941
5. b, p. 941
6. a, p. 939
7. f, p. 939
8. t, p. 939
9. t, p. 941
10. f, p. 941
11. f, p. 941
12. f, p. 944
13. t, p. 941
14. t, p. 944

Prenatal Period
15. a, p. 944
16. b, p. 944
17. a, p. 944
18. b, p. 953
19. c, p. 949
20. t, p. 946
21. f, p. 944
22. f, p. 954

23. t, p. 944
24. t, p. 944

Birth, or Parturition, and the Postnatal Period
25. c, p. 954
26. c, p. 956
27. d, p. 957
28. b, p. 959
29. b, p. 957
30. t, p. 955
31. t, p. 955
32. f, p. 954
33. f, p. 957
34. t, p. 958

Effects of Aging
35. d, p. 961
36. d, p. 961
37. t, p. 959
38. f, p. 961

Mechanisms of Disease
39. c, p. 963
40. a, p. 962
41. d, p. 963
42. b, p. 962
43. h, p. 963
44. f, p. 963
45. j, p. 962
46. g, p. 963

Applying What You Know
47. Only about 40% of the taste buds present at age 30 remain at age 75.
48. Identical twins have the same genetic code.

One Last Quick Check
49. g, p. 944
50. f, p. 953
51. c, p. 952
52. b, p. 948
53. a, p. 944
54. h, p. 954
55. e, p. 955
56. d, p. 954
57. i, p. 949
58. j, p. 952
59. d, p. 959

60. d, p. 961
61. d, p. 961
62. a, p. 958
63. b, p. 953
64. d, p. 961
65. e, p. 958
66. a, p. 959
67. c, p. 959
68. b, p. 958

CHAPTER 34

The Science of Genetics; Chromosomes and Genes; Gene Expression

1. c, p. 969
2. c, p. 969
3. d, p. 972
4. c, p. 974
5. a, p. 969
6. d, p. 975
7. c, p. 975
8. d, p. 968
9. f, p. 971
10. t, p. 972
11. f, p. 972
12. f, p. 974
13. t, p. 974
14. t, p. 974
15. f, p. 969
16. f, p. 972

Medical Genetics; Prevention and Treatment of Genetic Diseases

17. b, p. 976
18. b, p. 981
19. a, p. 981
20. c, p. 978
21. c, p. 981
22. b, p. 983
23. d, pp. 978 and 981
24. d, p. 985
25. c, p. 984
26. b, p. 984
27. f, p. 977
28. t, p. 972
29. f, p. 977
30. t, p. 983
31. t, p. 985
32. f, p. 977
33. t, p. 979
34. t, p. 984
35. t, p. 976

Applying What You Know

36. In a form of dominance called *co-dominance*, the effect will be equal, causing "light brown" to occur.
37. One in four or 25%

One Last Quick Check

38. a, p. 971
39. d, p. 983
40. c, p. 978
41. b, p. 972
42. a, p. 969
43. c, p. 969
44. b, p. 974
45. c, p. 974
46. a, p. 984
47. b, p. 982
48. h, p. 981
49. k, p. 984
50. c, p. 977
51. e, p. 969
52. a, p. 977
53. d, p. 972
54. j, p. 978
55. l, p. 968
56. g, p. 972

SOLUTIONS TO CROSSWORD PUZZLES

CHAPTER 1

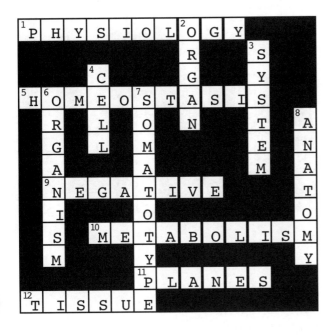

CHAPTER 2

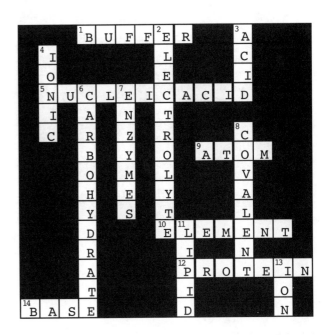

CHAPTER 3

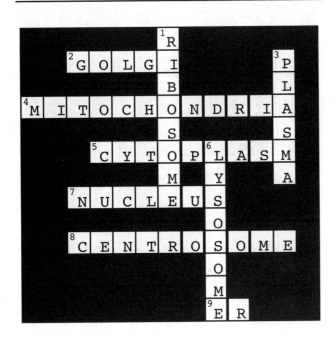

CHAPTER 4

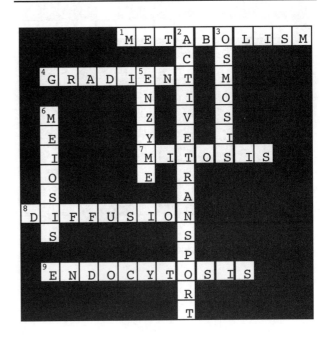

CHAPTER 5

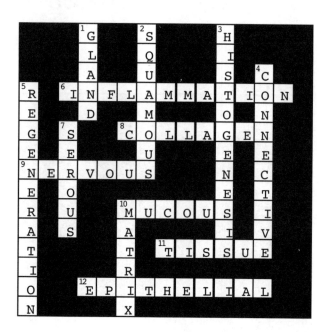

CHAPTER 6

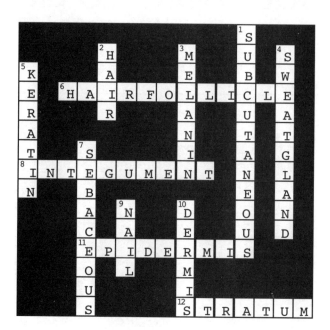

CHAPTER 7

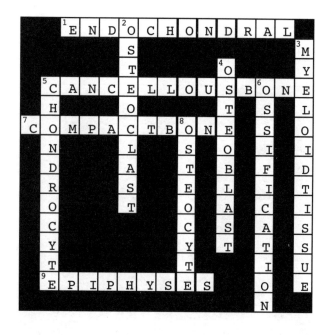

CHAPTER 8

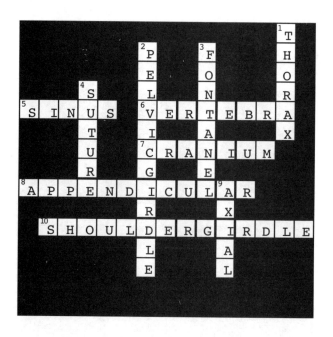

CHAPTER 9

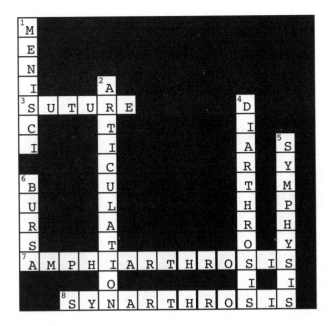

CHAPTER 10

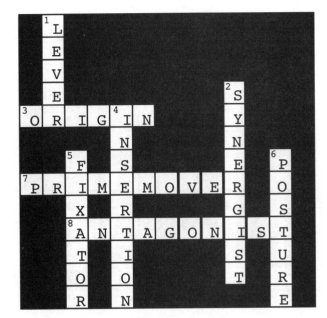

CHAPTER 11

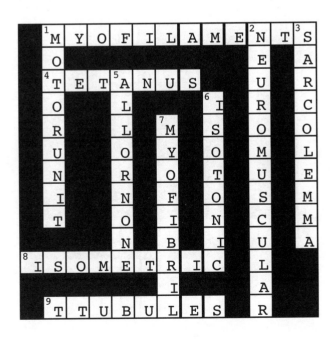

CHAPTER 12

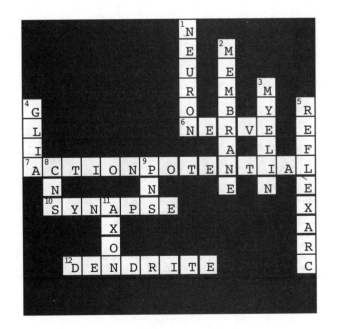

CHAPTER 13

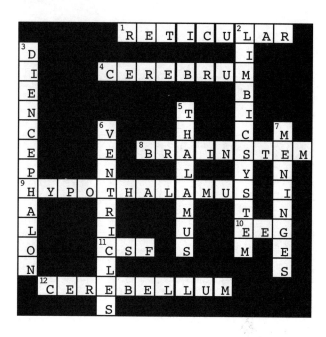

CHAPTER 14

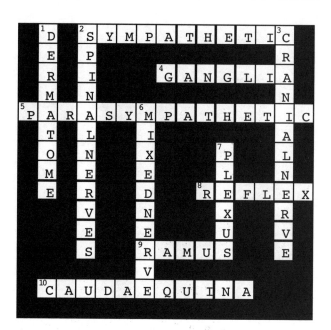

CHAPTER 15

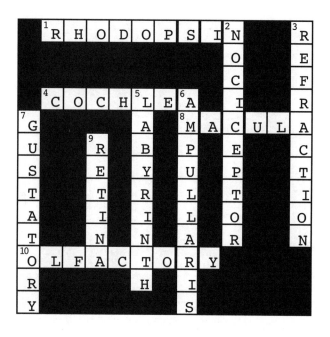

CHAPTER 16

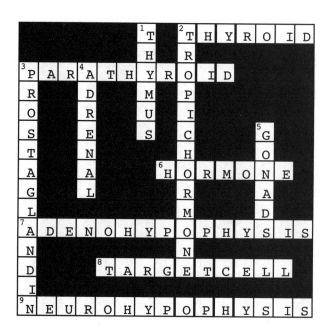

CHAPTER 17

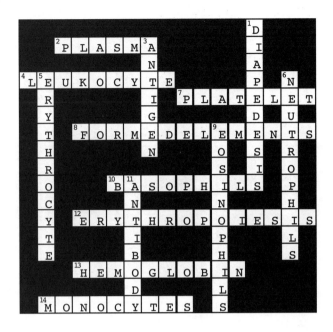

CHAPTER 18

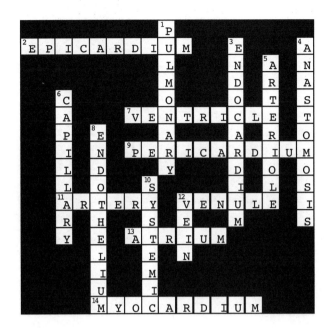

CHAPTER 19

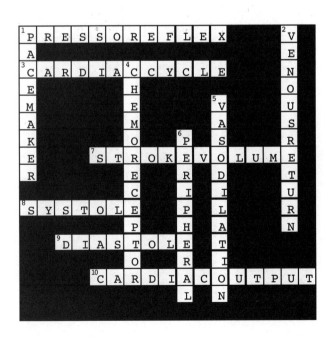

CHAPTER 20

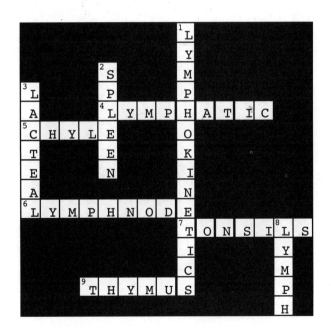

CHAPTER 21

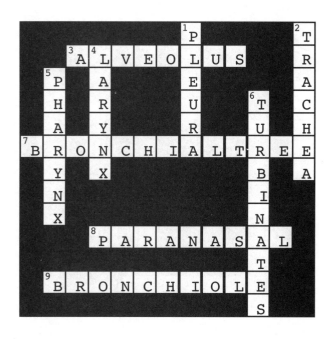

CHAPTER 22

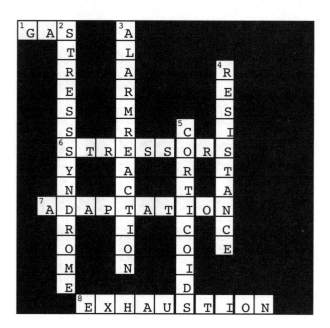

CHAPTER 23

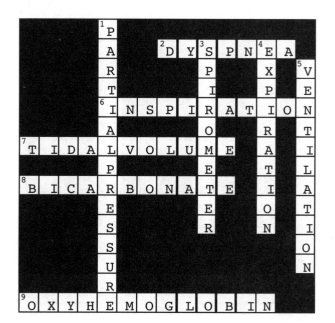

CHAPTER 24

CHAPTER 25

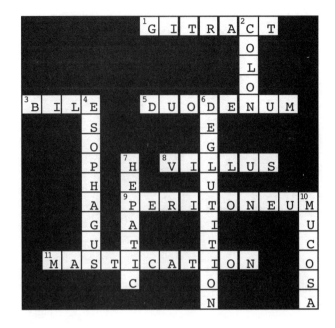

CHAPTER 26

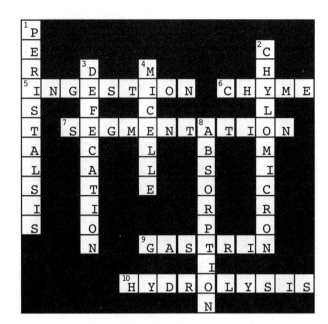

CHAPTER 27

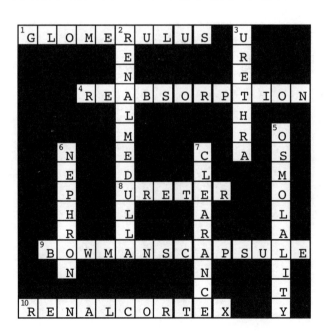

CHAPTER 28

CHAPTER 29

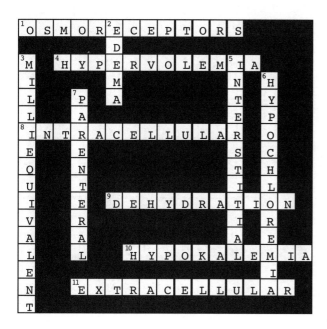

CHAPTER 30

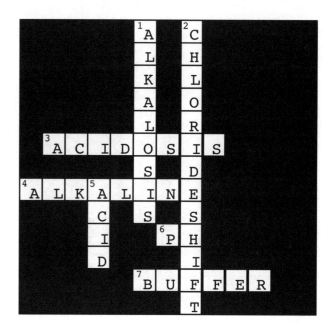

CHAPTER 31

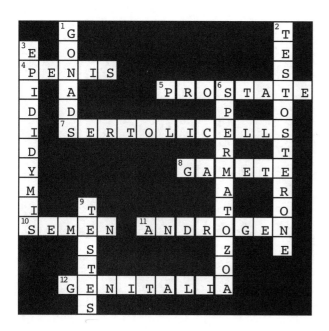

CHAPTER 32

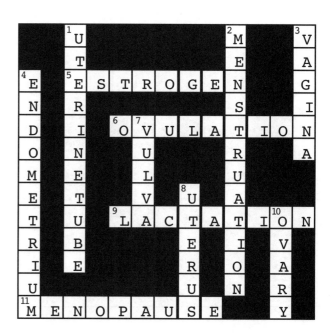

CHAPTER 33

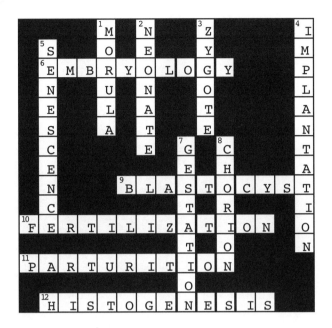

CHAPTER 34

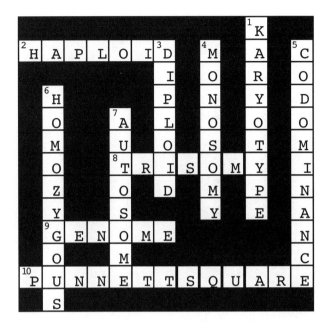